DRUGS AND PREGNANCY

DRUGS AND PREGNANCY

A HANDBOOK

Bertis B Little PhD
Associate Vice-President for
Academic Research and Professor
Tarleton State University
Stephenville, Texas
USA
Texas A&M University System

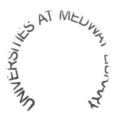

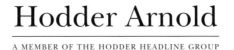

Hodder Arnold

A MEMBER OF THE HODDER HEADLINE GROUP

First published in Great Britain in 2006 by
Hodder Arnold, an imprint of Hodder Education and a member of the Hodder Headline Group,
338 Euston Road, London NW1 3BH

http://www.hoddereducation.com

Distributed in the United States of America by
Oxford University Press Inc.,
198 Madison Avenue, New York, NY10016
Oxford is a registered trademark of Oxford University Press

Hodder Headline's policy is to use papers that are natural, renewable and recyclable products
and made from wood grown in sustainable forests. The logging and manufacturing processes are
expected to conform to the environmental regulations of the country of origin.

Whilst the advice and information in this book are believed to be true and accurate at the date of
going to press, neither the author[s] nor the publisher can accept any legal responsibility or
liability for any errors or omissions that may be made. In particular, (but without limiting the
generality of the preceding disclaimer) every effort has been made to check drug dosages;
however it is still possible that errors have been missed. Furthermore, dosage schedules are
constantly being revised and new side-effects recognized. For these reasons the reader is strongly
urged to consult the drug companies' printed instructions before administering any of the drugs
recommended in this book.

British Library Cataloguing in Publication Data
A catalogue record for this book is available from the British Library

Library of Congress Cataloging-in-Publication Data
A catalog record for this book is available from the Library of Congress

ISBN-10 0 340 809 175
ISBN-13 978 0 340 809 174

1 2 3 4 5 6 7 8 9 10

Commissioning Editor: Sarah Burrows
Project Editor: Francesca Naish
Production Controller: Joanna Walker
Cover Design: Amina Dudhia
Indexer: Laurence Errington

Typeset in 9/12 pt Sabon by Phoenix Photosetting, Chatham, Kent
Printed and bound in Spain by Graphycems

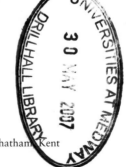

What do you think about this book? Or any other Hodder Arnold title? Please see our
website at www.hoddereducation.com

Dedication

Dr. Gilstrap and I dedicated *Drugs and Pregnancy* second edition to our mothers. Dr. Yonkers and I dedicated *Treatment of Psychiatric Disorders in Pregnancy* to our spouses. Present and past generations were thus recognized. Accordingly, *Drugs and Pregnancy – A Handbook* is dedicated to the future generation:

Christian Carroll
Ian Carroll
Lauren DelHomme
Leslie DelHomme
Luke DelHomme
Catherine DelHomme
Madeline DelHomme
Nicole Hery, Pharm.D. (Candidate)
William Hery
B. Britt Little, II
Alexis Reynolds
Zachary Reynolds
Christa Little White, R.N.
Raven Little White
Savannah White

Contents

Preface

The purpose of this volume was originally to condense and update *Drugs and Pregnancy* second edition. However, the book has evolved into a larger project since its inception in 2000. The total length of the original typescript was approximately three times the number of pages for which the publisher contracted. First strategy suggested was to eliminate the large number of references, but this was not acceptable. The final compromise developed was to post the full bibliography and supporting materials on a website for the book – http://www.drugsandpregnancy.com.

It is intended for the content of this book to be updated and corrected – as necessary – approximately four times per year. These additions to the book will be posted to the website above, which will be maintained by the publisher. In addition, a searchable index of proprietary and generic names is provided on the website.

In addition, a link to TERIS is provided on the website, and the reader is strongly encouraged to use TERIS in counseling patients who have been exposed to a medication during pregnancy. The information in TERIS has been vetted by leading authorities in the field, and is tantamount to high quality peer reviewed literature. It was through working on the development of TERIS (writing agent summaries, knowledgebase design) from 1985 to 1989 that I became deeply interested in human teratology.

Links to other sites that may be of use to readers of this book will also be included on the website. A feature under development for http://www.drugsandpregnancy.com is a current literature alert window. We have developed an automated search agent that will identify new publications (journal articles, books, etc.) relevant to human teratology, and will post those to the website under CURRENT LITERATURE ALERTS. This will assist the reader in maintaining access to up-to-date information. The main advantage of having a website accompany the published book is currency of information. Books usually take a year or longer to reach the reader after the author has completed the typescript, and may already be out-of-date by the time of release.

I thank the publisher for providing this option to (1) maintain scholarly references for the book's content, (2) provide readers the most recent information available, and (3) refer readers to other authoritative sources such as TERIS.

BBL
July 2006

Acknowledgements

My friend and colleague, Rick Weideman, PharmD of the VA Medical Center, Dallas even gave vacation time to help with the completion of this volume. Beverly A DelHomme, JD, my wife, has read and edited the typescript of this book more than a couple of times over the past several years. Marie Kelly, MD, friend and colleague, made significant contributions to the completion of this volume through editing, updating sources, and information during her personal holiday time. My Staff Assistant, Nona Williamson, did computer MEDLINE searches, typed chapters, checked bibliography, and sought out difficult-to-find literature. Eva Malina, PhD also assisted in production of this volume during her summer vacation by reading and marking page proofs. Donna Savage, University Librarian, and her staff have patiently worked with Nona and me to acquire numerous uncommon reference sources.

Finally, I wish to thank the Illinois Poison Control Board for allowing reproduction of their comprehensive list of antidotes, and to Saunders/Elsevier Publishing for allowing the adaptation of Figure 14.1.

1

Introduction to drugs in pregnancy

Birth defects occur among 3.5–5 percent of infants examined at birth or neonatally (Polifka and Friedman, 2002) but prevalence of birth defects may be as high as 8 percent, according to a universal disease registry from British Columbia (Baird *et al.*, 1989). Using the estimated teratogenic causes of birth defects in Fig. 1.1, it may be extrapolated that as many as 1 percent of congenital anomalies are caused by drugs, chemicals and other exogenous agents (i.e., approximately one in 400 infants has a birth defect with a teratogenic etiology). These estimates have not changed over the past decade and a half, perhaps because genomic research eclipses research in clinical teratology, as suggested by a recent review (Polifka and Friedman, 2002). Nonetheless, much research remains to be done because the magnitude of the problem of medication use during pregnancy may be somewhat underestimated because 65–70 percent of birth defects have an unknown etiology. This may include unreported medically prescribed medication with teratogenic potential, use of alcohol and/or drugs of abuse, and other preventable causes of birth defects (i.e., congenital anomalies and other pregnancy complications due to drug and chemical exposure are unique because they are potentially preventable). Knowledge of the effects of prenatal exposure and the window of opportunity for intervention are the key factors in evaluation and prevention of morbidity and mortality due to drug and chemical exposure during pregnancy. Chapters 2–15 summarize information currently available regarding drug exposure during pregnancy, with detailed

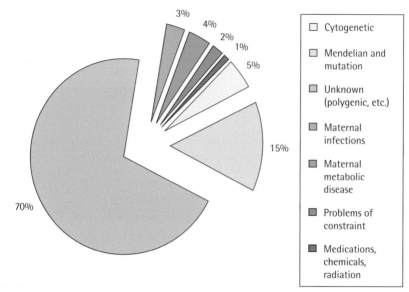

Figure 1.1 *Causes of birth defects*

drug-specific information obtained from the current medical literature, clinical experience, and science.

Clinicians find it difficult to use the narrow window of opportunity to intervene in
medication use during pregnancy because pregnant women do not present for prenatal
care until embryogenesis is complete (i.e., after 58 days postconception). Intervention
is further complicated because many women are not aware of the potential adverse
affects of drugs and chemicals on pregnancy. For example, more than 60 percent of
gravidas had never heard of fetal alcohol syndrome and were not aware of the adverse
effects of alcohol on pregnancy in several surveys. Patient education prior to conception is obviously the best intervention, but very little funding is available for this. In
addition, social and cultural barriers must also be overcome for the patient education
process to be successful.

Even the most well-educated obstetrical patients have culturally based 'folk etiologies'
that they believe explain the occurrence of birth defects and other adverse pregnancy
outcomes that are usually not correlated with medically founded causes. The author has
counseled gravid physicians who were not entirely correct in their understanding of prenatal development and how the environment can be a disruptive influence. Folk or cul-
ture-specific explanations and educational background must therefore be considered
when counseling the obstetrical patient of specific risks to pregnancy, including exposures to medications, drugs, and chemicals.

MAGNITUDE OF THE PROBLEM

Women ingest a variety of medications or drugs during pregnancy, usually related to a
medical condition that was being treated before the pregnancy was recognized.
Prevalence of medication use varied from less than 10 percent of pregnant women to

more than 95 percent. Frequently, more than one medication will be used. For example, in one comprehensive study in the United States of tens of thousands of patients, women received an average of 3.1 prescriptions for medications other than vitamins or iron during their pregnancies. Similar prevalences were observed in Brazil, Australia, New Zealand, and Egypt. The high end estimates are probably closer to the prevalence in 2004, and this is an international pattern and problem. Medication use during pregnancy is clearly a frequent event. However, safety may be questionable or simply unknown in many instances (Polifka and Friedman, 2002), primarily because of the paucity of clinical teratology research conducted over the last two decades (Lo and Friedman, 2002).

Three scenarios describe inadvertent drug exposure during pregnancy: (1) some medications are taken before the pregnancy is recognized; (2) some medications are taken without the physician's advice once the pregnancy is recognized; and (3) some are taken with physician's advice. In practice, the predominant case is for physicians to be faced with determining whether or not a medication or drug may be harmful to a pregnant woman or her unborn child after the exposure has occurred.

Also of concern are nonmedical exposures to drugs. Nonmedical exposures to drugs during pregnancy occur in suicide gestures (technically a subcategory of substance abuse) and substance abuse (i.e., recreational use). Suicide gestures occur among approximately 1 percent of pregnant women. Substance abuse during pregnancy is much more prevalent than suicide gestures, and is discussed in Chapter 15. Briefly, an estimated 10–20 percent of pregnant women use an illicit substance and/or alcohol during their pregnancies. Cocaine seems to be the most frequently used substance in 2004.

CLINICAL EVALUATION

Clinical evaluation of potentially teratogenic and/or toxic exposures during pregnancy must consider three separate components of normal pregnancy: maternal, embryonic, and fetal. Marked differences in the physiology of these components exist because of differences in the purposes of the cells, or the end points of cell division (replacement versus morphogenesis versus hyperplastic growth) and the metabolic capabilities of the mother and the developing conceptus. In the embryo, organs are being formed, and drugs cannot be metabolized at adult or fetal rates, if at all. The embryo is not a little fetus. The fetus is not a little adult. Most of the fetal period is occupied with growth in size of organs, not usually their formation, and these are growing very rapidly. Exceptions exist (e.g., thyroid, sexual organs, brain cell 'arrangement'), but this is generally true for the fetus. Fetal enzyme systems involved in drug metabolism are only beginning to function, and some will not be active until after the neonatal period (e.g., cholinesterase). Pregnant women have the full enzyme complement for metabolizing drugs, but most such systems have lower activity during pregnancy, as does cholinesterase (Pritchard, 1955), which metabolizes cocaine. In addition, gender differences in the nonpregnant state also exist [e.g., alcohol dehydrogenase (ADH) among adult females is only 55 percent of adult males' activity]. Therefore, the responses of adults, fetuses, embryos, and pregnant women to drugs (pharmacodynamics, pharmacokinetics) differ markedly (Little, 1999). Therefore, it is important to differentiate the effects of drugs and chemicals upon these distinctly different components of pregnancy. We shall repeatedly observe that many drugs and chemicals have different effects on these three components of pregnancy.

HUMAN TERATOLOGY – PRINCIPLES

A teratogen is usually defined as any agent, physical force, or other factor (e.g., maternal disease) that can induce a congenital anomaly through alteration of normal development during any stage of embryogenesis (Polifka and Friedman, 2002). Agents include drugs and other chemicals. Physical forces include ionizing radiation and physical restraint (e.g., amniotic banding). Teratogenic maternal diseases include disorders such as diabetes mellitus and phenylketonuria. Agents that cause defects during the postembryonic (fetal) period are termed to have the potential for producing adverse 'fetal effects.' However, not all agents or factors that are teratogens have adverse fetal effects, and vice versa.

A simplified overview of the differences between the embryonic and fetal periods should be presented during consultation to clarify status for the patient. The period of the embryo should be described as the growth of cells that all look alike (i.e., are undifferentiated) into specialized cells that are arranged in special ways (i.e., organs, specialized tissues). These specialized cell lines or lineages grow in number and change in structure and arrangement, giving rise to organs and tissues. Some organs and tissues are formed earlier than are others. For example, the brain and spine form earlier than do the face and endocrine system. After embryogenesis (58–60 days postconception) is completed, the conceptus is a fetus (Fig. 1.2). With few exceptions, the morphological architecture for a normal (or abnormal) human is laid down during the embryonic period, and these structures simply grow in size and develop normal physiologic function during the fetal period.

Congenital anomalies can be induced during the fetal period through a fetal effect, although they are usually induced during the critical embryonic period. For example, a structure that was formed normally during embryogenesis can be damaged during the fetal period, and the resulting malformation may appear to have arisen during morphogenesis. A classic example of a fetal effect is hemorrhaging due to Coumadin exposure, which may induce brain or eye defects despite the fact that these structures were formed normally during the embryonic period.

Of all the human teratogens, thalidomide is the most notorious and heuristic example of how such agents might not be identified. In the case of thalidomide, the animal models normally used in drug screening failed to identify this drug as a dangerous substance for use during pregnancy before it was released to the market. In the human experience, it was one of the most potent teratogens ever discovered. Although laboratory studies cannot replace large, well-controlled, human epidemiologic studies, they do play an important role in screening drugs and chemicals for their potential to cause human birth defects during pregnancy. Isotretinoin (Accutane) is the only human teratogen ever discovered through laboratory research. It was known before isotretinoin was ever released on the market that this drug had a high potential for inducing congenital anomalies and pregnancy loss, and this fact was clearly displayed on the manufacturer's package insert. Unfortunately, inadvertent exposures to isotretinoin during early human pregnancy have confirmed laboratory findings. More than 100 pregnancies have been exposed to date, and a pattern of anomalies known as isotretinoin embryopathy has been observed in more than 40 percent of the offspring. Other human teratogens were discovered by astute clinicians who recognized patterns or constellations of anomalies

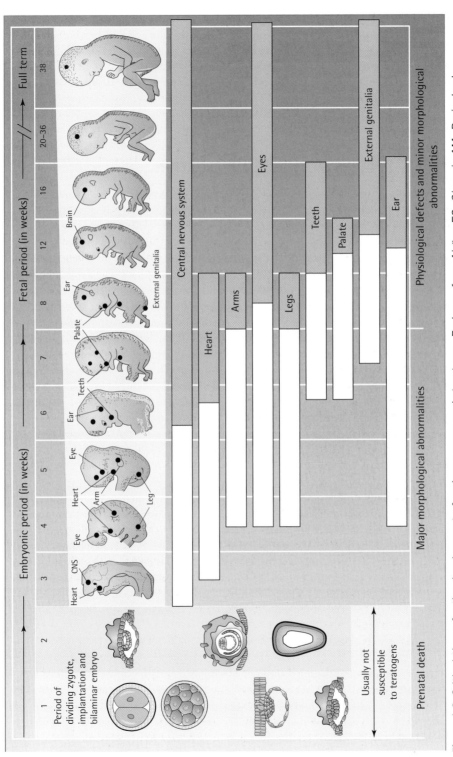

Figure 1.2 Critical times for the development of various organs and structures. Redrawn from Airёns ES, Simonis AM. De invlsed Chemischestoffen op het angebaren kind. Natuuren Technieke 1974; **43**.

in small clinical series of infants whose mothers used or were exposed to certain drugs or chemicals during early pregnancy. Epidemiological studies of infants whose mothers used certain drugs or chemicals during embryogenesis, as well as research with pregnant animals, have served primarily to confirm clinical observations.

Maternal complications and fetal effects due to drug or chemical exposures are not considered under the rubric of classical teratology, but the discovery of drugs and other agents with such potential adverse effects parallels the pattern of the discovery of human teratogens.

ANIMAL STUDIES IN CLINICAL EVALUATION

Animal models are poor predictors of whether or not a drug or chemical is teratogenic in humans. The accuracy and precision (sensitivity and specificity) of animal models in the prediction of human teratogenicity is dependent upon how close the experimental animal species is to humans. Nonhuman primates are better predictors of human teratogenicity and fetotoxicity than are rodent models because primates are genetically more closely related to humans. Animal teratology experiments are further complicated because doses used are many times greater than those given to humans, even approaching maternally toxic doses. Extremely high doses and toxic effects on the mother confound the interpretation of fetal outcome. Metabolism and absorption of drugs and chemicals are different between species because of differences in placentation, pharmacokinetics, pharmacodynamics, embryonic development timing, and innate predisposition to various congenital anomalies. Sensitivity and specificity of rodent studies are less than 60 percent (Schardein, 2000). Rodent animal teratology studies are undertaken by the US Food and Drug Administration (FDA) as part of an accepted drug-approval process to evaluate the safety of medications for use during human pregnancy, despite their very poor ability to predict human teratogens. Nonhuman primate teratology studies are considerably better predictors of which medications may be harmful when given during human pregnancy, with sensitivity and specificity of 90 percent or greater. Nonhuman primate studies are, however, orders of magnitude more expensive than rodent teratology studies, and few drugs are evaluated in primates. Unfortunately, the ultimate assessment of the safety of medication use in pregnancy must come from human studies (Schardein, 2000; Shepard, 2004). Human teratogens are discovered only after numerous children have been damaged, and an astute clinician recognizes a pattern (syndrome) of congenital anomalies, and makes the link to an exposure during pregnancy. These differences are well recognized. For example, of approximately 2000 drugs and chemicals tested in animal models, 55 percent were found to have teratogenic effects (Shepard, 2004). But the number of human teratogens is approximately 50.

HUMAN STUDIES

Human teratogens are identified through careful interpretation of data obtained from case reports, clinical series, and epidemiologic studies. A recurrent pattern of anomalies in babies who experienced similar well-defined exposures at similar points during embryogenesis are suggestive that the agent in question may be teratogenic. Case reports are important in raising causal hypotheses; however, most hypotheses are subsequently proven incorrect. For example, a high incidence of environmental exposure to spermicides by pregnant women and congenital anomalies in offspring is a coincidental occurrence, despite what the legal literature states.

An example of a teratogen that was identified through epidemiologic studies, case reports, and animal studies is carabamazepine. For several decades, carabamazepine was assumed to be safer for the treatment of epilepsy during pregnancy than phenytoin or the other hydantoins. In 1993, a case report was published that reported a suicide attempt by a nonepileptic gravida during the period of spinal closure. The result was a fetus with a very large meningomyelocele (Little *et al.*, 1993). In 1989, Jones *et al.* published a case–control study of carabamazepine and concluded that the study drug was the cause of an increased frequency of birth defects. Other epidemiologic studies throughout the 1990s were conducted, and in 2006 the association of neural tubes defects with carabamazepine exposure during early pregnancy is generally accepted as causal, and the risk is quantified at about 1 percent, compared to about 0.1 percent in the general population.

Quantitative estimates of risks for birth defects (strength and statistical significance of associations between agent exposures in pregnant women and abnormalities in their offspring) are obtained only through epidemiological studies. Human investigations are necessary to demonstrate that an agent is teratogenic. Unfortunately, such studies are not informative until the agent has already damaged a number of children. There are two types of epidemiology studies: cohort studies and case–control studies. In cohort studies the frequencies of certain anomalies in the offspring of women who are exposed are compared to the frequencies in those who are unexposed to the agent in question. A higher frequency of anomalies among exposed pregnancies indicates that the drug or agent should be scrutinized as a teratogen. In case–control studies the frequency of prenatal exposure to the agent is compared among children with and without a specific birth defect. If malformed children were more frequently exposed to a drug or agent than unaffected controls, then the drug or agent may be a teratogen. If an agent increases the risk of anomalies in the offspring only slightly, very large studies over a protracted period may be necessary to demonstrate that the increase is causal.

Epidemiologic studies have several limitations. Spurious associations often occur because many epidemiologists lack medical or biological training, and fail to scrutinize their 'statistical associations' for biological plausibility. Other confounders are sample size, investigations that involve small numbers of exposed or affected subjects, or situations in which the maternal disease or situation that led to the exposure may be responsible for an observed association with a congenital anomaly, rather than the agent itself. Of paramount importance is that the observed association makes biological sense. Exposures that produce malformations in the embryo should do so only during organogenesis or histogenesis. Affected structures should be susceptible to the teratogenic action of an agent only at specific gestational times. Systemic absorption of the agent by the mother and its presence at susceptible sites in the embryo or placenta should be demonstrable. Exposure to a greater quantity of the agent should be associated in a dose–response fashion with an increased frequency of abnormalities. Finally, a causal inference is supported if a reasonable pathogenic mechanism can be established for the observed effect. For example, lower birth weight is associated with maternal antihypertensive therapy, but maternal hypertension is itself strongly associated with decreased birth weight. Is lower birth weight associated with the blood pressure medication, or the disease of hypertension, or some combination?

KNOWN HUMAN TERATOGENS

The list of known human teratogens is surprisingly small (Box 1.1). The most notorious human teratogen is thalidomide. It is currently available in the USA on a limited basis for treatment of several infectious diseases such as acquired immune deficiency syndrome (AIDS), tuberculosis, and leprosy. In 1996, a new thalidomide embryopathy epidemic was reported in Brazil and other South American countries (Castilla *et al.*, 1996).

The astute reader will note that some of the putative teratogens do not fit precisely the definition of teratogen (i.e., exposure is not strictly confined to the period of organogenesis).

Box 1.1 Known human teratogens

ACE inhibitors	Coumarin derivatives	Retinoids (oral)
Amiodarone	Cyclophosphamide	Tetracycline derivatives
Aminopterin	Danazol	Thalidomide
Antiepileptic drugs	Diethylstilbestrol	Fluconazole
Carbamazepine	Lithium	Methimazole
Clonazepam	Methotrexate	Misoprostol
Primidone	Methylene blue	Trimethadione,
Phenobarbital	Penicillamine	paramethadione
Phenytoin/fosphenytoin	Quinine	Trimethoprim
Valproic acid	Radioiodine	

ACE, Angiotensin converting enzyme
Adapted from Schardein (2000), Shepard (2004), and Polifka and Friedman (2002).

CRITICAL TIME PERIODS

In utero development is divided into three time periods of development: (1) preimplantation; (2) period of the embryo; and (3) time of the fetus. Exposure to drugs during pregnancy must be separated into these time periods because the conceptus responds differently in each of the three stages of development.

Preimplantation

No physiologic interface between the mother and the conceptus exists at conception (ovum penetration by the spermatid to form a single diploid cell). Traditionally, the first week postconception (until the blastocyst attaches to the wall of the uterus forming chorionic villi) was considered protected from drugs or medications that may be in the maternal circulation because there is no formal biological interface between the blastocyst and the mother. However, recent evidence (e.g., mitomycin) indicates that the preimplantation embryo may not be as protected as previously thought.

Embryonic development

The most critical stage of development for the induction of birth defects is the period of the embryo. The period of the embryo extends the time of implantation until 58–60 days postconception. The organs and tissues of the unborn baby are being formed (i.e., organogenesis) during this period. Mistakes which occur during the period of the embryo result in malformations (congenital anomalies) and are called birth defects. Teratogens are agents that cause abnormal embryonic physical or physiological development by acting during the period of the embryo, or organogenesis (Jones, 1988). Malformations lethal to the embryo present as spontaneous abortion, sometimes before pregnancy is recognized. Similarly, some substances that are directly toxic to the embryo, e.g., methotrexate, also present as spontaneous abortions. The critical times for the development of various organs and structures of the human embryo are given in Fig. 1.2 (p. 5).

Fetal development

Important changes occur during the embryonic development that can also be damaged outside the period of the embryo. Traditionally, things that happened to a fetus were not considered a teratogenic effect, but some authorities have begun lumping fetal effects into this category. Changes in cellular structures such as the brain cell arrangements during neuronal migration occur during the fetal period. However, the predominant fetal event is hyperplastic growth (increase in cell number) with organs and other tissues becoming larger through cellular proliferation, and only secondarily through hypertrophy. An important example is the thyroid, which appears early in the fetal period, as does fetal endocrine function. Most of the potential adverse effects during fetal development are maldevelopment due to interrupted cell migration and growth retardation (Jones, 1988). If blood flow to an organ or structure is interrupted or obstructed, structures that were normally formed during embryogenesis may be malformed during the fetal period (e.g., vascular disruption and fetal cocaine or warfarin exposure). The structure deprived of blood flow would undergo necrosis and be resorbed. This would produce a defect that may mimic an embryonic effect. However, the true origin of the defect would be fetotoxicity.

The embryo and fetus are exposed to drugs through the placenta which can: (1) metabolize certain drugs before they reach the conceptus; (2) allow 99 percent of drugs to cross by simple diffusion; (3) not transport large molecules (i.e., larger than 1000 molecular weight), unless there is an active transport system (e.g., antibodies); (4) transport neutrally charged molecules; (5) easily transport lipid-soluble drugs; and (6) not transport charged (+ or –) molecules. Poor potential for transfer back to the maternal circulation occurs for some drugs (e.g., water-soluble drugs transfer back to the mother's circulation poorly), resulting in accumulation in the embryofetal compartment.

POTENTIAL ADVERSE EFFECTS

Spontaneous abortion

As many as 50 percent of early pregnancies (0–58 days) end in spontaneous abortion. Recent findings from *in vitro* fertilization studies suggest that the majority of these spontaneous abortuses are chromosomally abnormal. The risk of spontaneous abortion is 15–20 percent among fetuses surviving 59–126 days of gestation. The risk of spontaneous abortion/fetal death decreases to 1–2 percent by 18–20 weeks (127–140 days). Up to 28 weeks (196 days) postconception the risk for spontaneous abortion is approximately 2 percent.

Congenital anomalies

The frequency of congenital anomalies detected at birth is approximately 3.5–5 percent (Brent and Beckman, 1990). This figure is thought to underrepresent the true frequency of anomalies by as much as twofold because 100 percent detection of anomalies is not usually reached until about 5 years of age. The frequency of congenital anomalies is severalfold higher among stillbirths and miscarriages than live births, and is especially high among early (i.e., first-trimester) miscarriages.

Fetal effects

Fetal effects are of four primary types: (1) damage to structures or organs that are formed normally during embryogenesis; (2) damage to systems undergoing histogenesis during the fetal period; (3) growth retardation; or (4) fetal death or stillbirth. Any or all of these fetal effects can occur concomitantly. Fetal effects may be caused by a teratogen, but may also be caused by agents that have no apparent potential to produce abnormal embryonic development. Organs, structures, or functions formed normally during embryogenesis can be damaged by some environmental exposures during the fetal period.

Fetal growth retardation is the most frequently observed effect of agents given during pregnancy and outside the period of embryogenesis. Sometimes it is difficult to distinguish between the effects of the agents from those of the disease entity being treated. Propranolol, for example, is associated with fetal growth retardation, but the maternal disease for which the drug is given (hypertension) is also associated with fetal growth retardation in the absence of antihypertensive therapy. Some agents that are teratogenic may be associated with fetal growth retardation. Fetal growth retardation may also occur without embryonic damage. Risks of fetal death, stillbirth, and other adverse effects are increased with exposure to some agents during pregnancy (Table 1.1).

Neonatal and postnatal effects

Prenatal exposure to some drugs is associated with adverse neonatal effects, such as difficulty in adaptation to life outside the womb. Drugs associated with adverse neonatal are not usually associated with teratogenic effects. Transient metabolic abnormalities, withdrawal, and hypoglycemia are well-documented neonatal effects of certain medications and nonmedical drugs. Examples of other adverse neonatal effects are the floppy infant syndrome with the use of benzodiazepines near term, patent ductus arteriosus with the use of prostaglandin synthestase inhibitors (non-steroidal anti-inflammatory agents – or NSAIDs) such as aspirin or indomethacin, and gray baby syndrome with high-dose chloramphenicol near the time of delivery (Table 1.1). Developmental delay is frequently associated with the action of teratogens, but is also observed in association with the fetal effects of drugs that are apparently not teratogenic.

Table 1.1 Adverse effects other than birth defects on the human fetus associated with drugs

Maternal medication	Fetal/neonatal effect
Acetaminophen	Renal failure
Adrenocortical hormones	Adrenocortical suppression; electrolyte imbalance
Alcohol	Muscular hypotonia: hypoglycemia (?); withdrawal; intrauterine growth restriction (IUGR); blood changes; affect mental ability
Alphaprodine	Platelet dysfunction
Amitriptyline	Withdrawal
Ammonium chloride	Acidosis
Amphetamines	Withdrawal
Antihistamines	Infertility(?)
Antineoplastics	Transient pancytopenia IUGR
Antithyroid drugs	Hypothyroidism
Barbiturates/diphenylhydantoin	Coagulation defects; withdrawal (barbiturates only); IUGR
Chloral hydrate, excess	Fetal death
Chloramphenicol	Death ('gray baby syndrome')
Chlordiazepoxide	Withdrawal(?)
Chloroquine	Death(?)
Chlorpropamide	Prolonged hypoglycemia; fetal death
Cocaine	Vascular disruption, withdrawal, IUGR
Coumarin anticoagulants	Hemorrhage, death, IUGR
Diazepam	Hypothermia; hypotonia; withdrawal
Diphenhydramine	Withdrawal
Ergot	Fetal death
Erythromycin	Liver damage(?)
Gold salts	Complications; kernicterus
Glutethimide	Withdrawal
Heroin/morphine/methadone	Withdrawal; neonatal death
Hexamethonium bromide	Neonatal ileus
Hykinone	Blood changes; jaundice
Immunosuppressants	Transient immune system depression, danger of infection
Insulin (shock)	Fetal loss
Intravenous fluids, excess	Fluid and electrolyte abnormalities
Iophenoxic acid	Evaluation of serum protein-bound iodine (PBI)
Lithium	Cyanosis, flaccidity, polyhydramnios, toxicity
Magnesium sulfate	Central depression and neuromuscular block
Meperidine	Neonatal depression
Mepivacaine	Fetal brachycardia and depression
Meprobamate	Retarded development(?)
Nitrofurantoin	Hemolysis
Novobiocin	Hyperbilirubinemia(?)
Oral progestogens, androgens, and estrogens	Advanced bone age
Phenformin	Lactic acidosis(?)
Phenobarbital, excess	Neonatal bleeding; death
Phenothiazines	Hyperbilirubinemia(?), depression, hypothermia(?), withdrawal
Polio vaccine, live	Fetal loss(?)

continued

Table 1.1 *Continued*

Maternal medication	Fetal/neonatal effect
Prednisolone	Acute fetal distress, fetal death (?)
Primaquine, pentaquine	Hemolysis(?)
Primidone	Withdrawal(?)
Propoxyphene	Withdrawal
Quinine	Thrombocytopenia
Reserpine	Nasal congestion, lethargy, respiratory depression, brachycardia
Salicylates, excess	Bleeding, fetal death
Sedatives	Behavioral changes
Smoking	Premature births, IUGR, perinatal loss(?)
Sulfonamides	Kernicterus(?), anemia(?)
Tetracyclines	Deposition in bone, inhibition of bone growth in premature infants, discoloration of teeth
Thiazide diuretics	Thrombocytopenia, salt and water depletion, neonatal death(?)
Thioureas	Blood changes, affect mental ability
Tolbutamide	Thrombocytopenia, fetal death
Vaccinations	Fetal vaccinia
Verapamil	Transient fetal-neonatal cardiovascular
Vitamin K analogs, excess	Hyperbilirubinemia

Adapted from Schardein, 2000.

MATERNAL PHYSIOLOGY DURING PREGNANCY

Profound physiological changes occur during pregnancy. Maternal enzymes, particularly cholinesterases (Pritchard, 1955), have lowered activity. Maternal blood volume increases dramatically during pregnancy, by perhaps 40–50 percent, to support the requirements of the developing fetus (Cunningham *et al.*, 2001). Distribution of drugs in this increased blood volume may lower serum concentrations. Absorption of drugs occurs with about the same kinetics as in the nonpregnant adult; however, renal clearance is increased and enzyme activity is downregulated. Decreased enzyme activity levels are exacerbated somewhat by the increased blood volume, decreasing the overall effective serum concentration of a given dose. In turn, increased renal output may effect an increased clearance index for most drugs. Drugs that are tightly bound to the serum proteins have little opportunity to cross the placenta or enter breast milk. Consequently, increased demands are placed on cardiovascular, hepatic, and renal systems. In addition, the gravid uterus is vulnerable to a variety of effects not present in the nonpregnant state, such as hemorrhage, rupture, or preterm contraction.

Increased demands imposed on these physiological systems by pregnancy may, under normal conditions, be dealt with in an uncomplicated manner. However, conditions of disease or other stress weaken these key systems and they may be unable to function normally. For example, cocaine abuse during pregnancy actually targets these key systems that are already stressed from the gravid state of the woman. Hence, it would be expected that cocaine use during pregnancy would place cardiovascular, renal, and hepatic systems at greater risk than those of the nonpregnant adult. Indeed, these expectations are borne out in the observations of cocaine use during pregnancy.

PHARMACOKINETICS IN PREGNANCY

The quantity of pharmacokinetic data during pregnancy is extremely limited. Only two investigations examined for this review made explicit quantitative recommendations for dose or schedule during pregnancy (Caritis et al., 1989; Wisner et al., 1993). Frequently, results are conflicting between studies of the same drug. Across all investigations reviewed, area under the curve was decreased in 41 percent of the studies, volume of distribution was increased in 30 percent, and peak plasma concentration was decreased in 34 percent. Steady-state plasma concentration was decreased in 44 percent of the studies, as was half-life in 41 percent. Clearance was increased in 55 percent of the studies (Table 1.2).

No general statement about pharmacokinetic changes during pregnancy can be made. The individual drug must be considered. These changes in pharmacokinetics cause decreases in drug plasma concentrations. When pharmacokinetic data are altered in this way, increased doses or schedules are needed to maintain effective systemic drug levels. However, this summary information is biased by a lack of information on many therapeutic agents used during pregnancy and because some drugs are represented more than once among the investigations reviewed. Still, the physiologic changes during pregnancy and their effects on the disposition of medications given during gestation found in this review are consistent with previous surveys of the literature (Amon and Hüller, 1984a, b; Cummings, 1983; Kafetzis et al., 1983; Mattison et al., 1992; Philipson 1978; Reynolds 1991). Multiple confounders make it difficult to interpret available pharmacokinetic data in pregnancy. Many studies have had very small sample sizes, frequently fewer than 10 pregnant women. Comparison groups have varied in composition. Studies have used nonpregnant women, adult males, the same patients 6–8 weeks postpartum, or published pharmacokinetic data. None of the studies reviewed gave maternal weight-

Table 1.2 Pharmacokinetics in pregnancy

Index	Studies reporting pharmacokinetic data changes associated with pregnancy			
	n	Decrease	No change	Increase	Studies not reporting pharmacokinetic data (%)
AUC	17	7	5	5	44 (72.1)
V_d	23	3	11	9	38 (62.3)
C_{max}	30	10	17	3	31 (50.8)
C_{ss}	42	19	4	19	19 (31.1)
$t_{1/2}$	39	16	17	6	22 (36.1)
t_{max}	9	3	4	2	52 (85.2)
Cl	44	5	15	24	17 (27.9)
PPB	7	6	1	0	54 (88.5)

Source: Little BB. *Obstet Gynecol* 1999; **93**: 858.

AUC, area under the curve; V_d, volume of distribution; C_{max}, maximum concentration; C_{ss}, steady state concentration; $t_{1/2}$, half-life; t_{max}, time to plasma concentration; Cl, clearance; PPB, plasma protein bound.

adjusted values, despite the strong influence this variable might have on area under the curve, volume of distribution, peak plasma concentration, steady-state plasma concentration, half-life, and time to peak plasma concentration. Route of administration also varied, even with the same drug, and is also known to be an important influence on peak plasma concentration, steady-state plasma concentration, half-life, time to peak plasma concentration, and area under the curve. Another important confounder is estimated gestational age. Most pharmacokinetic measures differ by the stage of gestation, and the method of determining estimated gestational age was not reported in any of the studies reviewed. A lack of consistency in the method of quantitative assay of drug levels and interlaboratory variation further confound the studies. The empiric effect of pharmacogenetic variation on drug disposition during pregnancy has been reported by only one group of investigators (Bardy *et al.*, 1982). Polymorphisms in enzymes are known to exist and might result in lower enzyme activity in 10–20 percent of the population, including pregnant women (Vesell, 1997). No data are available to address this variation directly among gravidas, although pharmacogenetic differences must affect drug disposition during pregnancy.

PRENATAL DIAGNOSIS

Medication exposure or substance use during pregnancy, including that which is chronic, is not necessarily an indication for pregnancy termination, although this is a common reaction among patients and physicians. Such exposure is, however, an indication for prenatal diagnosis. Prenatal diagnosis cannot rule out defects that are not related to gross structural abnormalities, but major congenital anomalies, such as spina bifida, structural heart defects, and limb reduction, can usually be determined prenatally.

Prenatal diagnosis can be used to screen for congenital anomalies and other fetal complications following use of medications or drugs during pregnancy. Commonly available prenatal diagnosis procedures include: (1) high-resolution ultrasound; (2) maternal serum alpha-fetoprotein (MSAFP); and (3) fetal echocardiography. Ultrasound studies are informative in assessment of fetal growth and in possible detection of specific structural anomalies of major organs. MSAFP is important for screening pregnancies for open neural tube or other open defects (e.g., gastroschisis). Amniocentesis may be performed to assess an abnormal alpha-fetoprotein level, but a karyotype study is not indicated by drug or alcohol exposure *per se*, except for colchicine. Fetal echocardiography is used to screen for cardiovascular defects that cannot be detected with the basic ultrasound four-chamber view of the heart, for example, valvular defects and vascular stenosis.

The patient should be advised of the limitations of prenatal diagnosis not only in the constraints on what can be detected (i.e., gross structural abnormalities), but also in its reliability in detecting defects prenatally (ranging from 40 to 90 percent).

COUNSELING AND EVALUATION OF THE DRUG-EXPOSED PREGNANT PATIENT

Counseling patients who have been exposed to drugs or other environmental agents during pregnancy is difficult for several reasons. Many patients have anxiety regarding the exposure because they fear their child will be born with birth defects. Anxiety is heightened because the mother frequently feels guilt, believing she may have damaged her baby through some action of her own. Cultural beliefs regarding the causes of congenital anomalies differ from scientific explanations, placing blame on the mother. Other factors, such as the patient's educational background, socioeconomic status, and ethnic-specific folklore, may also pose an obstacle to communication during counseling. These influences come into play when counseling patients exposed to potential teratogens.

Rapport with the patient is important, assuring confidentiality and establishing a basis for the patient's trust. The counselor must convey to the patient his or her understanding of the patient's concerns, and explain that the purpose of the consultation is to deal directly with those concerns by ascertaining the magnitude of the risk for an adverse pregnancy outcome arising from the drug exposure.

General principles of counseling

Many patients are not satisfied with the counseling they receive for exposure to potential teratogens during pregnancy. Dissatisfaction stems largely from two major issues that both cause patient anxiety. First, the physician is frequently unable to obtain adequate information to make meaningful statements regarding the medical risks of whether the pregnancy was adversely affected by the drug exposure. Second, most patients do not understand the difference between an embryo and a fetus. Consequently, patients may not be able to grasp the importance of the concept of 'critical periods' unless they have been given a proper briefing during the consultation.

It is our policy to explain that there are two distinct phases involved in the growth of a baby, as shown in Fig. 1.2. The first phase is the embryonic development, and it is during this period that the structure or architecture for the baby is laid down. Embryonic age should be differentiated from menstrual age, which is 2 weeks greater than embryonic age. Briefly, we explain to our patients that organs take shape and the body assumes the form it will have thereafter by day 58 postconception. All major structures, such as the heart, brain, liver, kidneys, and limbs, have formed by this time. Fetal development during the remainder of pregnancy, the second phase of development, is primarily devoted to the growth of these organs and structures, and to augmenting their function.

It is through this heuristic approach to counseling that the patient understands that most congenital anomalies are caused by early exposures, often before the pregnancy was recognized. This ameliorates anxiety and guilt. This component is included early in the consultation; patients then understand why certain questions are important and having such knowledge increases their cooperation and rapport.

Preconceptional counseling

Ideally, all counseling regarding drug or medication use during pregnancy should occur before conception, because the opportunity to prevent possible adverse effects is then optimal. Preconceptional counseling should include all the components of a consultation during the pregnancy, with one exception. Recommendations regarding medication or drug use during pregnancy will be *prospective* for a preventive purpose, and only medically indicated drugs and medications known to be safe will be recommended for continued use while attempting to conceive.

Counseling the exposed gravida

Counseling for drug or medication exposures during pregnancy should follow a protocol as laid out in Fig. 1.3. The concept of background risk for major congenital anomalies should be explained in a manner tailored to the patient's level of understanding.
This concept is especially important because it conveys to the patient that, even if the
drug exposure is harmless, no guarantee can be given that the fetus she carries will not
have a congenital anomaly. Notwithstanding other risk factors, the risk for major congenital anomalies is approximately 3.5–5 percent. Other identified risks are generally
considered to be additive to background risk.

A usual component of counseling is the determination of exactly what drugs were
taken, the dosage, the timing and duration of the exposure(s), the patient's health history
and present state of health. A thorough physical examination should be used to determined the present state of health. Also, a medical genetic pedigree, including the patient's

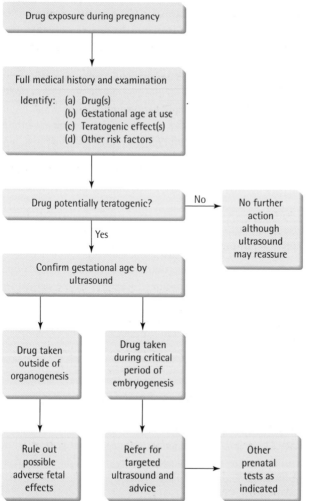

Figure 1.3 *Flow diagram*

parents as well as the baby's father's parents, brothers and sisters, and nieces and nephews, should be constructed. The current state of health of all people in the pedigree should also be elicited. For those individuals in the pedigree who are no longer living, whether death was due to a birth defect or to a heritable disorder should be determined. It is also important to ask whether the patient's family or the baby's father's family has any member who was mentally retarded, or has a chromosomal abnormality, Down syndrome, congenital heart disease, spina bifida or another neural tube defect, or any other inherited disease. When such risk factors are discovered, it is important to explore these avenues further. It is desirable to refer the patient for a medical genetic consultation and evaluation when a risk increase above background is other than zero.

The next step in the consultation is to determine whether or not the agent(s) has known teratogenic potential. This is the most difficult part of the evaluation because there is insufficient information to make such a determination for more than 60 percent of medications. Currently, the most reliable source of information regarding drug or medication use during pregnancy is TERIS (Teratogen Information System), a computerized database available for use either on IBM-compatible personal computers or

Box 1.2 Sources of information on drugs and medications during pregnancy

Databases

TERIS, Department of Pediatrics, University of Washington, Seattle, WA 206-543-4365
http://depts.washington.edu/~terisweb/
Note: Individual summaries may be purchased for clinical use

REPROTOX, An independent non-profit organization: reprotox@reprotox.org; http://reprotox.org/

Hotlines

MotheRisk Program   +1-416-813-6780
Teratogen Information Service (TIS) +1-800-532-3749 or +1-619-294-6084
Organization of Teratology Information Services (OTIS) +1-888-285-3410

Textbooks

Catalog of Teratogenic Agents. 10th edn. T.H. Shepard. Baltimore: Johns Hopkins University Press, 2001.
Drugs in Pregnancy and Lactation. 6th edn. G.G. Briggs, R.K. Freeman, S.J. Yaffe. Baltimore: Williams & Wilkins, 2002.
Chemically Induced Birth Defects. 3rd edn. J.L. Schardein. New York: Marcel Dekker, 2002.
Drugs and Pregnancy. 2nd edn. L.C. Gilstrap, B.B. Little. New York: Chapman and Hall, 1998.
Management of Psychiatric Disorders in Pregnancy. K.A. Yonkers, B.B. Little. London: Arnold Press, 2001.
The Effects of Neurologic and Psychiatric Drugs on the Fetus and Nursing Infant: A Handbook for Health Care Professionals. J.M. Friedman, J.E. Polifka. Baltimore: Johns Hopkins University Press, 1998.
Teratogenic Effects of Drugs: A Resource for Clinicians, 2nd edn. J.M. Friedman, J.E. Polifka. Baltimore: Johns Hopkins University Press, 2000.

online by subscription (Box 1.2). If it can be documented that the agent has no terato-genic risks or adverse fetal effects associated with its use during pregnancy, then no fur-ther action is required except to document this in the medical record and counsel the patient accordingly. Some patients may benefit from reassurance offered by high-resolu-tion ultrasound to confirm fetal well-being, and this procedure should be offered if the patient's anxiety is not relieved through counseling. The limitations of diagnostic ultra-sound should also be included in the consultation.

If the drug is known not to be safe for use during pregnancy, or if there are reasons to suspect that a drug with unknown risks is associated with congenital anomalies, then gestational age should be confirmed by ultrasound. It is of utmost importance to base the risk assessment and counseling upon embryonic age, not menstrual age. If the expo-sure occurred during embryogenesis, then it is necessary to undertake high-resolution ultrasound in an attempt to detect damage to specific organ systems or structures that were being formed during the time of the exposure. If the ultrasound scan is normal, then it is reasonable to reassure the patient of normal fetal structure within the limits of the sensitivity and specificity of ultrasound, which range from 40 to 90 percent for gross structural abnormalities when the procedure is performed by an experienced sonogra-pher. If the exposure occurred during the fetal period, it is likewise important to evalu-ate the possible fetal effects of the medication.

If defects are detected, it is necessary to describe them in detail to the patient and to give a prognosis, as far as available medical knowledge will allow, regarding the out-come of pregnancy and postnatal development. To assist the patient in making a deci-sion on the disposition of the pregnancy, prognostication should include medically doc-umented risk figures. Ethically, pregnancy termination should not be a recommendation made to the patient and her family and significant others. This option should be dis-cussed, but the ultimate decision of whether to continue the pregnancy should be left to the patient and her family and significant others. The role of teratogen counseling is ulti-mately to provide the patient with as much information as possible and encourage her to make her own decision regarding whether to continue the pregnancy.

Drug- or chemical-related causes of maternal complications, congenital anomalies, and fetal toxicity are almost unique among adverse pregnancy outcomes because they are potentially preventable, given the window of opportunity to do so. These problems are also exceptional among obstetric complications in that they are often the focus of malpractice litigation. Attorneys recognize that such adverse outcomes could have been prevented, and litigation ensues despite the fact that the window of opportunity to inter-vene prudently may not have existed for the physician and, more importantly, the drug exposure may not be teratogenic at any time during the pregnancy.

FOOD AND DRUG ADMINISTRATION CLASSIFICATION OF DRUGS AND INFORMED CONSENT

Until 1979, most drugs and medications were accompanied by disclaimers, the most common of which were the 'safe use in pregnancy has not been established' and such a medication 'should not be used in pregnant women unless, in the judgment of the physi-cian, the potential benefits outweigh the possible hazards' (Brent, 1982). The major drawback with such disclaimers was that there existed little to no information upon which to 'weigh the possible hazards'. Such disclaimers would make defense of a litigation case involving a drug or medication extremely difficult for the physician because benefits are not easily weighed against unknown possible hazards. With no scientific data relating a specific malformation to a given drug, it is nearly impossible to 'prove' in the courtroom that a drug is not a teratogen and is safe for use during pregnancy. Thus a jury may be asked to consider the important question of why a physician would utilize a medication that carried the warning 'safe use in pregnancy has not been established'. The disclaimer itself implies that a medication may indeed be a teratogen, although the warning is actually little more than legally formulated rhetoric designed to protect the pharmaceutical company (Brent, 1982). There have been many efforts to encourage the FDA to change the nature of the labeling on the package insert and to change the manner in which drugs are classified with regard to their reproductive risks (Brent, 1982).

In 1979, the FDA attempted to improve labeling policies for the use of medications during pregnancy. Five risk categories that addressed potential adverse fetal effects, including congenital anomalies, were developed. Although an improvement over the previous labeling disclaimers, this classification is less than perfect (Brent, 1982).

According to the *Physicians' Desk Reference* (2005), the categories devised by the FDA are 'based on the degree to which available information has ruled out risk to the fetus, balanced against the drug's potential benefits to the patient'. Although intended to provide management guidance about teratogenic risks, a recent study found that FDA categories have little, if any, correlation to teratogenic risk. Friedman and colleagues (1990) compared the teratogenic risk of 157 most frequently prescribed drugs according to TERIS, a computerized database of clinical teratology information, to the FDA pregnancy categories, where available. These authors pointed out that 'any classification of agents according to teratogenic risk is incomplete because the risk to a given patient is determined by all of the conditions of exposure'. Paramount importance must also be ascribed to drug dose, route of administration, and timing of exposure, as well as exposure to multiple agents during the pregnancy (Friedman *et al.*, 1990). The information on the package insert, a joint effort of the FDA and the pharmaceutical company, fails to provide information about risks that are known, does not discuss the option of pregnancy interruption, and provides anxiety-provoking information that is irrelevant, such as 'this drug crosses the placental barrier' (Brent, 1982).

INFORMED CONSENT AND POST-EXPOSURE COUNSELING

Before initiating informed consent regarding medication exposure during pregnancy, the factors of dose, route of administration, and timing must be ascertained as accurately as possible. Even if an agent is a potential teratogen of significant risk or even a proven teratogen such as thalidomide, the actual risk to the fetus may be minimal to none if the timing of exposure occurred during late pregnancy or after the period of organogenesis. In contradistinction, some teratogens, such as radioactive iodine or the angiotensin-converting enzyme inhibitors may be harmful only after early organogenesis (Brent and Beckman, 1990).

After a detailed history is obtained, the patient should be given 'full disclosure' regarding the known or suspected risk of the agent, as well as the various therapeutic and diagnostic options available. This information should be accurate, yet easily understandable. All such information and counseling should be well documented in the patient's chart.

All counseling regarding a drug or medication exposure should be performed by a clinician knowledgeable in both teratology and in counseling. Taking the whole clinical picture into account, one should utilize a resource such as TERIS as well as other teratogen information resources as sources of the most recent and accurate information on the potential teratogenic effects of a specific agent.

The TERIS summaries are available for a nominal fee by fax from the Department of Pediatrics, University of Washington, Seattle, WA, USA. The contact is Dr. Janine Polifka at +1-206-543-2465. The TERIS website is http://www.depts.washington.edu/~TERISweb/TERIS.

Experienced counselors may also have their own personal reprint collection dealing with teratogens. We include all such information, especially the TERIS summary in exposure cases, in the patient's chart, and it is used as an adjunct in counseling of each drug- or chemical-exposed pregnant patient.

In counseling, one could also make this statement: 'Although this agent may be associated with an increased risk of malformation when utilized in the first 8–10 (menstrual) weeks of pregnancy, it would not be expected to be associated with significant risk when given in the latter half of pregnancy'. In the case of an agent such as tetracycline, one might state: 'It is logical to conclude that tetracycline would not be expected to cause yellow-brown discoloration of the teeth when given during the first 16–20 weeks of pregnancy'.

Another suggested statement would be as follows: 'Although the actual teratogenic risk of this agent is unknown, given the dose and route of administration, the fetal risk of this preparation is negligible to nonexistent, since little to none of it reaches the fetus'.

Other sources of information regarding the teratogenic risk of specific agents that may be useful in counseling patients, in addition to the present text and TERIS, include Shepard's *Catalog of Teratogenic Agents, Drugs in Pregnancy and Lactation: A Reference Guide to Fetal and Neonatal Risk, Chemically Induced Birth Defects* and other similar texts.

SUMMARY

The clinician must be cognizant of the fact that many patients, as well as attorneys, believe that most congenital malformations must be secondary to a drug or medication taken during gestation. Counseling of such patients requires a significant degree of both knowledge and skill. Physicians must also realize that erroneous counseling by inexperienced health professionals is one of the leading stimuli for nonmeritorious litigation (Brent, 1977). Moreover, the clinician must be aware that drugs and medications represent a bountiful field for litigation, since there is a reasonable likelihood that, once the family and the attorney have concluded that there is merit to their allegation, they can locate experts who will support the nonmeritorious allegation. Thus, physicians may focus their attention on attorneys as the cause of the plethora of litigation, when in reality they could not proceed without the assistance of unknowledgable or unscrupulous experts.

Key references

Baird PA, Anderson TW, Newcombe HB, Lowry RB. Genetic disorders in children and young adults. A population study. *Am J Hum Genet* 1989; **42**: 677.

Castilla EE, Ashton-Prolla P, Barreda-Mejia E et al. Thalidomide, a current teratogen in South America. *Teratology* 1996; **54**: 273.

Friedman JM, Little BB, Brent RL et al. Potential human teratogenicity of frequently prescribed drugs. *Obstet Gynecol* 1990; **75**: 594.

Little BB. Pharmacokinetics during pregnancy. Evidence-based maternal dose formulation. *Obstet Gynecol* 1999; **93**: 858–68.

Little BB, Santos-Ramos R, Newell JF, Maberry MC. Megadose carbamazepine during embryogenesis. *Obstet Gynecol* 1993; **82**: 705–8.

Lo WY, Friedman JM. Teratogenicity of recently introduced medications in human pregnancy. *Obstet Gynecol* 2002; **100**: 465–73.

Polifka JE, Friedman JM. Medical genetics. 1. Clinical teratology in the age of genomics. *CMAJ* 2002; **167**: 265–73.

Schardein JL. *Chemically Induced Birth Defects*, 3rd edn. New York: Marcel Dekker, 2000.

Shepard TH. *Catalog of Teratogenic Agents.* 11th edn, Baltimore: Johns Hopkins University Press, 2004.

Further references are available on the book's website at http://www.drugsandpregnancy.com

2

Antimicrobials during pregnancy: bacterial, viral, fungal, and parasitic indications

This chapter is divided into five sections, four dealing with the major classes of antimicrobials, and a final section on special considerations deals with specific indications for antibiotic use (disease entities), and first-line therapies available for each indication:

- Antibiotics
- Antifungals
- Antivirals
- Antiparasitics
- Special considerations

Infections are commonplace during pregnancy. Treatment of infections occur during pregnancy brings up several important questions.

- Is immediate antimicrobial treatment necessary?
- Could therapy safely be withheld until after the first trimester?
- Could therapy possibly be delayed until after delivery?
- How does pregnancy affect the efficacy and safety of a particular antimicrobial agent, i.e., what are the effects on the mother and fetus?
- What scientific data are available regarding the use of various agents during pregnancy?
- How does pregnancy affect the pharmacokinetics and pharmacodynamics of various antimicrobial agents?

The nature and severity of the infection will contribute to the clinician's decision of when to treat and what the treatment should be. Infections such as trichomonal vaginitis or other parasitic infections usually do not require immediate treatment, and initiation of treatment can safely wait until after the first trimester. In contrast, urinary tract infections should be treated upon diagnosis because delay in therapy may have untoward consequences for both mother and fetus.

All antimicrobial agents cross the placenta. Therefore, potential adverse effects are not limited to the mother but extend to the fetus as well. Limited scientific data are available regarding the safety of most antimicrobial agents during pregnancy. Nonetheless, many of these agents have been used in pregnant women out of necessity.

Pregnancy causes physiologic changes that may alter the pharmacokinetics and pharmacodynamics of an antimicrobial agent (Little, 1999). Perhaps the most significant of pregnancy-associated changes is the marked increase in blood volume, 40–50 percent above the nonpregnant state at term. Blood volume increase begins during the first trimester, with marked changes occurring during the second and third trimesters. There is marked variation from patient to patient in the actual increase in blood volume. Additionally, endogenous creatinine clearance is increased, serum binding proteins are lowered in concentration, and gastrointestinal motility is lower compared to the nonpregnant state. These pregnancy-associated physiologic changes may affect the serum level through increased volume of distribution, altered (usually lowered) metabolism, reduced absorption and increased clearance of various antimicrobial agents. Ultimately, the therapeutic dose of an antimicrobial will be altered, usually making it necessary to adjust dosage during pregnancy. Importantly, certain pregnancy complications (e.g., hypertension, vascular disease, acute pyelonephritis) may alter 'normal' pregnancy-associated physiologic changes.

Limited information on pharmacokinetics of most antimicrobial agents during pregnancy is available. A comprehensive review of pharmacokinetics during pregnancy is published (Little, 1999), and Table 2.1 is adapted for antimicrobials.

Serum levels of most antimicrobial agents that have been studied are reduced during pregnancy, often by approximately 10–15 percent (Landers *et al.*, 1983). Ampicillin and gentamicin, for example, are known to result in lower serum levels during pregnancy compared to nonpregnant women given the same dose (Duff *et al.*, 1983; Philipson, 1977; Zaske *et al.*, 1980). Increased blood volume (i.e., increased volume of distribution) is probably the cause of lowered serum drug concentrations. Lower serum drug concentrations are probably not caused by strong dissociation of ampicillin at physiological pH, which should theoretically interfere with placental transfer. Although ampicillin and methicillin are strongly dissociated, their maternal–fetal concentration ratios are 1:1, suggesting uninhibited transfer across the placenta (Pacifici and Nottoli, 1995).

Physicians are also at risk from the use of antimicrobial agents during pregnancy with the litigation crisis in obstetrics, and the many cases that involve drugs and medications. A particular agent may not be a teratogen (i.e., a cause of birth defects), but it may still be a 'litogen' (i.e., cause law suits) (Brent, 1985).

ANTIBIOTICS

Antibiotics are prescribed during pregnancy and the postpartum period to treat bacterial infections (e.g., urinary tract infections, chorioamnionitis, endometritis). There has been a proliferation of antibiotics over the last decade. Unfortunately, there have been few, if any, scientific studies regarding the use of these antibiotics during pregnancy.

Penicillins

The penicillins are bactericidal by virtue of interference with cell wall synthesis. Virtually all the agents in this class cross the placenta, resulting in significant detectable serum

Table 2.1 Pharmacokinetic study of antibiotic agents during pregnancy: pregnant compared with nonpregnant

Agent	n	EGA (weeks)	Route	AUC	V_d	C_{max}	C_{ss}	$t_{1/2}$	CI	PPB	Control group[a]
Arnikacin	11	40	IM			=	=				Yes (3)
Ampicillin	14	26–34	IM		↑	↓	↓	↓	↑		Yes (1)
Ampicillin	26	9–36	IV, PO		↑	↓	↓	=	↑		Yes (2)
Ampicillin	13	32	IV			=	=	=			Yes (1)
Azlocillin	7	30–40	IV		↓	=	=	=			Yes (1)
Azlocillin	20	32–40	IV	=							No
Cefazolin	6	10–27	PO	=	=	↓	↓	↓	↑		Yes (2)
Cefuroxime	7	11–35	PO		↓	=	↓	↓	↓	↑	Yes (2)
Cephradine	12	10–27	PO		↓	↑	↓	↓	↓	↑	Yes (2)
Piperacillin	5	30–40	IV		=	↑	=	=	=	=	No

Source: Little BB. *Obstet Gynecol* 1999; 93: 858.

EGA, estimated gestational age; AUC, area under the curve; V_d, volume of distribution; C_{max}, peak plasma concentration; C_{ss}, steady-state concentration; $t_{1/2}$, half-life; CI, clearance; PPB, plasma protein binding; PO, by mouth; ↓ denotes a decrease during pregnancy compared with nonpregnant values; ↑ denotes an increase during pregnancy compared with nonpregnant values; = denotes no difference between pregnant and nonpregnant values; IV = intravenous; IM = intramuscular.

[a]Control groups: 1, nonpregnant women; 2, same individuals studied postpartum; 3, historic adult controls (sex not given); 4, adult male controls; 5, adult male and female controls combined.

Table 2.2 Mean antibiotic concentration ratios for various penicillins

	Antibiotic cord blood to maternal blood ratio
Ampicillin	0.71
Ampicillin plus sulbactam	1.0
Mezlocillin	0.4
Ticarcillin plus clavulanic acid	0.8

From Gilstrap et al., 1988a; Maberry et al., 1990.

levels in the fetus (Gilstrap *et al.*, 1988a; Landers *et al.*, 1983; Maberry *et al.*, 1990). The ratios of cord blood to maternal blood concentration of several penicillins are shown in Table 2.2.

Although all penicillins (Box 2.1) would appear to cross the placenta readily, there is no evidence to date that they are teratogenic, and they have been used in pregnant women for many years without apparent adverse fetal effects.

Although they are not teratogenic, the penicillins may cause significant adverse effects in the mother, including hypersensitivity reactions, serum sickness, hematologic toxicity, renal toxicity, hypokalemia, gastrointestinal toxicity, and central nervous system toxicity (Box 2.2).

Box 2.1 The penicillins

Natural penicillins
Penicillin G
Penicillin V

Antistaphylococcal penicillins
Cloxacillin
Dicloxacillin
Methicillin
Nafcillin
Oxacillin

Derivatives of 6-aminopenicillanic acid
Amoxicillin
Ampicillin

Bucampicillin

Extended-spectrum penicillins
Azlocillin
Carbenicillin
Mezlocillin
Piperacillin
Ticarcillin

Penicillins with beta-lactamase inhibitors
Amoxicillin plus clavulanic acid (Augmentin)
Ampicillin plus sulbactam (Unasyn)
Piperacillin plus tazobactam (Zosyn)
Ticarcillin plus clavulanic acid (Timentin)

Adapted from Faro, 1989; PDR, 2004.

Box 2.2 Potential adverse fetal and maternal effects of penicillin

Fetal effects
None known, but fetal hypersensitivity is a
theoretical risk

Maternal effects
Hypersensitivity reactions

Hematologic toxicity
Renal toxicity
Central nervous system toxicity
Gastrointestinal toxicity

From Faro, 1989.

Macrolide antibiotics

The macrolide antibiotics as a group are effective against a variety of aerobic organisms and have poor activity against most Gram-negative organisms. The major antibiotics in this group are erythromycin, azithromycin, and clarithromycin.

Erythromycin

Erythromycin is a bacteriostatic agent which interferes with bacterial protein synthesis. Unlike most antibiotics, erythromycin crosses the placenta poorly, achieving very low levels in the fetus. This latter fact is exemplified by the observation that erythromycin provides inadequate treatment for the fetus when given to the mother for the treatment of syphilis, as is discussed in detail later in this chapter. The major preparations are listed in Box 2.3.

Box 2.3 The erythromycins

Erythromycin	Erythromycin gluceptate
Erythromycin estolate	Erythromycin lactobionate
Erythromycin ethylsuccinate	Erythromycin stearate

From PDR, 2004 (trade names too numerous to list).

There are no reports linking erythromycin and congenital anomalies or adverse fetal effects. Likewise, there have been few maternal adverse effects (Box 2.4) reported with the use of this antibiotic during pregnancy, with the exception of gastrointestinal upsets (which may be worse in pregnancy), hypersensitivity reactions, and hepatitis (Hautekeete, 1995).

Box 2.4 Potential adverse fetal and maternal effects of erythromycin

Fetal effects
None known
Maternal effects
Gastrointestinal intolerance
Hepatitis
Hypersensitivity reactions

Hautekeete, 1995.

Azithromycin

Azithromycin (Zithromax) belongs to the azalide class of antibiotics and is similar to the macrolide erythromycin. It is effective against many of the same organisms as erythromycin and especially useful against *Neisseria gonorrhoeae* and *Chlamydia trachomatis*.

It is well absorbed orally and has the advantage of single-dose therapy for chlamydial infections. Although there are no large epidemiological studies in pregnant women, it is listed as a category B drug by its manufacturer. This antibiotic has been utilized as single-dose therapy for chlamydial infections during pregnancy (Allaire *et al.*, 1995; Bush and Rosa, 1994; Rosenn *et al.*, 1995, Turrentine *et al.*, 1995).

Clarithromycin

Clarithromycin (Biaxin) belongs to the macrolide group of antibiotics. Although it is effective against a wide variety of aerobic organisms, it is most commonly used for treatment or prophylaxis against *Mycobacterium avium* complex (MAC) in patients who are human immunodeficiency virus (HIV)-positive. It also has good activity against *Ureaplasma urealyticum* (Reisner, 1996). There are no large randomized studies of clarithromycin in pregnant women, and it is listed as a category C drug by its manufacturer.

Cephalosporins

As a group, the cephalosporins are probably the most commonly used antibiotics in obstetrics and gynecology. They are very similar in structure to the penicillins, both containing a four-member beta-lactam ring. They are also bactericidal and inhibit cell wall synthesis. Cephalosporins are generally classified into first, second, and third generation (Box 2.5).

All of the cephalosporins cross the placenta (Bawdon *et al.*, 1982; Dinsmoor and Gibbs, 1988; Giamarellou *et al.*, 1983; Gilstrap *et al.*, 1988b; Kafetzis *et al.*, 1983; Maberry *et al.*, 1990; Martens 1989), although their half-lives $(t_{1/2})$ may be shorter and their serum levels lower than in nonpregnant women (Landers *et al.*, 1983). The ratio of cord blood to maternal blood for cefoxitin in one study was 0.35 and for cefotaxime was 1.0 (Gilstrap *et al.*, 1988a; Maberry *et al.*, 1990). Cephalosporins as a group are

---

Box 2.5 The cephalosporins

First generation
Cephalothin
Cephaprin
Cephradine
Cefazolin

Second generation
Cefamandole
Cefoxitin
Cefotetan
Cefuroxime
Cefonicid
Cefaclor

Third generation
Cefotaxime
Ceftizoxime
Cefoperazone
Ceftriaxone
Moxalactam
Cefmenoxime
Cefmetazole
Cefuroxime
Cefixime
Ceftazidime
Cefpodoxime proxetil
Cefprozil

Adapted from Martens, 1989; PDR, 2004.

apparently not teratogenic in humans, although few scientific studies have been done with these antibiotics during pregnancy. However, animal studies with cephalosporins containing the N-methylthiotetrazole (MTT) side chain have revealed potential adverse fetal effects (Martens, 1989). When given to rats at doses 1.5 to 8 times the human dose, these types of cephalosporins resulted in testicular toxicity manifested by the failure of seminiferous tubule and spermatozoa development. The consequences of this finding for the human fetus is unknown at this time. Since the majority of second- and third-generation cephalosporins contain the MTT side chain, they should be used with caution during pregnancy. Cefoxitin, a second-generation cephalosporin, does not contain this side chain and at least theoretically would appear to be a better choice when a broad-spectrum cephalosporin is indicated during pregnancy (Martens, 1989).

Cephalosporins may also cause adverse effects in the mother, such as hypersensitivity reactions, hematologic toxicity, renal toxicity, hepatic toxicity, diarrhea, and pseudomembranous colitis (Box 2.6). In addition, clinically significant bleeding dyscrasias may occur secondary to the MTT side chain, which in turn may cause hypothrombinemia (Agnelli et al., 1986; Martens, 1989). This complication has been reported to be more common with moxalactam and very uncommon with other MTT-containing cephalosporins, such as cefamandole, cefoperazone and cefotetan (Martens, 1989).

Box 2.6 Potential fetal and maternal adverse effects with cephalosporins

Fetal effects	Gastrointestinal
Testicular toxicity[a]	Hematologic
	Hepatic
Maternal effects	Hypersensitivity reactions
Bleeding dyscrasia[a]	Renal

[a]Animal studies only; has not been reported in humans.

Tetracyclines

The tetracyclines (Box 2.7) inhibit protein synthesis and are bacteriostatic. They cross the placenta readily and, when utilized in the latter half of pregnancy, may cause yellow-brown discoloration of the deciduous teeth (Kline et al., 1964; Kutscher et al., 1986; Rendle-Short, 1962). Tetracyclines may also be deposited in the long bones of the developing fetus, although there is no scientific evidence that they inhibit fetal or neonatal growth.

The tetracyclines may also cause adverse maternal effects (Box 2.8). Whalley and colleagues (1964) reported an association between tetracycline use during pregnancy and liver toxicity manifested by azotemia, jaundice and acute fatty degeneration. Pancreatitis has also been reported to occur in these patients. As with erythromycin, tetracycline may cause significant gastrointestinal disturbances manifested by severe nausea and vomiting.

Box 2.7 The tetracyclines

Demeclocycline (Declomycin)
Doxycycline (Vibramycin, Vira-Tabs, Doryx, Doxy Caps or Tabs, Mondox)
Minocycline (Minocin, Dynacin)
Oxytetracycline (Terramycin, Urobiotic, Bio-Tabs)
Tetracycline (Achromycin)

From PDR, 2004.

Box 2.8 Potential adverse fetal and maternal effects of the tetracyclines

Fetal effects	Gastrointestinal intolerance
Yellow-brown discoloration of the deciduous	Hypersensitivity
teeth[a]	Pancreatitis
	Photosensitivity
Maternal effects	Vestibular disturbances[b]
Fatty degeneration of the liver	

[a]When given in the latter half of pregnancy.
[b]Minocycline only.

Because of potential adverse fetal effects, the tetracyclines are rarely indicated during pregnancy, except for penicillin-allergic patients who need treatment for syphilis and for whom desensitization is not available.

Aminoglycosides

The aminoglycosides interfere with protein synthesis but, unlike erythromycin and tetracycline, they are bactericidal. The various antibiotics in the class are listed in Box 2.9. All of the aminoglycosides cross the placenta. Yoshioka and associates (1972), as well as Weinstein and coworkers (1976) reported cord levels of gentamicin of 33 and 42 percent, respectively, of maternal levels. Gilstrap and colleagues (1988a) reported a mean concentration ratio between cord blood and maternal blood for gentamicin of 0.62. It is important to note that serum levels of various aminoglycosides may be subtherapeutic in the fetus and mother.

Streptomycin was one of the first members of this group and for many years was the primary drug for the treatment of tuberculosis. It has been reported to result in eighth-nerve damage of the fetus with protracted maternal therapy (Conway and Birt, 1965; Donald and Sellars, 1981). However, the risk of ototoxicity with streptomycin or any of

Box 2.9 The aminoglycosides

Amikacin (Amikin)	Netilmicin (Netromycin)
Gentamicin (Garamycin)	Streptomycin (Streptomycin)
Neomycin	Tobramycin (Nebcin)

Box 2.10 Potential adverse fetal and maternal effects of aminoglycosides

Fetal effects	Maternal effects
Eighth cranial nerve damage[a]	Neuromuscular blockage
	Ototoxicity
	Renal toxicity

[a]Uncommon and not reported for all aminoglycosides.

the other aminoglycosides is extremely low when these agents are used in therapeutic doses over a short period of time. Excluding possible eighth cranial nerve damage, there is no scientific evidence to date that the aminoglycosides as a group are teratogenic.

Aminoglycosides may cause significant adverse effects in the mother, such as neuro-muscular blockade, renal toxicity and ototoxicity (Box 2.10). Again, it should be noted that it may be very difficult to maintain therapeutic levels of aminoglycosides in the mother (or fetus) with usual or standard doses.

Clindamycin

Clindamycin is a derivative of lincomycin, and interferes with protein synthesis. It is a bacteriostatic antibiotic and is used primarily for serious anaerobic infections. Thus, it is used infrequently during pregnancy. Clindamycin crosses the placenta readily, with detectable levels in the fetus (Gilstrap *et al.*, 1988a; Weinstein *et al.*, 1976). In one study, the mean concentration ratios of clindamycin for cord blood versus maternal blood was 0.15 (Gilstrap *et al.*, 1988a). In other reports, the serum levels of this antibiotic approached 50 percent of maternal serum levels (Philipson *et al.*, 1973; Weinstein *et al.*, 1976).

Although clindamycin crosses the placenta readily, it causes no known adverse fetal effects. There are no adequate studies in humans, but clindamycin was not shown to be teratogenic in laboratory animals (Gray *et al.*, 1972). However, clindamycin may be associated with adverse maternal effects, the most serious of which is pseudomembra-nous colitis (Box 2.11). This latter complication is associated with a toxin produced by *Clostridium difficile* (George *et al.*, 1980).

Lincomycin

Lincomycin is rarely used today in obstetrics and has been mostly replaced by clin-damycin, at least in obstetrics and gynecology. However, it has been used in the past on large numbers of pregnant women without apparent adverse fetal effects (Mickal and Panzer, 1975).

Metronidazole

Metronidazole is a nitroimidazole that was first introduced as an antiparasitic and utilized primarily for the treatment of trichomoniasis. Subsequently, it was shown to be

Box 2.11 Potential adverse fetal and maternal effects of aminoglycosides

Clindamycin (Cleocin)	Hypersensitivity reaction
Gastrointestinal intolerance	Leukopenia
Diarrhea	
Pseudomembranous colitis	*Chloramphenicol (Chloromycetin)*
	Aplastic anemia
Metronidazole (Flagyl)	Hypersensitivity reaction
Antabuse-like effects (disulfiram-like)	Blood dyscrasias
Peripheral neuropathy	Neurotoxicity
Gastrointestinal intolerance	

From PDR, 2004.

very useful for the treatment of serious anaerobic infections. Its usage in pregnancy has been limited primarily to the treatment of trichomonal vaginitis. Metronidazole interferes with nucleic acid synthesis and causes cell death. It is a relatively small molecule and crosses the placenta readily, with levels in cord blood reaching significant concentrations (Heisterberg, 1984). Although this drug crosses the placenta readily, there is no evidence that it is teratogenic in humans. In one study reported by Rosa and colleagues (1987a) of over 1000 women with first-trimester exposure to this drug, the frequency of fetal anomalies was not increased. In addition, the frequency of congenital anomalies has been shown not to be increased in animal reproduction studies in which metronidazole was given in doses five times the human dose (Hammill, 1989).

However, metronidazole has been reported to be carcinogenic in mice and rats (Hammill, 1989) and to be mutagenic in certain bacteria. To date, metronidazole has not been shown to be carcinogenic in humans. Because of the tumorigenic effects in animals, however, metronidazole is not recommended for use in the first trimester.

Unfortunately, this nitroimidazole provides the only effective treatment for trichomoniasis. Most pregnant women with this infection can be treated with betadine solution or other similar agents until they are past the first trimester, and then started on metronidazole as necessary. In a recent meta-analysis on the use of metronidazole in pregnant women, no increase in malformations was found (Burtin *et al.*, 1995).

Metronidazole does concentrate in the breast milk and results in concentrations close to those found in maternal serum (Simms-Cendan, 1996). Potential adverse maternal effects of metronidazole are summarized in Box 2.11, and include central nervous system manifestation, peripheral neuropathy, gastrointestinal intolerance (nausea, vomiting), and a disulfiram-like reaction (Hammill, 1989) associated with alcohol use (nausea, abdominal cramps, and headaches). It may also be associated with a metallic aftertaste.

Chloramphenicol

Chloramphenicol interferes with protein synthesis and is bacteriostatic. It is rarely used today and generally is not recommended for use in pregnant women, although there is little or no scientific evidence to suggest that it is teratogenic. In a review from the Collaborative Perinatal Project of approximately 100 infants exposed to chloramphenicol in the first trimester, there was no evidence of an increased frequency of congenital malformations (Heinonen *et al.*, 1977). It has been associated with the 'gray baby syndrome' (cyanosis, vascular collapse, and death) in the premature neonate given large doses of this drug. Although chloramphenicol does cross the placenta readily (Scott and Warner, 1950), transplacental passage of the drug rarely, if ever, causes gray baby syndrome in the fetus or newborn (Landers *et al.*, 1983). The most significant potential adverse maternal effect is aplastic anemia, which has been reported in approximately one of 100 000 cases. Other potential maternal side effects are summarized in Box 2.11.

Sulfonamides

The sulfonamides inhibit folate synthesis and are analogs of para-aminobenzoic acid, which is necessary for production of folic acid by bacteria (Landers *et al.*, 1983). As a group, they are bacteriostatic. The most common sulfonamides are listed in Box 2.12.

Box 2.12 Sulfonamides, trimethoprim, and nitrofurantoin

Sulfonamides
Sulfisoxazole (Gantrisin)
Sulfamethoxazole (Gantanol)
Sulfacytine (Renoquid)
Sulfamethizole (Thiosulfil)

Trimethoprim
Trimethoprim (Proloprim, Trimpex)
Trimethoprim plus sulfamethoxazole (Bactrim, Septra, plus many others)

Nitrofurantoin
Nitrofurantoin macrocrystals (Macrodantin)

The sulfonamides cross the placenta readily and reach significant levels in the fetus, although the levels may be lower in the fetus than in the mother (Reid *et al.*, 1975). There are no scientific reports of an association between congenital malformations and the use of sulfonamides during pregnancy. Although the sulfonamides are not teratogenic, they do compete for bilirubin binding sites and, if used near delivery, may cause hyperbilirubinemia, especially in the premature infant (Landers *et al.*, 1983). Maternal side effects include hypersensitivity, photosensitivity, blood dyscrasias, and gastrointestinal intolerance.

Trimethoprim

Although trimethoprim crosses the placenta, it has not been shown to cause adverse fetal effects. In one report of over 100 women treated with a combination of trimethoprim and sulfamethoxazole, there was no increase in the frequency of fetal anomalies (Williams *et al.*, 1969). In another study of 186 pregnant women receiving either a placebo (66 patients) or trimethoprim plus sulfamethoxazole (120 patients), the incidence of fetal malformations was actually lower in the group receiving the antibiotics (3.3 versus 4.5 percent) (Brumfitt and Pursell, 1973). However, because trimethoprim is a folate antagonist (at least in bacteria!), it is generally not recommended for use in pregnancy. Like sulfonamides, trimethoprim is associated with few adverse maternal effects (skin rash, gastrointestinal intolerance, and possible hematologic abnormalities).

Nitrofurantoin

Nitrofurantoin macrocrystals, commonly used for urinary tract infections during pregnancy, have not been reported to be associated with adverse fetal effects. In a randomized prospective study of 100 women treated with nitrofurantoin versus 100 controls, there were no significant differences in birth weight, head circumference, or body length of the offspring (Lenke *et al.*, 1983). The incidence of congenital malformations was not reported. Nitrofurantoin has been reported to cause hemolytic anemia in women with glucose-6-phosphate dehydrogenase deficiency (Powell *et al.*, 1963), and because this drug crosses the placenta, this side effect could theoretically also occur in the fetus with this enzyme deficiency. However, in the authors' experience of approximately 1000 pregnant women receiving this medication for urinary tract infections, hemolytic anemia has not occurred in either the mother or the fetus. A pneumonitis has also been reported with this antibiotic. However, this is rare.

Vancomycin

Vancomycin is an antibiotic which does not belong to any other class of antimicrobial agents. It is both bactericidal and bacteriostatic, and is effective against a wide variety of Gram-positive organisms, including the *Enterococci* (Hermans and Wilhelm, 1987). It is the drug of choice for *Clostridium-difficile*-associated pseudomembranous colitis. It is also used in penicillin-allergic pregnant women for bacterial endocarditis prophylaxis.

There is no available scientific information linking this agent with adverse pregnancy outcomes, including congenital malformations. However, vancomycin may be associated with significant maternal side effects, such as nephrotoxicity and ototoxicity. Although there are no such reports, vancomycin could theoretically result in the same toxicity in the fetus, since this drug readily crosses the placenta.

Aztreonam

Aztreonam belongs to a relatively new class of antibiotics: the monobactams. It is effective against most of the aerobic Gram-negative rods or Enterobacteriaceae, and is used as an alternative to the aminoglycosides. There are no well-controlled studies in pregnant humans. However, according to its manufacturer, aztreonam has not been shown to be teratogenic in several animal models given several times the human dose. Moreover, a particular advantage of this antibiotic over the aminoglycosides is that it is not associated with either nephrotoxicity or ototoxicity in either the mother or the fetus.

Imipenem

Imipenem is a carbapenem antibiotic that is derived from thienamycin. It is presently combined with cilastatin, which inhibits the renal metabolism of imipenem. Cilastatin has no intrinsic antimicrobial activity. Imipenem is effective against a wide variety of

Gram-positive and Gram-negative aerobic and anaerobic organisms. It has the potential to be very effective as single-agent therapy for polymicrobial pelvic infections in women. There are no available human reproductive studies, but the imipenem–cilastatin combination has not been shown to be teratogenic in rats or rabbits, according to its manufacturer. There are few indications for the use of this very 'potent' antibiotic in pregnant women. Potential maternal side effects include hypersensitivity, central nervous system toxicity, and pseudomembranous colitis.

Quinolones

Ciprofloxacin, norfloxacin, and ofloxacin belong to the fluoroquinolone group of antibiotics. They are very effective against the aerobic Gram-negative bacilli, and hence are especially useful for the treatment of urinary tract infections. They also exhibit good activity against a variety of aerobic Gram-positive organisms, although most anaerobes are resistant to both antibiotics. They may also be effective against *C. trachomatis* and *N. gonorrhoeae*.

Among 549 pregnancies that were exposed to quinolones during the first trimester, there were the following exposures: 318 norfloxacin, 93 oflaxacin, 70 ciprofloxacin, and 57 pefloxacin (Schaefer *et al.*, 1996). Analyses controlled for various confounding factors, and it was found that the frequency of congenital anomalies was not increased above background (3.5 percent) for first-trimester exposure to quinolones except for ofloxacin.

However, two of the defects associated with ofloxacin exposure were secondary to prematurity (undescended testicle and inguinal hernia). When these two infants were excluded from the analysis, the frequency of congenital anomalies was not increased above background. Hence it appears that quinolones do not pose a teratogenic risk. Norfloxacin was not found to be teratogenic when given to monkeys during the critical period of organogenesis (Cukierski *et al.*, 1989). However, according to the manufacturer, quinolones may cause lameness or irreversible arthropathy in immature dogs

---

Box 2.13 Potential adverse fetal and maternal effects of quinolones

Fetal effects
None known
Irreversible arthropathy in immature animals[a]
Maternal effects
Central nervous system toxicity
- headache
- dizziness
- insomnia
Gastrointestinal intolerance
- nausea
- vomiting
- anorexia
Hypersensitivity

[a]Cukiersi *et al.*, 1989; Christian, 1996.

secondary to lesions in the cartilage (Box 2.13). Thus, this class of drugs is not recommended for use during pregnancy. The few serious maternal side effects are summarized in Box 2.13. It should be noted that approximately 2 percent of women taking these drugs experienced a reversible skin rash and photosensitivity (Christian, 1996).

Naldixic acid, another quinolone, was associated with pyloric stenosis but the relationship is apparently not causal. Although data are not adequate to exclude a risk of birth defects following exposure during the first trimester, it seems unlikely that naldixic acid poses a substantial risk of birth defects (Friedman and Polifka, 2006). Other quinolones have not been investigated for use during pregnancy: moxifloxacin (Avalox), gatifloxacin (Tequin), levofloxacin (Levaquin), garebixacin, and gemifloxacin.

Azithromycin

No epidemiological studies of azithromycin use during pregnancy have been published. Although, it does not seem to be associated with a high risk of congenital anomalies following first-trimester exposure, a small risk cannot be excluded (Friedman and Polifka, 2006).

Antituberculosis drugs

There are several drugs utilized to treat tuberculosis. These are summarized in Box 2.14. In a review of 15 studies involving 446 pregnancies exposed to rifampin, Snider and coworkers (1980) reported a malformation rate of 3–4 percent, similar to that of the general population. There were also over 600 pregnancies exposed to ethanbutol and almost 1500 exposed to isoniazid without evidence of an increase in congenital malformations (Snider *et al.*, 1980). There is no information regarding the drug pyrazinamide during pregnancy. The maternal side effects are also listed in Box 2.14. More recently, thalidomide has been utilized for the treatment of tuberculosis, especially in HIV-infected patients (Kaplan, 1994; Klausner *et al.*, 1996; Peterson *et al.*, 1995; Tramontana *et al.*, 1995). This most potent teratogen should obviously be avoided in pregnant women or those likely to become pregnant.

ANTIFUNGALS

The more commonly used antifungal agents are summarized in Box 2.15. Many of these are for topical application.

Nystatin, clotrimazole, and miconazole

These agents are utilized primarily for the treatment of candidiasis. In at least two recent reports there were no increases in malformations from their use (Jick *et al.*, 1981; Rosa *et al.*, 1987a).

Butoconazole, terconazole, and ketoconazole

There are no large studies of the use of these three antifungal agents during pregnancy. Butoconazole is a category B drug, and the other two are listed as category C by their

Box 2.14 Potential adverse fetal and maternal effects of rifampin, ethambutol, isoniazid and pyrazinamide

Rifampin
Fetal effects
None known

Maternal effects
Discoloration of urine, feces, sweat, sputum, tears
Gastrointestinal intolerance
Headache, fatigue, myalgia, fever
Hypersensitivity

Ethambutol
Fetal effects
None known

Maternal effects
Hypersensitivity
Hyperuricemia
Optic and peripheral neuritis

Isoniazid
Fetal effects
None known

Maternal effects
Gastrointestinal disturbance
Hepatitis
Hypersensitivity
Peripheral neuritis

Pyrazinamide
Fetal effects
Unknown

Maternal effects
Arthralgias
Elevated liver enzymes
Gastrointestinal disturbance
Rash

Adapted in part from the *USP DI* (United States Pharmacopeial Convention, 2003); PDR, 2004.

manufacturers. It seems unlikely that these agents would have significant, if any, teratogenic risks.

Fluconazole

Fluconazole is an azole antifungal similar to ketoconazole and is utilized for both local and systemic fungal infections (Hollier and Cox, 1995). It is useful in the treatment of vaginal, oral, and systemic candidiasis, as well as for prophylaxis and treatment of cryptococcal infections in immunocompromised patients (i.e., HIV-infected). Among 239 women who took single low doses of fluconazole, 60 took it during the first trimester of pregnancy. None of the infants had any congenital anomalies (Inman *et al.*, 1994).

Box 2.15 Antifungals

Amphotericin B	Ketoconazole
Butoconazole	Miconazole
Ciclopirox	Nystatin
Clotrimazole	Terconazole
Fluoconazole	Tolnaftate
Griseofulvin	Undecylenic acid

From PDR, 2004.

However, four cases of craniosynostosis with radial-humeral bowing and tetrology of Fallot have occurred following repeated high-dose fluconazole for cocci meningitis (Aleck and Bartley, 1996; Lee *et al.*, 1992; Pursley *et al.*, 1996), although normal healthy children have been delivered following high-dose fluconazole treatment (Krcmery *et al.*, 1995). In one study of 226 pregnancies exposed to fluconazole during the first trimester, the frequency of congenital anomalies was not increased (Mastroiacovo *et al.*, 1996). However, it should not be withheld in HIV-infected pregnant women who require cryptococcal prophylaxis. Maternal side effects may include headache, dizziness, or gastrointestinal upset.

Ciclopirox

This is a relatively new, topical antifungal agent effective against various dermatophytes such as *Trichophyton* species and *Candida albicans*. There is little, if any, information regarding its use during pregnancy but, according to its manufacturer, it was not teratogenic in various animal studies. It is a category B drug.

Tolnaftate, undecylenic, and terbinafine

Both tolnaftate (Tinactin) and undecylenic acid (Desenex) are utilized for dermatophyte infections such as tinea pedis and tinea corporis, but are not effective against yeast (Davis, 1995). Terbinafine (Lamisil) is a topical antifungal that is effective against most dermatophytes as well as most *Candida* species (Davis, 1995; PDR, 2004). There are no reports of these agents being teratogenic, and it would seem reasonable to classify them as category B agents at the present time.

Amphotericin B

Amphotericin B is an antifungal agent that is used primarily to treat systemic mycotic infections. There are no adequately controlled studies of this agent during pregnancy. However, in a review of case reports by Ismail and Lerner (1982), there was no evidence of teratogenicity of amphotericin B.

The potential adverse maternal effects of amphotericin B are summarized in Box 2.16.

Griseofulvin

Griseofulvin is an antifungal agent used primarily to treat mycotic infections of the skin, nails, and hair. It is incorporated in the keratin of the epidermis and nails and is fungistatic (Davis, 1995). There are no adequately controlled studies of this antifungal agent during pregnancy. However, Rosa and associates (1987b) reported two cases of conjoined twins born to mothers who took griseofulvin during early pregnancy. A variety of central nervous system malformations and skeletal anomalies have been observed in the offspring of animals treated with several times the human dose of griseofulvin during pregnancy (Klein and Beall, 1972; Scott *et al.*, 1975). Because of these reports, griseofulvin is not recommended for use during pregnancy. The potential maternal adverse effects are summarized in Box 2.16.

Box 2.16 Potential adverse fetal and maternal effects of antifungal agents

Nystatin, Clotrimazole, Miconazole, Butoconazole, Terconazole, Ketoconazole
Fetal effects
None known

Maternal effects
Local irritation

Ciclopirox, Tolnaftate, Undecylenic acid, Terbinafine
Fetal effects
None known

Maternal effects
Skin irritation

Fluoconazole
Fetal effects
None known; case reports of skeletal abnormalities

Maternal effects
Headache
Hypersensitivity
Liver dysfunction

Gastrointestinal disturbance

Amphotericin B
Fetal effects
None known

Maternal effects
Anemia, agranulocytosis
Hypokalemia
Hypersensitivity
Polyneuropathy
Central nervous system toxicity
Renal failure

Griseofulvin
Fetal effects
None known (humans)

Maternal effects
Headaches, confusion
Hepatitis
Hypersensitivity
Leukopenia
Peripheral neuropathy
Photosensitivity

Adapted in part from the *USP DI* (United States Pharmacopeial Convention, 2003); PDR, 2004.

ANTIVIRALS

Some of the more common antiviral agents are summarized in Box 2.17. Many of these agents are given for life-threatening illnesses.

Acyclovir and valacyclovir

Acyclovir is an antiviral agent used primarily in the treatment and prophylaxis of herpes simplex infections. The active metabolite of valacyclovir is acyclovir, and the use of valacyclovir during pregnancy will have risks similar to those of acyclovir. It has also been used in the treatment of other herpes infections, including varicella. There are no well-controlled studies in pregnant humans. However, in one review of seven women who received acyclovir during the second half of pregnancy, there were no congenital abnormalities detected (Leen *et al.*, 1987). Moreover, according to the manufacturer, acyclovir was not teratogenic in a variety of animals tested. In a review of 239 pregnancies in which acyclovir was utilized in the first trimester (Andrews *et al.*, 1992), there

Box 2.17 Antiviral agents

Amantadine	Osteltamivir
Acyclovir	Penciclovir
Cidofovir	Ribavirin
Didanosine (ddl)	Stavudine (d4T)
Docosanol	Valacyclovir
Famciclovir	Vidarabine
Famvir	Zalcitabine (ddC)
Foscarnet	Zanamivir
Ganciclovir	Zidovudine
Idoxuradine	

Box 2.18 Potential adverse fetal and maternal effects of antiviral agents

Acyclovir and valacyclovir

Fetal effects
None known

Maternal effects
Hypersensitivity
Acute renal failure
Hematuria
Arthralgia
Gastrointestinal intolerance
Dizziness
Insomnia
Anorexia

Famvir

Fetal effects
None known

Maternal effects
None known

Ribavirin

Fetal effects
Unknown in humans

Maternal effects
Conjunctivitis
Hypotension

Zidovudine

Fetal effects
None known

Maternal effects
Anemia, granulocytopenia
Gastrointestinal intolerance
Headache, dizziness, insomnia
Agitation, confusion, anxiety
Hypersensitivity

Idoxuridine

Fetal effects
None known (humans)

Maternal effects
Hypersensitivity

Amantadine

Fetal effects
None known

Maternal effects
Anticholinergic effects
Leukopenia
Orthostatic hypotension
Gastrointestinal intolerance
Central nervous system toxicity

Vidarabine

Fetal effects
None known (humans)

Maternal effects
Hypersensitivity

Adapted from Gilstrap *et al.*, 1991.

were 47 induced and 24 spontaneous abortions. Of 168 liveborn neonates, 159 had no congenital anomalies and of the nine neonates who did, no distinctive pattern of anomalies could be identified (Andrews et al., 1992). Acyclovir has also been used successfully during pregnancy to treat varicella pneumonia, disseminated herpes infection, and herpes hepatitis (Johnson and Saldana, 1994; Petrozza et al., 1993; Zambrano et al., 1995). Recently, acyclovir has been used during the last 4 weeks of pregnancy to prevent recurrent herpes infections and prevent the need for cesarean delivery (Scott et al., 1996). The potential adverse maternal effects are summarized in Box 2.18.

Ganciclovir

Ganciclovir is a nucleoside analog similar to acyclovir. It has been shown readily to cross the human placenta (Gilstrap et al., 1994; Henderson et al., 1993). Ganciclovir is more toxic than acyclovir, and there is no information regarding its use during pregnancy.

Zidovudine (AZT)

Zidovudine (Retrovir) is a thymidine analog that inhibits viral replication by inhibiting DNA synthesis. It is used primarily in the treatment of the acquired immunodeficiency syndrome (AIDS) and may also be used as a 'prophylactic agent' to delay the onset of clinical disease or after accidental exposure to the AIDS virus. Zidovudine was not teratogenic in human or animal studies. Some of the maternal side effects secondary to the drug are difficult to distinguish from those caused by the disease process itself. The antepartum (as early as 14 weeks gestation) and intrapartum prophylactic use of this agent is currently recommended to reduce the frequency of perinatal HIV transmission to the fetus (ACOG, 1994; CDC, 1993). The risk of fetal HIV infection is substantially reduced in women carrying this virus who are treated with zidovudine during pregnancy (Lyall et al., 2001; Minkoff, 2001; Mofenson et al., 2002; Mueller and Pizzo, 2001; Watts, 2001). Zidovudine seems unlikely to be associated with an increased risk of congenital anomalies and should be given for the treatment of HIV.

OTHER ANTI-HIV DRUGS

Other anti-HIV drugs include nucleoside/nucleotide reverse transcriptase inhibitors (lamivudine, emtricitabine, zalcitabine, abacavir, tenofovir), protease inhibitors (aprenavir, indinavir, saquinavir, fosamprenavir, ritonavir, darunavir, atazanavir, nelfinavir), and non-nucleoside reverse transcriptase inhibitors (delaviridine, efavirenz, nevirapine). A new type of anti-HIV drug is the 'entry inhibitors' that block HIV virus entry into the cell, and there is one currently available: enfuvirtide.

None of these drugs has been adequately studied during human pregnancy, but clearly the benefit (life-saving) of their use outweighs any theoretical risk.

Idoxuridine

Idoxuridine is an ophthalmic antiviral agent used primarily for the treatment of herpes simplex eye infections. To date, there have been no reports of congenital anomalies in infants born to women treated with this agent during pregnancy, but there have been no adequately controlled scientific studies in humans. Idoxuridine has been reported to be associated with both eye and skeletal malformations in the offspring of pregnant rabbits who received this local antiviral agent in usual human doses (Itoi *et al.*, 1975).

Amantadine

Amantadine is an antiviral agent used in the treatment and prophylaxis of influenza. There are no adequately controlled human studies. However, this particular agent was not shown to be teratogenic in rats or rabbits. Amantadine is rarely, if ever, indicated for use during pregnancy. Pandit and associates (1994) did report that one of four fetuses exposed to amantadine had tetralogy of Fallot.

Vidarabine

Vidarabine is a DNA inhibitor used systemically to treat disseminated herpes simplex infections and locally to treat herpetic ophthalmic infections. There are no adequate human studies available. However, Schardein *et al.* (1977) and Kurtz and associates (1977) reported congenital anomalies in rats given several times the usual human dose. Hillard and colleagues (1982) reported on the use of this drug late in pregnancy for disseminated herpes simplex infections.

Ribavirin

Ribavirin is used primarily as an inhalation aerosol to treat respiratory syncytial virus (RSV) infection in infants and young children. Although there are no reports of congenital abnormalities in well-controlled human studies, ribavirin has been reported to cause a variety of congenital anomalies in commonly used laboratory animals (Ferm *et al.*, 1978; Kilham and Ferm, 1977; Kochhar *et al.*, 1980). Since RSV infections in pregnant women are generally self-limited and do not normally require treatment, and because of the significant teratogenicity of ribavirin in a variety of animals, this drug is listed as FDA Category X and is not recommended for use during pregnancy.

Other antivirals

Other antivirals (idofovir, docosanol, famciclovir, penciclovir, foscarnet, valganciclovir, osteltamivir, zabamivir) have not been studied during pregnancy, or assessed for the possible association with birth defects following use during the first trimester.

ANTIPARASITICS

Although parasitic infections are relatively common during pregnancy, therapy (with a few exceptions) can usually be withheld until after pregnancy since many such infections are mild and asymptomatic. Metronidazole, the only effective antiparasitic agent for trichomoniasis, has already been discussed (p. 30).

Box 2.19 Pediculicides

Lice infestation	Mite infestations
Lindane (Kwell, Scabene)	Crotamiton (Eurax)
Pyrethrins and piperonyl butoxide (RID, A-200)	Lindane (Kwell, Scabene)
	Sulfur (6%) in petrolatum

Pediculicides

Both lice (*Pediculosis pubis*) and mite (scabies) infestations during pregnancy generally require some form of therapy. Several agents are available for treatment and are summarized in Box 2.19.

Of these, lindane (cream, lotion, or shampoo) is probably the most commonly used agent for both mites and lice. According to its manufacturer, lindane was not teratogenic in a variety of animals, although there are no adequate human reproduction studies. Lindane may be related to an increase in stillbirths in some animal studies (Faber, 1996). However, lindane may be absorbed systemically, which on rare occasions may lead to central nervous system toxicity (Feldman and Maibach, 1974; Orkin and Maibach, 1983). Although this adverse effect could also theoretically occur in the fetus, it would appear to be very unlikely and to date has not been reported. There is no information to suggest that any of the other agents listed in Box 2.19 cause adverse fetal effects, and thus all are apparently safe for use during pregnancy.

Antihelmintics

Several antihelmintics are available to treated infested women, although it is usually not necessary to treat helminth infections during pregnancy. Both mebendazole (Vermox) and thiabendazole (Mintezol) are effective for a variety of helminths, including pinworms (enterobiasis), whipworm (trichuriasis), roundworm (ascariasis), and hookworm (uninariasis). According to their manufacturer, none of these drugs was teratogenic in laboratory animals, although there are no adequate human reproduction studies.

Pyrantel pomoate (Antiminth) is used primarily for the treatment of roundworm and pinworm. It may also be of use in treatment of whipworm infestations. Although this agent has not been shown to be teratogenic in animals, there are no adequate studies in humans.

Antimalarials

The two major antimalarial drugs are chloroquine and quinine. Chloroquine is the primary drug used for the treatment of malaria, as well as for chemoprophylaxis in pregnant women who must travel to endemic areas (Diro and Beydoun, 1982). Although there have been no studies of infants whose mothers were treated for malaria during pregnancy with chloroquine, one study reported no increased frequency of congenital anomalies among 169 infants whose mothers received weekly low doses of the drug for malaria prophylaxis during pregnancy (Wolfe and Cordero, 1985). Quinine is used primarily for chloroquine-resistant falciparum malaria. Although there are no large studies regarding its use during pregnancy, increased malformations have been reported when large doses were used to attempt abortion (Nishimura and Tanimura, 1976). Quinine sulfate tablets have also been utilized for leg cramps, but their efficacy is unproven. Although not recommended for the treatment of leg cramps during pregnancy, the antimalarial quinines should not be withheld in the seriously ill pregnant woman with chloroquine-resistant malaria.

Pyrimethamine, spiramycin, and sulfadiazine

These agents are used primarily to treat toxoplasmosis. Pyrimethamine, a folic acid antagonist, is also used to treat malaria. There are no adequate scientific studies of its use during pregnancy, but Hengst (1972) reported no increase in the malformation rate in 64 newborns whose mothers had taken this drug during the first half of pregnancy. Spiramycin has been used extensively in Europe during the first trimester with no apparent adverse fetal effects. Sulfadiazine, a sulfonamide, has not been reported to be teratogenic when used in the first trimester. However, as with all sulfonamides, it could potentially be related to hyperbilirubinemia in the newborn, especially in the premature infant.

SPECIAL CONSIDERATIONS

There is a paucity of information regarding the most efficacious and safe antimicrobial regimens for the treatment of specific infection-related conditions during pregnancy (Table 2.3). The recommendations given in this section are derived from the author's experience or opinion.

Urinary tract infections

Urinary tract infections are among the most common infections encountered in pregnant women (Duff, 1994). For example, asymptomatic bacteriuria occurs in 2–10 percent of all pregnant women (Whalley, 1967). The majority of these infections are caused by the Enterobacteriaceae or enteric group of organisms, with *Escherichia coli* being the single most commonly isolated organism. Although it is often not necessary to treat these infections in nonpregnant women, it is of paramount importance to screen for and, if possible, eradicate bacteriuria in the pregnant woman, since acute pyelonephritis will develop in as many as 25 percent of untreated pregnant women with bacteriuria (Kass, 1978). The majority of pregnant women with asymptomatic bacteriuria can be treated successfully with a short course (3–5 days) of the antimicrobial regimens listed in Box 2.20.

An alternative regimen is to use nitrofurantoin macrocrystals, 100 mg given once a day at bedtime, for 7–10 days (Leveno *et al.*, 1981). Single-dose regimens, as listed in Box 2.21, may also prove useful. Regardless of the antimicrobial regimen used, approximately two-thirds of the patients will be cured and remain bacteriuria-free for the remainder of the pregnancy; approximately one-third of the patients will experience a recurrence and require further therapy.

Symptomatic infection of the lower urinary tract (acute cystitis) can be treated with a variety of antimicrobial regimens similar to that used for asymptomatic bacteriuria, with

Table 2.3 Summary of antimicrobial drugs: Teratogen Information System (TERIS) and Food and Drug Administration (FDA) risk estimates

Drug	TERIS risk	FDA risk rating
Acyclovir	Topical: undetermined	B_m
	Systemic: unlikely	
Amantadine	Undetermined	C_m
Amoxicillin	Unlikely	B_m
Amphotericin B	Undetermined	B_m
Ampicillin	None	B
Azithromycin	Undetermined	B_m
Aztreonam	Undetermined	B_m
Butoconazole	Undetermined	C_m
Cefamandole	Undetermined	B_m
Cefixime	Undetermined	B_m
Chloramphenicol	Unlikely	C
Chloroquine	Daily therapeutic dose: minimal	C
	Weekly prophylactic dose: none to minimal	
Ciclopirox	Undetermined	B_m
Ciprofloxacin	Unlikely	C_m
Clarithromycin	Undetermined	C_m
Clindamycin	Undetermined	B_m
Clotrimazole	Unlikely	B
Erythromycin	None	B_m
Famvir		B
Fluconazole	Undetermined	C_m
Gentamicin	Undetermined	C
Griseofulvin	Undetermined	C
Idoxuridine	Undetermined	C
Imipenem/cilastatin	Undetermined	C_m
Ketoconazole	Undetermined	C_m
Lindane	Undetermined	B_m
Metronidazole	None	B_m
Nitrofurantoin	Unlikely	B_m
Norfloxacin	Unlikely	C_m
Nystatin	None	C_m
Penicillin	None	B_m
Pyrazinamide	Undetermined	C_m
Pyrimethamine	Minimal	C_m
Quinine	Very large doses: moderate	D^*
	Low therapeutic doses: unlikely	
Ribavirin	Undetermined	X_m
Spectinomycin	Undetermined	B
Spiramycin	Undetermined	C
Streptomycin	Deafness: small	D_m
	Malformations: none	
Sulfadiazine	Unlikely	NA
Sulfamethoxazole	Unlikely	NA
Terconazole	Undetermined	C_m

Continued

Table 2.3 Continued

Drug	TERIS risk	FDA risk rating
Tetracycline	Unlikely	D
Thalidomide	High	X_m
Tolnaftate	Undetermined	NA
Trimethoprim	Minimal to small	C_m
Valacyclovir		B
Vancomycin	Undetermined	B_m
Vidarabine	Undetermined	C_m
Zidovudine	Unlikely	C_m

NA, not available.

Compiled from: Friedman *et al., Obstet Gynecol* 1990; **75**: 594; Briggs *et al.,* 2005; Friedman and Polifka, 2006.

Box 2.20 Outpatient antimicrobial regimens for treatment of asymptomatic bacteriuria or cystitis during pregnancy[a]

Ampicillin 250–500 mg qid	Nitrofurantoin 50–100 mg qid
Cephalosporins 250–500 mg qid	Sulfonamides 500 mg to 1 g qid

[a]Oral dose for 3–5 days.

Box 2.21 Single-dose antimicrobial regimens for the treatment of uncomplicated bacteriuria during pregnancy

Amoxicillin 2 g[a]	Nitrofurantoin 200 mg
Ampicillin 2 g[a]	Sulfisoxazole 2
Cephalexin 2 g	

[a]With or without 1 g probenecid.

---

the exception that there is little information regarding the treatment of pregnant women with single-dose regimens, which are thus not recommended. These women can generally be treated as outpatients with an oral antimicrobial agent for 3–5 days (Box 2.20). As with asymptomatic bacteriuria, recurrence in women with cystitis is common. Therefore, it is important to have frequent surveillance cultures.

Symptomatic infection of the upper urinary tract or acute pyelonephritis is a relatively common complication occurring in approximately 1 percent of all pregnant women. Many of these women experience nausea and vomiting, are dehydrated, and are unable to tolerate oral antimicrobial therapy. These women should be hospitalized for intravenous antibiotic therapy with one of the regimens listed in Box 2.22. As many as 25 percent of women with acute pyelonephritis during pregnancy will experience another such episode during either the antepartum or postpartum periods. Because of the attendant risks associated with acute pyelonephritis during pregnancy, such as septic shock and premature labor, consideration should be given to continuous suppressive antimicrobial therapy following an initial episode of pyelonephritis. One particularly useful regimen is nitrofurantoin macrocrystals, 100 mg orally every night (Hankins and Whalley, 1985).

Box 2.22 Inpatient antimicrobial regimens for the treatment of pregnant women with acute pyelonephritis

Ampicillin 500 mg IV q 6 h

Cefoxitin 1–2 g IV q 6 h

Cephalosporin (first generation) 500 mg IV q 6 h

Mezlocillin 3–4 g IV q 6 h

Piperacillin 3–4 g IV q 6 h

Aminoglycoside plus antibiotic listed below:

Gentamicin 3 mg/kg.day IV in divided doses

Tobramycin 3 mg/kg.day IV in divided doses

Cefazolin 1–2 g q 8 h is also useful.

Adapted from Duff, 1994.

Box 2.23 Antimicrobial regimens for the treatment of acute chorioamnionitis

Ampicillin plus 500 mg to 1 g IV q 6 h

Cefoxitin 1–2 g IV q 6 h

Gentamicin 3 mg/kg.day IV in divided doses

Piperacillin/Mezlocillin 3–4 g IV q 6 h

Ampicillin plus gentamicin or plus clindamycin for women with chorioamnionitis requiring Caesarean delivery

Acute chorioamnionitis

Acute chorioamnionitis occurs in approximately 1 percent of all pregnancies (Gibbs *et al.*, 1980; Hauth *et al.*, 1985). The majority of cases occur in the third trimester, although such infections may occur, secondary to invasive procedures such as amniocentesis or chorionic villus sampling, in the late first or early second trimester. There is no unanimity of opinion regarding specific antimicrobial regimens for the treatment of acute chorioamnionitis during pregnancy. Suggested regimens are summarized in Box 2.23. The combination of ampicillin and gentamicin is probably the most often used regimen in the USA (Gibbs *et al.*, 1980; Gilstrap *et al.*, 1988b; Maberry *et al.*, 1991).

Vaginitis

The two most common forms of vaginitis during pregnancy are fungal and protozoan. Pregnant women with vaginitis secondary to fungi, such as *Candida* species, can be treated with a variety of antifungal agents which are listed in Box 2.24. Women with trichomoniasis present an unusual therapeutic dilemma. Although there is no scientific evidence that metronidazole is either teratogenic or causes adverse effects in the embryo/fetus, the manufacturer has issued a stern warning regarding its use during the first trimester of pregnancy. Fortunately, many of the patients with trichomoniasis can be treated with antimonilial agents until they are past the first trimester and then treated with metronidazole – the only effective treatment for this protozoan infection.

Sexually transmitted diseases

Syphilis is a relatively common sexually transmitted disease in pregnant women, especially in the indigent population. Such women should be treated according to the

Box 2.24 Antifungal agents for the treatment of *Candida* vaginitis during pregnancy

Butoconazole   Nystatin
Clotrimazole   Terconazole
Miconazole

Centers for Disease Control (CDC) guidelines, as outlined in Box 2.25. Pregnant women with syphilis who are allergic to penicillin present another therapeutic dilemma. For example, erythromycin may eradicate the infection in the pregnant woman, but may not prevent congenital syphilis (Preblud and Williams, 1985; Wendel and Gilstrap, 1990; Wendel *et al.*, 1985; Ziaya *et al.*, 1986). Another agent, tetracycline, may be associated with significant yellow-brown discoloration of the fetal deciduous teeth and is currently not recommended for use in the latter half of pregnancy (Genot *et al.*, 1970). The current recommended approach to the pregnant patient with syphilis who is allergic to penicillin is to utilize penicillin desensitization, as outlined in Box 2.26, after skin testing to confirm allergy. Penicillin is the ideal antibiotic choice for the treatment of syphilis during pregnancy (Bofill and Rust, 1996).

Box 2.25 Antimicrobial regimens for the treatment of syphilis during pregnancy

Early syphilis (less than 1 year)
Benzathine penicillin G 2.4 million units IM as a single injection

Syphilis of more than 1 year's duration
Benzathine penicillin G 2.4 million units IM weekly for 3 doses

Neurosyphilis
- Aqueous crystalline penicillin G 2.4 million units IV every 4 h for at least 10 days, followed by benzathine penicillin G 2.4 million units IM weekly for 3 doses.
- Aqueous procaine penicillin G 2.4 million units IM daily, plus probenecid 500 mg orally 4 times daily, both for 10 days, followed by benzathine penicillin G 2.4 million units IM weekly for 3 doses
- Benzathine penicillin G 2.4 million units IM weekly for 3 doses (not recommended for HIV-infected adults)

CDC, 2002.

Box 2.26 Penicillin desensitization in pregnant women allergic to penicillin

- Requires hospitalization for at least 24 h
- Intravenous access, resuscitation medications, and equipment
- Oral protocol – graduated oral doses of phenoxymethyl penicillin (penicillin V suspension)
- Parenteral protocol – graduated intravenous doses of aqueous crystalline penicillin G

Adapted from Wendel and Gilstrap, 1990.

Gonorrhea is a common sexually transmitted disease encountered during pregnancy, and complicated infections may be treated with amoxicillin, ampicillin, aqueous procaine penicillin G, or ceftriaxone. For women with known strains of *Neisseria gonorrhoeae* that are penicillinase-producing, therapy should consist of either ceftriaxone, 250 mg intramuscular (IM) as a single dose, spectinomycin, 2 g IM as a single dose, or cefixime, 400 mg orally in a single dose. In fact, these last three regimens are recommended for the treatment of uncomplicated gonococcal infections during pregnancy by the CDC (1993).

Chlamydia trachomatis may be isolated in up to 30 percent of women of lower socioeconomic status (unpublished observations, 1990). Erythromycin base or stearate in a dose of 500 mg four times a day for 7–10 days will generally prove satisfactory for the treatment of chlamydial infections during pregnancy. Tetracycline is generally not recommended for use in pregnant women. Other antimicrobial agents such as amoxicillin (with or without clavulanic acid), clindamycin, or azithromycin (1 g single oral dose), may prove satisfactory in eradicating chlamydial infections in pregnant women who are unable to tolerate erythromycin because of its gastrointestinal side effects.

Viral infections

Fortunately, the majority of viral infections encountered during pregnancy do not require any specific therapy. Patients with life-threatening disseminated viral infections, such as varicella zoster or herpes infections, should be treated with acyclovir, as the benefits clearly outweigh any potential risk. The same is true for pregnant women with AIDS, who should be treated with zidovudine (Retrovir). Zidovudine is also recommended from 14 weeks gestation onward as prophylaxis for the prevention of perinatal viral transmission in HIV-positive women (Box 2.27). Acyclovir is not recommended for the routine treatment of localized genital tract herpes simplex virus infections (Scott *et al.*, 1996). Valacyclovir and famvir are also effective and are category B drugs (Table 2.3).

Vaccines

Fortunately, most pregnant women do not require vaccination during pregnancy. However, as with drugs and medications, occasionally a woman will be given an immunization when she does not realize she is newly pregnant. Probably the two most common immunizations given in this instance are rubella and influenza. The four types of immunizing agents are toxoids, killed microbial vaccines, viral vaccines, and immune globulins (ACOG, 1991).

Box 2.27 Recommended protocol for prophylactic zidovudine to decrease risk of perinatal HIV transmission

Zidovudine 100 mg five times daily or 200 mg three times daily, beginning at 14–34 weeks and continued throughout pregnancy
plus
Zidovudine intrapartum given as a loading dose of 2 mg/kg IV followed by an infusion of 1 mg/kg
and
Zidovudine syrup orally to the newborn in a dose of 2 mg/kg every 6 h for the first 6 weeks of life

From CDC 2002 and Connor *et al.*, 1994.

Toxoids

The major agent in this class is a combination tetanus–diphtheria that is recommended for pregnant women with no primary immunization or who have not had a booster within 10 years (ACOG, 1991). Needless to say, the mortality to both mother and neonate from tetanus is extremely high, and active immunization to the mother will provide protection to the neonate in the range of 80–95 percent or greater if the mother has received at least two doses 2 weeks before delivery (Faix, 1991; Hayden et al., 1989). This vaccine has no known adverse effects on the fetus.

Inactivated bacterial vaccines

The inactivated bacterial vaccines include cholera, meningococcus, plague, pneumococcus, and typhoid, and it is recommended that they not be utilized except for travel requirements or for high-risk close exposure (ACOG, 1982). There are no reports of adverse fetal effects from any of these inactivated bacterial vaccines.

Immune globulins

The immune globulins include hepatitis B, rabies, tetanus, and varicella, which are recommended for postexposure prophylaxis (ACOG, 1991). There are no adverse fetal effects reported with the use of any of these agents.

The dose schedule recommended for hepatitis B immune globulin and for vaccination is summarized in Table 2.4. Although there is general agreement that newborn infants of mothers who develop clinical varicella within 4–5 days before or within 2 days after delivery should receive varicella–zoster immune globulin (VZIG), the efficacy of VZIG in the exposed mother is less than clear. However, several authors have recommended its use in susceptible pregnant women if it can be given within 96 h (Enders, 1985; Faix, 1991; MacGregor et al., 1987; Miller et al., 1989). Enders (1985) has published the most compelling data to support this recommendation. In this study, in which 25 susceptible pregnant women were given VZIG in a dose of 0.2 mg/kg within 96 h of exposure, 20 (80 percent) did not develop varicella.

The immune globulins are used primarily for hepatitis A and measles. The recommended dose for hepatitis A exposure is 0.2 ml/kg in one dose for the mother and 0.5 ml to susceptible newborns (ACOG, 1991). The dose of immune globulin for measles is discussed below.

Table 2.4 Hepatitis B vaccines and hyperimmune globulin prophylaxis

Vaccine			
	Hepatovax-B	Recombivax HB	Engerix-B
Adult	1.0 mL	1.0 mL	1.0 mL
Infant of HBV carrier	0.5 mL	0.5 mL	0.5 mL
Prophylaxis, hepatitis B immune globulin (HBIG)			
Adult	0.6 mL/kg initially and 1 month later		
Newborn	0.5 mL initially and at 3 and 6 months		

From ACOG, 1982; Pastorek, 1989.

Table 2.5 The viral vaccines

	Use in pregnancy	Fetal risk
Live attenuated viruses		
Measles	Contraindicated	None known
Mumps	Contraindicated	None known
Poliomyelitis	Only for increased risk of exposure	None known (Fetal death?)
Rubella	Contraindicated	None confirmed
Yellow fever	Only for high-risk exposure	Unknown
Inactivated viruses		
Influenza	Pregnant women with other significant illnesses	None known
Rabies	Same as for nonpregnant women	Unknown

Viral vaccines

In general, live attenuated viral vaccines are not recommended for pregnant women, with few exceptions (Table 2.5). Of these vaccines, rubella has probably received the most attention. Although pregnancy is considered contraindicated in women within 3 months of receiving the rubella vaccine, the actual risk of congenital rubella syndrome from maternal vaccination would appear to be extremely small, if it exists at all (Preblud and Williams, 1985).

Measles and mumps vaccines are also considered contraindicated during pregnancy, although pooled immune globulin (0.25 mg/kg in a dose up to 15 ml) can be utilized for measles (ACOG, 1991).

The inactivated viruses include influenza and rabies. Obviously the benefits of rabies vaccination (considering the high mortality of rabies of nearly 100 percent) far outweigh any theoretical risk to the fetus, which is actually unknown. Although influenza vaccines are not routinely recommended for all pregnant women, they may be efficacious in certain pregnant women with significant medical complications.

Key references

Little BB. Pharmacokinetics during pregnancy: evidence-based maternal dose formulation. *Obstet Gynecol* 1999; **93**: 858.

Lyall EGH, Blott M, de Ruiter A *et al*. Guidelines for the management of HIV infection in pregnant women and the prevention of mother-to-child transmission. *HIV Med* 2001; **2**: 314.

Mofenson LM, Centers for Disease Control and Prevention, US Public Health Service Task Force. US Public Health Service Task Force recommendations for use of antiretroviral drugs in pregnant HIV-1-infected women for maternal health and interventions to reduce perinatal HIV-1 transmission in the United States. *MMWR Rec Rep* 2002; **51**: 1.

Mueller BU, Pizzo PA. Acquired immunodeficiency syndrome in the infant. In: Remington JS, Klein JO (eds). *Infectious Diseases of the Fetus and Newborn Infant*, 5th edn. Philadelphia: WB Saunders, 2001: 447.

Further references are available on the book's website at http://www.drugsandpregnancy.com

3

Cardiovascular drugs during pregnancy

Heart disease occurs among about 1 percent of pregnant women. Pregnant women with heart disease present several medical dilemmas. The physician is concerned with whether a specific medication is safe for the fetus, remaining cognizant that most cardiac medications are chronically used to treat life-threatening conditions, and that these therapeutics cannot be discontinued when pregnancy is first diagnosed (Little and Gilstrap, 1989). Hence, embryos/fetuses of women with cardiovascular disease are exposed to these medications during the critical period of organogenesis (i.e., the first eight embryonic weeks of pregnancy) and fetal development. Since heart disease may be inherited in a multifactorial or polygenic fashion, pregnant women with many forms of heart disease may give birth to a newborn with congenital heart disease, and this malformation may in turn be blamed by both the patient and her attorney on specific cardiac medications. Scientific studies regarding the efficacy and safety of most cardiac medications during pregnancy are not conclusive, but the life-threatening nature of cardiovascular disease mandates that treatment be provided, even during pregnancy.

Pharmacokinetic changes during pregnancy affect cardiovascular drug disposition. The few investigations that are available indicate that dose and timing adjustment may be necessary because of (1) decreased drug serum concentrations (C_{max} and steady state); (2) decreased half-life; and (3) increased clearance (Table 3.1).

Cardiovascular medications may be classified into several categories: antiarrhythmic, cardiac glycosides, anticoagulants, diuretics, antihypertensives, and antianginals.

ANTIARRHYTHMICS

Cardiac arrhythmias are relatively common in women with cardiac disease, and the clinician providing care for such women is faced with a myriad of medications for the treatment of arrhythmias during pregnancy. Arrhythmias may also occur in pregnant

Table 3.1 Pharmacokinetic studies of cardiovascular agents during pregnancy: pregnant compared with nonpregnant

Agent	n	EGA (weeks)	Route	AUC	V_d	C_{max}	C_{ss}	$t_{1/2}$	CI	PPB	Control group[a]	Authors
Labetalol	8	25–34	PO	=		=	=	↓			No	Rogers et al. (1990)
Labetalol	10	33–38	IV			=	=	=	=		Yes (1,2)	Rubin et al. (1983b)
Labetalol	7	30–36	PO			=	=	=	=		No	Saotome et al. (1993)
Metoprolol	5	35–38	IV	↓		↓	↓	↓	=	=	Yes (2)	Hogstedt et al. (1985)
Propranolol	6	32–36	PO, IV	↓	=		=	=	=		Yes (2)	O'Hare et al. (1984)
Sotalol	6	32–36	PO, IV	↓	=		=	=	=		Yes (2)	O'Hare et al. (1983)
Digoxin	15	3rd trimester	PO				↑		↑		Yes (2)	Luxford and Kellaway (1983)
Digoxin	7	Term	PO				↓		↑		Yes (2)	Rogers et al. (1972)

Source: Little BB. *Obstet Gynecol* 1999; **93**: 858.

EGA, estimated gestational age; AUC, area under the curve; V_d, volume of distribution; C_{max}, peak plasma concentration; C_{ss}, steady-state concentration; $t_{1/2}$, half-life; CI, clearance; PPB, plasma protein binding; PO, by mouth; ↓ denotes a decrease during pregnancy compared to nonpregnant values; ↑ denotes an increase during pregnancy compared with nonpregnant values; = denotes no difference between pregnant and nonpregnant values; IV, intravenous; IM, intramuscular.

[a]Control groups: 1, nonpregnant women; 2, same individuals studied postpartum; 3, historic adult controls (sex not given); 4, adult male controls; 5, adult male and female controls combined.

Table 3.2 Classification of antiarrhythmic agents

Class	Action
I	Interferes directly with depolarization
I_A	Prolongation of action-potential duration
I_B	Shortening of action-potential duration
I_C	No effect
II	Antisympathetic effects
III	Markedly prolonged duration of action potential
IV	Blockade of slow inward (calcium–sodium channel) depolarization current

Brown and Wendel, 1989; Vaughan-Williams EM, 1984.

This classification may prove useful in predicting both the efficacy and the toxicity of a specific agent (Brown and Wendel, 1989).

Table 3.3 Classification of antiarrhythmic agents

Drug	Brand names	Vaughan Williams classification
Amiodarone	Cardarone	III
Bretylium	Bretylol	III
Disopyramide	Norpace	I
Encainide	Enkaid	I_C
Esomolol[a]	Brevibloc	II
Flecainide	Tambocar	I_C
Lidocaine	Xylocaine, LidoPen	I_B
Mexiletine	Mexitil	I_B
Mibefradil[a]	Posicor	IV
Procainamide	Procan, Pronestyl, Promine, Rhthmin	I
Propranolol	Inderal	II
Quinidine	Cardioquin, Quindex, Quinaglute	I_A
Sotalol[a]	Betapace	II, III
Tocainide	Tanocard	I_B
Verapamil	Isoptin, Calan	IV

From Vaughan Williams, 1984.

[a]No data on use of esomolol, sotalol, or mibefradil during pregnancy have been published.

women without known heart disease. Antiarrhythmics have been classified into six classes according to their major mode of action or effect (Vaughan Williams, 1984), as shown in Tables 3.2 and 3.3.

Lidocaine

Commonly used as an amide local anesthetic, lidocaine is also effective in the treatment of ventricular and supraventricular tachycardias. Lidocaine rapidly crosses the placenta and fetal levels reach about 50 percent of maternal levels within less than an hour

(Rotmensch et al., 1983). Lidocaine's half-life is twice as long in the fetus/neonate (3 h) than in the mother (1.5–2 h) (Brown et al., 1976). Lidocaine persists for as long as 48 h after birth (Garite and Briggs, 1987). Importantly, most information available regarding pharmacokinetics of lidocaine in pregnant and postpartum women and newborns is from studies of regional or local anesthesia (Rotmensch et al., 1983). No published data are available on lidocaine from women who received the drug for cardiac arrhythmias. However, local anesthetics given in toxic doses may result in central nervous system and cardiac side effects in both the mother and the fetus. Lidocaine is not known to be teratogenic at acute therapeutic levels in humans or in chronic doses in animals (Fujinaga and Mazze, 1986; Heinonen et al., 1977; Rotmensch et al., 1983). Toxicity risk is minimal when maternal lidocaine levels are maintained at less than 4 mg/mL (Bhagwat and Engel, 1995). Amide-type local anesthetics given for paracervical block are associated with spasm of the uterine arteries, causing decreased uterine blood flow.

Procainamide

Another amide compound, procainamide, is used to treat ventricular tachycardia. There is little information regarding the pharmacokinetics of this drug during pregnancy. However, it has been estimated that fetal levels are approximately one-fourth the maternal levels (Garite and Briggs, 1987). Scientific evidence of the safety of procainamide for use during pregnancy does not address possible human teratogenicity. However, given the safety profile of a closely related drug (lidocaine), procainamide seems to not pose a great risk when used during pregnancy (Little and Gilstrap, 1989). Chronic use of this drug should be avoided, unless necessary for life-threatening conditions, because a lupus-like syndrome may occur (Rotmensch et al., 1987). Breastfeeding is not contraindicated in mothers on procainamide (American Academy of Pediatrics, 1994).

Encainide and flecainide

Two other lidocaine-related antiarrhythmic medications are encainide and flecainide. Encainide was not teratogenic in rats and rabbits when given at doses up to 9 and 13 times the human dose (data from the manufacturer's insert). Flecainide has been reported to cause teratogenic and embryotoxic effects in some species of rabbits when given in doses four times the usual adult dose. It was not, however, teratogenic in rats, mice, and other species of rabbits when given in the usual adult dose, according to its manufacturer. One case report suggested an association with birth defects with flecainide. Flecainide has been used to treat fetal arrhythmias, but fetal deaths have occurred with this treatment. Given the alternative related medications available, flecainide should be avoided, or at least the drug of last resort when others have failed.

Tocainide

Tocainide is another amide antiarrhythmic agent, closely related to lidocaine. It was not teratogenic in animals at doses several times the usual adult dose, but it may be embryotoxic. There are no human studies during pregnancy, but it is closely related to lidocaine and its data may be extrapolated to tocainide.

Disopyramide

Similar in action to quinidine, disopyramide is used to treat supraventricular and ventricular arrhythmias. Dysopyramide crosses the placenta readily, with fetal levels approximately half those of the mother (Rotmensch *et al.*, 1983). The drug was embryotoxic in laboratory animals when given at several times the human dose, but no pattern or specific malformations were noted (data from the manufacturer's insert). Disopyramide use during the third trimester has been associated with premature onset of labor (Leonard *et al.*, 1978; Rotmensch *et al.*, 1983).

Bretylium

This drug is primarily indicated for life-threatening ventricular arrhythmias, such as ventricular tachycardia and ventricular fibrillation. No human data are published regarding safety of the drug during pregnancy. Bretylium was reported to be 'without effect' in one rat study published by West (1962).

Amiodarone

This drug is used primarily to treat life-threatening ventricular arrhythmias (e.g., ventricular fibrillation, tachycardia). Amiodarone has limited ability to cross the placenta, with newborn concentrations reaching only 10–25 percent of maternal serum levels (Rotmensch *et al.*, 1987). Of six pregnancies exposed to amiodarone after 10 weeks gestation, hypothyroidism (n = 2) and small size for gestational age (n = 4) was observed (Magee *et al.*, 1995). Amiodarone contains a large amount (37 percent by weight) of iodine. Learning disabilities were unusually frequent in two small series of children exposed to amiodarone during gestation (Bartalena *et al.*, 2001; Magee *et al.*, 1999). When administered chronically during pregnancy, fetal goiter is a major risk after 10 weeks gestation. Fetal death is consistently reported in animal studies of the drug during pregnancy. A possible association between fetal cretinism has also been suggested, especially from direct fetal injection (Pinsky *et al.*, 1991). Otherwise, the frequency of congenital anomalies was not increased among 30 infants exposed to amiodarone during the first trimester (Bartalena *et al.*, 2001).

Mexiletine

Similar in action to lidocaine, mexiletine is a local anesthetic type of antiarrhythmic agent (Zipes and Troup, 1978). Mexiletine is used primarily to treat ventricular arrhythmias (ventricular tachycardia, premature ventricular contractions). No studies of congenital anomalies in infants exposed to mexiltene have been published. A few anecdotal case reports suggest no adverse effects on the fetus or on labor, but the importance of such observations is not clear. Mexiletine was not teratogenic in various laboratory animals (data from the manufacturer's insert). Cord blood concentrations of this drug were similar to maternal levels, and therapeutic levels may be found in breast milk (Timmis *et al.*, 1980). However, breastfeeding is not contraindicated when the mother is using mexiletine (American Academy of Pediatrics, 1994).

Verapamil

A calcium channel blocker that is used as an antiarrhythmic, antihypertensive, and antianginal treatment, verapamil is especially efficacious for the treatment of paroxysmal supraventricular tachycardia.

Verapamil is used to transplacentally treat fetal supraventricular tachycardia (Klein and Repke, 1984; Rey et al., 1985; Wolff et al., 1980). Verapamil should be used with caution in pregnant patients because it might reduce uterine blood flow by 25 percent or more (Murad et al., 1985). Importantly, 10–20 percent of neonates who received this drug intraveneously for supraventricular tachycardia and congestive heart failure developed cardiac depression and cardiac arrest (Kleinman and Copel, 1991). Therefore, verapamil is not recommended for use in infants of less than 1 year (Garson, 1987). Verapamil might have adverse effects in the fetal heart, especially in the presence of heart failure and hydrops (Shen et al., 1995). Among 33 infants exposed to verapamil in the first trimester, no increase in congenital anomalies was reported (Magee et al., 1996). Verapamil is not contraindicated in breastfeeding mothers (American Academy of Pediatrics, 1994).

Propranolol

Propranolol is a beta-adrenergic blocker used to treat supraventricular and ventricular tachycardias, hypertension, hyperthyroidism, and migraine headaches. It is also used in the intrauterine treatment of fetal arrhythmias (Bhagwat and Engel, 1995; Eibeschitz, 1975). Propranolol is probably the best studied of all the agents in this group. The majority of this information is derived from the treatment of hypertension during pregnancy. Nonetheless, no controlled human teratology studies of propranolol have been published. The drug was not teratogenic in at least two animal studies (Fuji and Nishimura, 1974; Speiser et al., 1983). No reports of malformations in either animals or humans have been published. Adverse fetal effects have been reported with the use of propranolol during pregnancy. Intrauterine growth retardation and use of propranolol were associated in one study (Pruyn et al., 1979). However, other studies have not found this association (Rotmensch et al., 1987). Importantly, it is also possible that the maternal hypertension, and not propranolol therapy per se, is responsible for decrease in fetal growth.

In addition to intrauterine growth restriction (IUGR), fetal effects of beta-blockers include apnea, bradycardia, and hypoglycemia (Bhagwat and Engel, 1995; Habib and McCarthy, 1977; Pruyn et al., 1979; Rubin, 1981; Turnstall, 1969), as summarized in Box 3.1.

Several other beta-adrenergic blocking agents are available but are used primarily for the treatment of hypertension. These are discussed below under Antihypertensives.

Box 3.1 Possible adverse fetal effects of maternal beta-blocker therapy

Apnea and respiratory depression	Intrauterine growth retardation
Bradycardia	Jaundice
Hypoglycemia	

Quinidine

Primarily ventricular arrhythmias and supraventricular tachycardias are treated with quinidine. It was successfully used for the intrauterine treatment of fetal tachycardias (Spinnato *et al.*, 1984). Quinidine was also used to treat fetal hydrops from reciprocating tachycardia that did not convert with maternal digitalization (Guntheroth *et al.*, 1985). There have been no controlled studies in human pregnancies. Among fewer than 20 pregnancies, quinidine exposure during the first trimester was not associated with an increased frequency of congenital anomalies (Rosa, personal communication, cited in Briggs *et al.*, 2002).

Adenosine

Adenosine is a purine nucleoside approved by the Food and Drug Administration (FDA) for the treatment of supraventricular tachycardia (Mason *et al.*, 1992). It has also been reported to be effective in the treatment of supraventricular tachycardia in pregnant women (Afridi *et al.*, 1992; Hagley and Cole, 1994; Mason *et al.*, 1992). There are no published studies regarding the teratogenic effects of this adenosine.

CARDIAC GLYCOSIDES

Cardiac glycosides are used to treat atrial fibrillation, other supraventricular tachycardias, and treatment of fetal tachycardias.

Cardiac glycosides are effective because of their inotropic effects on the heart and antiarrhythmic effects. Various digitalis preparations cross the placenta readily, resulting in significant fetal levels with cord levels that are 50–80 percent of maternal levels (Chan *et al.*, 1978; Rogers *et al.*, 1972). No scientific studies regarding the safety of cardiac glycosides in pregnant women have been published. Fetal digitalis toxicity has occurred, but this was secondary to maternal overdose (Sherman and Locke, 1960). In this latter report, it is estimated that the mother ingested 8.9 mg of digitoxin, resulting in significant fetal toxicity and neonatal death. Available information supports the view that cardiac glycosides are probably safe for use during pregnancy.

ANTICOAGULANTS AND THROMBOLYTICS

Heparin is used in pregnant women primarily for the treatment of thromboembolic disease or for prophylaxis in women with artificial heart valves. Low-molecular-weight heparin is also used to treat thromboembolism in pregnancy, and does not cross the placenta (Feijgin and Lourwood, 1994; Macklon *et al.*, 1995; Schneider *et al.*, 1995).

Warfarin derivatives are contraindicated for use during pregnancy

Coumarin derivatives, including warfarin, are contraindicated for use during pregnancy. The fetal warfarin syndrome is comprised of skeletal and brain defects. Use after the first trimester includes brain and eye defects, and other anomalies associated with vascular disruption.

No controlled trials investigating the use of thrombolytics, such as streptokinase or urokinase, during pregnancy have been published. However, in a review of 172 pregnant women from published reports, Turrentine and associates (1995) found no increase in congenital anomalies and a pregnancy loss rate of 5.8 percent. Hemorrhagic complications occurred in 8 percent of the women. Among more than 140 infants exposed to heparin during the first trimester, the frequency of congenital anomalies was not increased (Chan *et al.*, 2000). Similarly, in a literature review among more than 440 infants exposed to low molecular weight heparins during pregnancy, including nearly 200 infants whose mothers were treated during the first trimester, no congenital anomalies were noted (Sanson *et al.*, 1999). Seven to 10 infant defects would have been expected to occur in the absence of any drug exposure. Therefore, ascertainment bias may confound the detection of birth defects in their study.

Protamine sulfate is used to reverse the anticoagulant effects of heparin prior to surgery (e.g., Caesarean section). No studies regarding use of protamine in pregnancy have been published. One infant with neonatal depression following maternal protamine sulfate injection was reported Wittmaack *et al.*, 1994).

ANTIANGINAL AGENTS

Antianginal agents, potent vasodilators, are listed in Box 3.2. Organic nitrites are the most commonly used agents in this group, and nitroglycerin is the prototype organic nitrite agent. No human studies of organic nitrites in pregnant women have been published, although these agents were not teratogenic in animal studies.

Box 3.2 Antianginal agents

Organic nitrites
Amyl nitrate
Dipyramidole (Persantine)
Erythrityl tetranitrate (Cardilate)
Isosorbide dinitrate (Isordil, Sorbitrate)
Nitroglycerin
Pentaerythritol tetranitrate (Pentritol, Peritrate)

Calcium antagonists
Aminodipine[a]
Bepridil[a]
Diltiazem (Cardizem)
Feldopine[a]
Mibefradil[a]
Nicardipine (Cardene)

Nifedipine (Procardia Adalat)
Nisoldipine[a]
Posicor[a]
Verapamil (Calan, Isoptin)

Beta blockers
Atenolol
Bisoprolol[a]
Bucindolol[a]
Labetalol
Metoprolol
Propranolol

New class
Ranolazine[a]

Adapted in part from the *USP DI*, 2003.
[a]Not studied during pregnancy.

Intravenous nitroglycerin has also been utilized to blunt the hypertensive effect of endotracheal intubation in women with severe preeclampsia undergoing Caesarean section (Cheek and Samuels, 1996; Longmire *et al.*, 1991).

The calcium channel blocker verapamil has been discussed above. Other calcium antagonists, such as diltiazem, nicardipine, and nifedipine, may also be useful as antianginal agents and have not been reported to be associated with an increase in malformation rates in animal studies (Ariyuki, 1975). No studies of the use of other calcium channel antagonists use during pregnancy have been published.

No information has been published on the use of dipyramidole, a selective coronary vasodilator, in pregnant women. The beta-blockers are discussed above, as well as in the Antihypertensives section below.

ANTIHYPERTENSIVES

Methyldopa

Methyldopa (Aldomet) is a commonly utilized alpha-adrenergic blocking agent for the treatment of chronic hypertension in pregnant women. No epidemiologic studies are published on methyldopa use during pregnancy. Nonetheless, the available data suggest that methyldopa does not pose a significant risk of birth defects, and postnatal growth and development seems unaffected by prenatal exposure.

In summary, it would appear that methyldopa is not a human teratogen and is probably one of the safest antihypertensives for use during pregnancy.

Hydralazine

One of the commonly used antihypertensive drugs is hydralazine, especially for acutely lowering of blood pressure in women with severe preeclampsia. It is thought to work primarily as a peripheral vasodilator (i.e., smooth muscle relaxant). No epidemiological studies of congenital anomalies in children born to women who took hydralazine during pregnancy have been published. Transient neonatal thrombocytopenia was reported.

Box 3.3 Antihypertensive drugs

Acebutolol (Sectral)	Lisinopril
Atenolol (Tenormin)	Methyldopa (Aldomet)
Betaxolol (Kerlane)	Metoprolol (Lopressor)
Captopril (Capoten)	Nadolol (Corgard)
Carteolol (Cartol)	Penbutolol (Levatol)
Clonidine (Catapres)	Propranolol (Inderal)
Diazoxide (Hyperstat)	Quinapril
Enalapril	Ramipril
FosinaprilHydralazine (Apresoline)	Sodium nitroprusside (Nipride, Nitropress)
Hydralazine (Apresoline)	Timolol (Blocadren)
Labetolol (Normodyne, Trandate)	

Beta-adrenergic blockers

Several beta-blockers are available for the treatment of hypertension (Box 3.3) and have been used in pregnant women. Propranolol has been discussed above. Although there are no large human reproduction studies for labetolol, metaprolol, or atenolol use in pregnant women, there are reports of their use without apparent adverse fetal effects. There are no reports of human teratogenicity for any of the beta-adrenergic blockers.

LABETOLOL

Investigators who studied drug-free, methyldopa, and labetolol groups reported a higher frequency of fetal growth retardation in the labetolol group with no obvious improvement in neonatal outcome (Sibai *et al.*, 1987, 1990); neither was there an increase in congenital anomalies or any adverse effects in the offspring of 85 women with severe hypertension who were treated with labetolol during pregnancy (Michael, 1979). Comparing oral labetolol to intravenous diazoxide for hypertensive crisis during pregnancy, no significant maternal or fetal side effects were observed (Michael, 1986). Among 104 labetolol- versus methyldopa-treated women with pregnancy-induced hypertension, labetolol caused fewer side effects than methyldopa (el-Qarmalawi *et al.*, 1995). Labetolol is the agent of choice to blunt the hypertensive response to endotracheal intubation, with few maternal, fetal or neonatal side effects (Cheek and Samuels, 1996).

METOPROLOL AND ATENOLOL

Metoprolol (Lopressor) and atenolol (Tenormin) are beta-blockers that are used to treat hypertension during pregnancy. No studies on the use of these agents during the first trimester of pregnancy are published. No increase in adverse maternal or fetal effects, including no significant differences in birth weight, were reported in 120 women treated with atenolol or placebo during pregnancy (Rubin *et al.*, 1983a,b). Similarly, no adverse fetal effects or pregnancy outcomes associated with metoprolol or metprolol/hydralazine treatment in second and third trimesters of pregnancy were noted (Sundstrom, 1978). According to the manufacturer, it was not teratogenic in several animal studies.

Breastfeeding is allowed during maternal therapy with either metoprolol or atenolol (American Academy of Pediatrics, 1994), despite a case report of toxicity in a neonate whose mother was receiving atenolol while breastfeeding (Schmimmel *et al.*, 1989).

ACEBUTOLOL

No studies of acebutolol (Sectral) use in the first trimester of pregnancy have been published, but several reports of acebutolol treatment for hypertension during pregnancy (*n* = 56 infants) have been published that were without adverse maternal or fetal effects (Dubois *et al.*, 1980, 1982; Williams and Morrissey, 1983). Neonatal hemodynamic adaptation failure occurred in five of 11 infants whose mothers were treated with acebutolol during pregnancy (Yassen *et al.*, 1992). It seems unlikely that this drug is associated with an increased risk of congenital anomalies.

PINDOLOL

No studies regarding the use of pindolol during the first trimester of pregnancy have been published. Among 51 women with pregnancy-induced hypertension randomized to hydralazine, hydralazine and propranolol, or hydralazine and pindolol, pindolol was associated with fewer maternal and fetal side effects (Paran *et al.*, 1995). However, infants born to mothers who received propranolol had smaller birth weights. In a comparative study of atenolol or pindolol on uterine/fetal hemodynamics and fetal cardiac function, investigators found that pindolol was preferable to atenolol for the treatment of pregnancy-induced hypertension based upon maternal and fetal cardiovascular function (Rasanen and Jouppila, 1995).

BETAXOLOL, CARTEOLOL, NADOLOL, PENBUTOLOL, AND TIMOLOL

No human teratology or reproduction studies with betaxolol, carteolol, nadolol, penbutolol, or timolol have been published. No increase in congenital malformations was noted in the offspring of pregnant mice who received up to 150 mg/kg.day of carteolol (Tanaka *et al.*, 1979). Also, no increase in the frequency of malformations was found among the offspring of rats, rabbits, and hamsters that had received nadolol in doses several times higher than the usual human dose (Sibley *et al.*, 1978; Stevens *et al.*, 1984). No increased frequency of adverse fetal effects was found in the offspring of mice treated with penbutolol (Sugisaki *et al.*, 1981).

CLONIDINE

Clonidine (Catapres) is a centrally acting antihypertensive that blocks alpha-adrenergic receptors. No epidemiologic studies of the frequency of congenital anomalies and clonidine use during early pregnancy have been published. Anecdotal case reports of clonidine use during pregnancy suggest no adverse fetal effects (Horvath *et al.*, 1985). Head size and neurologic examination of 22 children whose mothers received clonidine during pregnancy were normal (Huisjes *et al.*, 1986; Raftos *et al.*, 1973). One rat teratology study found no increased frequency of birth defects (Angelova *et al.*, 1975), but one study found an increase in growth retardation and cleft palates in offspring of mice treated with large doses of this antihypertensive (Chahoud *et al.*, 1985). Clonidine is probably not associated with an increased risk of congenital anomalies when used therapeutically.

DIAZOXIDE

Diazoxide is a thiazide (Hyperstat) that is used parenterally as an antihypertensive. An oral form of this drug (Proglycem) is also used to treat hypoglycemia secondary to hyperinsulinism. No epidemiologic studies of diazoxide have been published. An anecdotal case report of abnormalities of body and scalp hair, including alopecia, in four neonates of women who received oral diazoxide during the last trimester of pregnancy has been published (Milner and Chonskey, 1972). Maternal diazoxide therapy was also reportedly associated with hyperglycemia in the neonate (Milsap and Auld, 1980). No animal teratology studies are available. Pancreatic islet cell damage was found in the offspring of sheep and goats treated with intravenous diazoxide (Boulos *et al.*, 1971). Diazoxide may inhibit uterine contractions (Landesman *et al.*, 1969) and was used in the past by some clinicians as a tocolytic agent.

SODIUM NITROPRUSSIDE

A potent vasodilator, sodium nitroprusside (Nipride, Nitropress), is used primarily for hypertensive emergencies. It is also used to induce hypotension during certain types of

Box 3.4 Loop and potassium-sparing diuretics

Loop diuretics
Bumetanide (Bumex)
Ethacrynic acid (Edecrin)
Furosemide (Lasix, Myrosemide)

Potassium-sparing diuretics
Amiloride (Midamor)
Spironolactone (Aldactone)
Triamterene (Direnium)

Box 3.5 Thiazide diuretics

Bendroflumethiazide (Naturetin)
Benzthiazide (Exna, Hydrex)
Chlorothiazide (Diuril)
Cyclothiazide (Anhydron)
Hydrochlorothiazide (Esidrix, Hydro-Chlor,
  Hydro-D, Hydrodiuril)

Hydroflumethiazide (Diucardin, Saluron)
Methyclothiazide (Aquatensen, Enduran)
Metolazone (Diulo, Zaroxolyn, Mykrox)
Polythiazide (Renese)
Quinethazone (Hydromox)
Trichlomethiazide (Metahydrin, Naqua,
  Trichlorex)

surgical procedures, especially neurosurgical procedures. No epidemiological studies of congenital anomalies in association with nitroprusside use during pregnancy have been published. Nitroprusside was reported to be associated with cyanide toxicity in animals (Lewis *et al.*, 1977), but this is apparently not a significant risk in the human fetus when recommended human doses are used in the mother (Shoemaker and Meyers, 1984). Nonetheless, it is prudent to avoid use of nitroprusside during pregnancy because of the theoretical accumulation of cyanide in the fetal liver. Chronic use of sodium nitroprusside is logically associated with a much higher risk than acute usage.

DIURETICS

Diuretics are used to treat hypertension, sometimes alone or in conjunction with another drug regimen. Three basic categories of diuretics are: (1) loop diuretics; (2) potassium-sparing diuretics; and (3) thiazide diuretics. Agents in these categories are listed in Boxes 3.4 and 3.5.

Loop diuretics

Loop diuretics act primarily by inhibiting sodium and water reabsorption by the loop of Henle. Loop diuretics include bumetanide, ethracrynic acid, and furosemide.

BUMETANIDE

No epidemiological studies of bumetanide (Bumex) during pregnancy have been published. No increase in malformations was found in offspring of animals receiving several times the usual adult human dose of bumetanide (McClain and Dammers, 1981).

ETHACRYNIC ACID

No animal or human teratology studies of ethacrynic acid (Edecrin) have been reported.

FUROSEMIDE

Among 350 infants born to women who used furosemide during pregnancy, the frequency of congenital anomalies was not increased (Rosa, personal communication, cited in Briggs *et al.*, 2002). Diuretics given after the first trimester of pregnancy may interfere with normal plasma volume expansion. An adverse effect on plasma volume, no improvement in perinatal outcome (Sibai *et al.*, 1987), and decreased placental perfusion were reported with the use of diuretics during pregnancy (Shoemaker *et al.*, 1973). Furosemide also displaces bilirubin from albumin, increasing the risk for fetal hyperbilirubinemia (Turmen *et al.*, 1982). In animal studies, furosemide exposure in pregnancy was associated with an increase in fetal loss and skeletal anomalies in offspring (Godde and Grote, 1975; Mallie *et al.*, 1985). Furosemide crosses the placenta and assists in assessing fetal urinary tract obstruction and fetal urine production (Barrett *et al.*, 1983; Wladimiroff, 1975). Furosemide is probably not associated with an increased risk of birth defects.

Potassium-sparing diuretics

Potassium-sparing diuretics include amiloride, spironolactone, and triamterene, and result in sodium and water loss while sparing potassium. Spironolactone is a competitive inhibitor of aldosterone, while ameloride and triamterene function at the level of the collecting tubules.

AMILORIDE

No epidemiological studies regarding the use of amiloride in pregnant women are published. No increase in malformations in offspring of pregnant hamsters that received small doses of ameloride was found (Storch and Layton, 1973).

SPIRONOLACTONE

No epidemiological studies of spironolactone (Aldactone) in pregnant women have been published. Spironolactone was not associated with an increased frequency of malformations in offspring of rats (Miyakubo *et al.*, 1977), but feminization of the genitalia in the male offspring of rats that received this diuretic in doses five times that normally used in humans was reported (Hecker *et al.*, 1980). This diuretic is not recommended for use during human pregnancy because of the theoretical risk of feminization of male genitalia. This specific complication has not been reported in humans. Spironolactone for the treatment of pregnant women with Bartter's disease (Groves and Corenblum, 1995; Rigo *et al.*, 1996) has been reported. None of the three male infants or two female infants had any demonstrable adverse effects, including undervirilization of the male infant.

TRIAMTERENE

Triamterene (Direnium) is another potassium-sparing diuretic. Of 271 pregnant women included in the Collaborative Perinatal Project who were treated with this diuretic (Heinonen *et al.*, 1977), only a few received this diuretic in the first months of pregnancy. The frequency of congenital malformations was not increased in the offspring of these women; neither was the frequency of malformations increased in the offspring of animals who received triamterene (Ellison and Maren, 1972).

Thiazides

Thiazides comprise the largest group of diuretics (Box 3.5). Thiazides function by preventing reabsorption of sodium at the distal renal tubules. No increase in frequency of congenital anomalies in the offspring of over 500 women who took thiazide diuretics in the first trimester of pregnancy was noted (Kraus et al., 1966).

BENDROFLUMETHIAZIDE

Among more than 1000 women included in the Collaborative Perinatal Project who received bendroflumethiazide (Naturetin), only 13 received this diuretic in early pregnancy (Heinonen et al., 1977). In a study of diuretics to prevent preeclampsia, no increase in the frequency of malformations or stillbirths was found in the offspring of over 1000 women who received this diuretic after the first trimester. No increased frequency of congenital anomalies was found among offspring of rats given hundreds of times the usual human dose (Stevens et al., 1984).

BENZTHIAZIDE

There are no epidemiological studies on the use of this diuretic in pregnant women. No animal teratology studies are available regarding benzthiazide.

CHLOROTHIAZIDE

Chlorothiazide (Diuril) is the most commonly used thiazide diuretic. The frequency of congenital anomalies was not increased over the expected rate reported among offspring of 63 women who took this diuretic in early pregnancy and of over 5000 women who took this drug after the first trimester of pregnancy (Heinonen et al., 1977).

Neonatal thrombocytopenia was reported in the offspring of several mothers who received chlorothiazide during pregnancy (Rodriguez et al., 1964), but not among infants in another series (Finnerty and Assali, 1964). An increased frequency of hypertension was reported in the offspring of rats treated with chlorothiazide at doses 30 times those employed in humans (Grollman and Grollman, 1962). No increase in malformations in offspring of rats treated with this agent in doses up to 12 times that used in humans was found by another group of investigators (Maren and Ellison, 1972).

HYDROCHLOROTHIAZIDE

Hydrochlorothiazide is a very commonly used thiazide diuretic. Birth defects were not increased in frequency among offspring of more than 200 women who received this diuretic in early pregnancy (Heinonen et al., 1977; Jick et al., 1981). Neonatal thrombocytopenia was observed with hydrochlorothiazide, as with other thiazide diuretics (Rodriguez et al., 1964). Hydrochlorothiazide was not teratogenic in the offspring of rats who received this agent in doses many times that of the human adult dose (George et al., 1995; Maren and Ellison, 1972).

HYDROFLUMETHIAZIDE

No human epidemiological studies or animal teratology studies are published for hydroflumethiazide (Diucardin, Saluron). It is reasonable to assume that the potential risks of this diuretic are similar to those of other thiazides.

METHYCLOTHIAZIDE, POLYTHIAZIDE, AND TRICHLORMETHIAZIDE

No information is available on which to base a risk estimate for these thiazide drugs. For example, the Collaborative Perinatal Project database included only three women treated with methyclothiazide (Aquatensen, Enduran), 10 women treated with polythiazide (Renese), and only two women treated with trichlormethiazide (Metahydrin, Naqua, Trichlorex) in the first 4 months of pregnancy (Heinonen et al., 1977). There are no available animal teratology studies with these three thiazide diuretics. Nonetheless, based upon information for a closely related and better-studied drug, chlorothiazide, it is reasonable to state that the risk of birth defects with these drugs is low, if it exceeds background risk.

Other thiazide-like diuretics

Chlorthalidone (Hygroton, Thalitone), metolazone (Diulo, Zaroxolyn), and quinethazone (Hydromox) are not true thiazide diuretics from the standpoint of chemical structure, although their mode of action is very similar to the thiazide group. There is little available information regarding the use of chlorthalidone in women in the first trimester of pregnancy. Over 1300 women who used thiazide diuretics were included in the Collaborative Perinatal Project database, but only 20 used chlorthalidone during the first trimester (Heinonen et al., 1977). Although there was an increased frequency of congenital dislocation of the hip in this latter group, it is difficult if not impossible to draw valid conclusions from such numbers. Tervila and Vartianen (1971) reported no significant differences in offspring of mothers exposed to chlorthalidone after 15 weeks gestation, compared to controls. Only eight pregnant women were exposed to quinethazone in the Collaborative Perinatal Project database, and none who received metolazone (Heinonen et al., 1977). No published reports are available on congenital anomalies in the offspring of women who took either of these two diuretics during pregnancy. Metolazone was not found to be teratogenic in one animal study (Nakajima et al., 1978), and no animal teratology studies are available for quinethazone.

CALCIUM CHANNEL BLOCKERS

Calcium channel blockers are used to treat hypertension and supraventricular tachycardia.

Verapamil

This calcium channel antagonist was discussed under Antiarrhythmics.

Nifedipine

Nifedipine was used 'off-label' as a tocolytic agent and an antihypertensive medication. Nifedipine was teratogenic in rats given 30 times the usual human dose (data from the manufacturer's insert). There are no studies of nifedipine use during the first trimester of pregnancy. No adverse maternal or fetal effects were reported for the use of nifedipine to treat preeclapmsia or hypertension, respectively (Sibai et al., 1992). The frequency of congenital anomlies was not increased among 64 infants born to women treated with nifedipine (or a related calcium channel blocker) (Magee *et al.*, 1996). It is regarded as the 'second line' antihypertensive therapy in pregnant women. Nifedipine use during pregnancy is probably safe with 'little teratogenic or fetotoxic potential' (Childress and Katz, 1994).

Nicardipine

Treatment of hypertension in pregnancy with nicardipine was more effective than metoprolol in decreasing blood pressure, and neonatal outcomes were not different (Jannet *et al.*, 1994). One study of 40 pregnant women with hypertension reported that intravenous nicardipine 'seems to be safe' (Carbonne *et al.*, 1993). Nicardipine was not teratogenic in rats given an oral dose many times the recommended human dose (Sato *et al.*, 1979).

Isradipine

Isradipine, a dihydropyridine calcium channel blocker, is used as an antihypertensive agent. Isradipine was not teratogenic in rats given several times the human dose (data from the manufacturer's insert). No human reproduction studies have been published on isradipine. This calcium channel blocker was evaluated for the treatment of hypertension in pregnancy and reported to be effective for the treatment of nonproteinuric hypertension. No adverse fetal effects were mentioned in this report (Wide-Swensson *et al.*, 1995).

Diltiazem, nimodipine, and amlodipine

There is little information regarding the use of these calcium channel blockers during pregnancy. Nimodipine was teratogenic in rabbits (data from the manufacturer's insert).

ANGIOTENSIN-CONVERTING ENZYME INHIBITORS

Angiotensin-converting enzyme (ACE) inhibitors are a class of drugs used to treat hypertension (see Table 3.4). The ACE inhibitor group should be considered contraindicated for use during pregnancy because of the risks discussed below (Shotan *et al.*, 1994). Risks associated with ACE inhibitors are second and third trimester events. First trimester exposures do not seem to present a significant risk for congenital anomalies, but this is an unknown area.

Captopril

Captopril (Capoten) is an ACE inhibitor used as an oral antihypertensive agent. No epidemiological studies of this antihypertensive agent in pregnant women have been published. There were no malformations among 22 infants born to mothers who received captopril during the first trimester (Kreft-Jais and Boutroy, 1988), but no controlled studies have addressed whether or not captopril is a potent human teratogen. Case report evidence strongly suggests that captopril and other ACE inhibitors may be associated with

Table 3.4 Summary of cardiovascular drugs: Teratogen Information Service (TERIS) and Food and Drug Administration (FDA) risk estimates

Drug	Risk	Risk rating
Acebutolol	Unlikely	B_m*
Amiloride	Undetermined	B_m*
Amiodarone	Neonatal thyroid dysfunction or goiter: small to moderate	D_m
	Congenital anomalies: undetermined	
Atenolol	Undetermined	D_m
Betaxolol	Undetermined	C_m*
Bendroflumethiazide	Undetermined	C_m*
Benzthiazide	Undetermined	C*
Bumetanide	Undetermined	C_m*
Captopril	First-trimester use: undetermined	C_m*
	Use later in pregnancy: moderate	
Chlorothiazide	Unlikely	C_m*
Chlorthalidone	Unlikely	B_m*
Clonidine	Undetermined	C_m
Diazoxide	Undetermined	C_m
Digoxin	Unlikely	C_m
Diltiazem	Undetermined	C_m
Disopyramide	Undetermined	C_m
Enalapril	First-trimester use: undetermined	C_m*
	Use later in pregnancy: moderate	
Encainide	Undetermined	B_m
Flecainide	Undetermined	C_m
Furosemide	Undetermined	C_m*
Heparin	Unlikely	C_m
Hydralazine	Undetermined	C_m
Hydrochlorothiazide	Unlikely	B_m*
Lidocaine	Local administration: none intravenous	B_m
	Administration: undetermined	
Lisinopril	First-trimester use: none to minimal	C_m*
	Second or third trimester: moderate	
Methclothiazide	Unlikely	NA
Methyldopa	Undetermined	B_m
Metolazone	Undetermined	B_m*
Nadolol	Undetermined	C_m*
Nifedipine	None to minimal	C_m
Pindolol	Unlikely	B_m*
Polythiazide	Undetermined	C*
Procainamide	Undetermined	C_m
Propranolol	Undetermined	C_m*
Quinethazone	Undetermined	D*
Quinidine	Undetermined	C_m
Spironolactone	Undetermined	C_m*
Streptokinase	Undetermined	C_m
Timolol	Undetermined	C_m*
Tocainide	Undetermined	C_m

Continued

Table 3.4 *Continued*

Drug	Risk	Risk rating
Triamterene	Undetermined	C_m*
Trichlormethiazide	Undetermined	C*
Urokinase	Undetermined	B_m
Verapamil	Undetermined	C_m

NA, not available.

Compiled from: Friedman *et al.*, *Obstet Gynecol* 1990; **75**: 594; Briggs *et al.*, 2005; Friedman and Polifka, 2006.

anuria, renal failure, and hypocalvaria, possibly contributing to perinatal death (Anonymous, 1989; Barr and Cohen, 1991; Boutroy, 1989; Boutroy *et al.*, 1984; Rosa and Bosco, 1991; Rothberg and Lorenz, 1984). Of 29 infants with neonatal renal failure, nine were born to women who had used captopril throughout pregnancy (Rosa and Bosco, 1991). The other 20 were born to women who used other ACE inhibitors. These antihypertensives are, therefore, contraindicated for use during pregnancy, and should be avoided if possible. No animal teratology studies have been published for captopril, but an increased frequency of fetal deaths was reported in two animal studies (Pipkin *et al.*, 1980, 1982).

Enalapril

This drug is an ACE inhibitor. Of 29 cases of perinatal renal failure, 18 occurred following maternal therapy with enalapril during pregnancy (Rosa and Bosco, 1991). This drug in contraindicated in the second and third trimesters.

Lisinopril

Lisinopril is another ACE inhibitor. Among 29 infants with neonatal renal failure, two were born to women who used lisinopril during pregnancy (Rosa and Bosco, 1991). This drug is contraindicated in the second and third trimesters.

Quinapril, ramipril, and fosinapril

These ACE inhibitors theoretically carry the same risks of adverse fetal/neonatal effects as the other ACE inhibitors. They should be contraindicated in the second and third trimesters.

Angiotensin II receptor blockers

Angiotensin II receptor blockers (ARBs) are a new class of ACE inhibitors used to treat hypertension. The ARBs include: valsartan, losartan, telmisartan, candesartan, omlesartan, tasosartan, and eprosartan. Based upon case reports, the ARBs have a collection of fetal complications strikingly similar to the ACE inhibitor fetopathy. The risk of congenital anomalies following use during the first trimester is unknown, but use during the second and third trimesters is associated with a significant risk of fetal-neonatal complications. The complications include: oligohydramnios, fetal/neonatal renal failure, and decreased calcification of the cranium (Friedman and Polifka, 2006).

SPECIAL CONSIDERATIONS

Cardiac arrhythmias and hypertension are the two most common cardiovascular diseases that require therapy during pregnancy. A complete review of these disorders is beyond the scope of this book. Only a few of the more common clinical problems are discussed below.

Cardiac arrhythmias

Fortunately, life-threatening cardiac arrhythmias are uncommon during pregnancy. However, certain less serious arrhythmias may actually be increased in frequency during pregnancy (Brown and Wendel, 1989).

Paroxysomal supraventricular tachycardia

Paroxysmal supraventricular tachycardia occurs among 1–2 per 500 young women, and frequently occurs in those without overt heart disease (Brown and Wendel, 1989). The disease frequently presents with heart rates of over 200 beats per minute. Symptoms include palpitations, light-headedness, and rarely, angina and syncope. Pregnancy may increase risk for this type of arrhythmia (Meller and Goldman, 1982; Szekely and Snaith, 1953). Most cases of paroxysmal supraventricular tachycardia are associated with AV-nodal reentry mechanisms, which can be managed in most patients with maneuvers of vagal stimulation to include carotid massage or Valsalva techniques (Brown and Wendel, 1989; Josephson and Kaster, 1977; Wu et al., 1978). If vagal stimulation is unsuccessful, verapamil at 5–10 mg intravenously will prove successful in most cases in pregnant women. Because of reports of adverse neonatal cardiac effects

---

Box 3.6 Treatment of acute episodes of paroxysmal supraventricular tachycardia in the pregnant patient without cardiac decompensation

Vagal stimulation
Carotid sinus massage
Valsalva
Verapamil, 5–10 mg IV[a]
Adenosine, 6 mg as a rapid intravenous bolus
Digoxin, 0.5–1.0 mg IV over 15 min (total dose not to exceed 1.5 mg in 24 h)
Propranolol, 0.5–1.0 mg/min (total dose not to exceed 3.0 mg)[b]
See manufacturer's recommendations for dosing.
[a]See text regarding possible fetal effects.
[b]Caution in patients with heart disease or asthma.

(including cardiac arrest), verapamil should be used with extreme caution during pregnancy, only after other agents have failed.

Cardioversion appears to be safe for the fetus (Clark *et al.*, 1994). Digoxin and propranolol may also be utilized (Box 3.6). Recently adenosine, in a dose of 6 mg given as a rapid intravenous bolus, has been recommended for the treatment of supraventricular tachycardia. As previously mentioned, there is little information regarding the safety of this agent during pregnancy. However, there are several reports regarding its efficacy in pregnant women (Afridi *et al.*, 1992; Hagley and Cole, 1994; Mason *et al.*, 1992). Electrical cardioversion should be reserved for patients with cardiac decompensation in whom medical therapy has failed.

Patients with frequent recurrences of this arrhythmia can usually be treated with digitalis and/or verapamil, quinidine, and propranolol as needed (Brown and Wendel, 1989; Zipes, 1988).

Atrial fibrillation

Atrial fibrillation is uncommon in pregnant women, and this event points to underlying cardiac or thyroid disease. Mitral valve disease, secondary to rheumatic heart disease, is the most commonly encountered underlying cause of atrial fibrillation in the pregnant patient. Chronic atrial fibrillation treatment is generally directed at slowing the ventricular rate through medical therapy, with such medications as digitalis, with or without verapamil or propranolol (Brown and Wendel, 1989). Such gravidas may also require heparinization to prevent embolization.

Electrical cardioversion is indicated for significant cardiac decompensation and has been utilized in pregnant women without apparent adverse effects (Schroeder and Harrison, 1971).

Ventricular arrhythmias

Premature ventricular contractions (PVCs) are relatively common and may actually be increased during pregnancy (Brown and Wendel, 1989). They generally do not require therapy, especially in asymptomatic pregnant women. Frequent PVCs should alert the clinician to possible organic heart disease, but medical therapy is rarely necessary for infrequent PVCs. Agents such as lidocaine, procainamide, quinidine, or disopyramide can be utilized for frequent or symptomatic PVCs.

Ventricular tachycardia is a life-threatening arrhythmia as it may lead to ventricular fibrillation, cardiac decompensation, and death. Fortunately, this arrhythmia is rarely encountered during pregnancy, especially in the absence of specific cardiac disease such as myocardial infarction. Therapy consists primarily of electric cardioversion, especially if the patient is hemodynamically unstable. Lidocaine, in a dose of 75–100 mg IV bolus followed by 1–4 mg/min infusion, should be utilized in conjunction with countershock and as initial therapy in the stable patient (Brown and Wendel, 1989). Lidocaine, procainamide, or bretylium may be used to prevent recurrence of tachycardia.

Ventricular fibrillation is a medical emergency of the highest magnitude. Treatment is primarily electrical cardioversion followed by lidocaine or bretylium to prevent further fibrillation.

Hypertension

Hypertension is one of the most common medical complications encountered during pregnancy and presents as chronic hypertension, pregnancy-induced hypertension, or preeclampsia. In the case of chronic hypertension, an underlying and potentially correctable etiology should be ruled out.

CHRONIC HYPERTENSION

Chronic hypertension is hypertension that was present before pregnancy or prior to 20 weeks gestational age, and occurs most frequently among multiparous patients. No unanimity of opinion has been reached regarding the most appropriate antihypertensive for use during pregnancy or the efficacy of such treatment with regard to pregnancy outcome.

Methyldopa (Aldomet) is one of the most commonly used antihypertensives in pregnant women. The initial dose of this agent is 250 mg twice a day with increases up to 2 g per day and a maximum recommended daily dose of 3 g (PDR, 2004).

Beta-adrenergic blockers such as atenolol, propranolol, or labetolol, as well as the calcium channel blockers and the centrally acting agent, clonidine, can also be used during pregnancy to treat hypertensions. However, no scientific evidence indicates that they offer any advantage over methyldopa during pregnancy.

A variety of thiazide diuretics may also be utilized as an adjunct in the treatment of hypertension. However, they should not be initiated after 20 weeks gestation because they may interfere with the 'normal' pregnancy expansion of blood volume and thus placental perfusion.

PREGNANCY-INDUCED HYPERTENSION

Antihypertensives are generally not indicated for the treatment of hypertension associated with preeclampsia except in severe preeclampsia. In the event of severe, acute hypertension (i.e., diastolic blood pressures greater than 110 mmHg) intravenous hydralazine in 5–10 mg doses will usually be effective. This dose can be increased and repeated every 15–20 min, as necessary. The treatment goal of medical therapy is to achieve a diastolic blood pressure less than 110 mmHg, and in the range of 90–100 mmHg. Caution must be exercised at the lower range to ensure adequate placental perfusion. Labetolol 10 mg IV may also be utilized every 10 min. Increasing doses (up to a total dose of 300 mg) may be necessary in some women.

Diuretics are generally contraindicated in women with preeclampsia because they may significantly interfere with utero-placental blood flow by further decreasing intravascular volume.

Prophylaxis of subacute bacterial endocarditis

Pregnant women with significant cardiac lesions should receive antibiotic prophylaxis for invasive procedures, including vaginal and Caesarean delivery, as prophylaxis for endocarditis (see Box 3.7).

Box 3.7 American Heart Association prophylaxis for bacterial endocarditis guidelines

Nonpenicillin allergic
Ampicillin 2.0 g IM or IV
Gentamicin 1.5 mg/kg IM or IV
To be given 30 min before delivery and repeated once 8 h later
Penicillin allergic
Vancomycin 1.0 g IV given over 60 min
Gentamicin 1.5 mg/kg IM or IV
To be given 60 min before delivery and repeated once 8–12 h later

Box 3.8 Fetal arrythmias

Tachycardia
Supreventricular tachycardia (sinus or atrial), rate >180 bpm
Atrial flutter, rate 400–500 bpm
Atrial fibrillation
Ventricular tachycardia, rate 180–400
Bradycardia
Sinus bradycardia
Complete heart block
Irregular rhythms
Premature atrial contractions
Premature ventricular contractions

From Kleinman and Copel, 1991; Pinsky *et al.*, 1991.

Fetal cardiac arrhythmias

A variety of fetal arrhythmias may be detected during pregnancy (Box 3.8). Not all such arrhythmias need to be or can be treated *in utero*. Factors that influence *in utero* therapy include the type and etiology of the arrhythmia, the potential for fetal compromise (i.e., heart failure or hydrops) and the gestational age of the fetus. Although virtually all antiarrhythmic drugs cross the placenta, it is often difficult to achieve adequate blood concentrations in both the mother and fetus with standard therapeutic doses.

Supraventricular tachycardia

Supraventricular tachycardia is probably the most common fetal arrhythmia associated with fetal congestive heart failure, especially if the condition is long-standing (Chitkara *et al.*, 1980; Kleinman *et al.*, 1985a,b; Pinsky *et al.*, 1991). The drug of choice for the initial treatment of supraventricular tachycardia is maternal digitalis therapy (Pinsky *et al.*, 1991). This drug crosses the placenta readily and is safe for the fetus, although it is sometimes difficult to achieve therapeutic levels in the fetus. Recommended maternal doses are summarized in Table 3.5.

Table 3.5 Maternal dose and serum level of medications for fetal supraventricular tachycardia

	Maternal dose	Serum level
Digoxin	0.25–0.75 mg (loading dose 1.0–2.5 ng pO) (or 0.5–2.0 ng IV)	0.5–2 ng/mL
Propranolol	20–160 ng q 6–8 h IV	20–100 ng/mL
Procainamide	6 mg/kg q 4 h IV	4–14 ng/mL
If above fail:		
Verapamil	80–120 mg q 6–8 h IV	50–100 ng/mL

From Kleinman et al., 1985a, 1985b; Pinsky et al., 1991.

Two other drugs that can be used are propranolol and procainamide. Verapamil, which has been utilized for this purpose, should be used with extreme caution and probably only after other therapeutic modalities have failed because of adverse events. Other agents that may used include quinidine, disopyramide, flecainide, and amiodarone, depending on the suspected etiology of the tachycardia (Kleinman and Copel, 1991).

Atrial flutter

Atrial flutter and fibrillation are uncommon during the fetal period and are often difficult to diagnose. The fetal heart rate may reach 400–500 bpm with atrial flutter. Control of the ventricular rate via atrioventricular nodal blocks with digoxin or verapamil may be inadequate and may actually worsen fetal hemodynamic status (Kleinman and Copel, 1991). Unless the atrial flutter itself is controlled, 'there will continue to be actual contractions against a closed or partially closed atrioventricular valve. ...' (Kleinman and Copel, 1991). A type I agent, such as procainamide or quinidine, should be included in the treatment regimen. Atrial fibrillation is even more rare than flutter and is treated similarly (Kleinman and Copel, 1991).

Key references

Bhagwat AR, Engel PJ. Heart disease and pregnancy. *Cardiol Clin* 1995; **13**: 163.

Chan WS, Anand S, Ginsberg JS. Anticoagulation of pregnant women with mechanical heart valves. A systematic review of the literature. *Arch Intern Med* 2000; **160**: 191–6.

Cheek TG, Samuels P. Pregnancy-induced hypertension. In: Datta S (ed.). *Anesthetic and Obstetric Management of High-Risk Pregnancy*, 2nd edn. St Louis: Mosby, 1996: 386–411 (Chapter 21).

Groves TD, Corenblum B. Spironolactone therapy during human pregnancy. *Am J Obstet Gynecol* 1995; **172**: 1655.

Little BB. Pharmacokinetics during pregnancy. Evidence-based maternal dose formulation. *Obstet Gynecol* 1999; **93**: 858–68.

Magee LA, Schick B, Donnenfeld AE *et al*. The safety of calcium channel blockers in human pregnancy. A prospective, multicenter cohort study. *Am J Obstet Gynecol* 1996; **174**: 823–8.

Paran E, Holzberg G, Mazor M, Zmora E, Insler V. Beta-adrenergic blocking agents in the treatment of pregnancy-induced hypertension. *Int J Clin Pharmacol Therap* 1995; **33**: 119.

Rigo J Jr, Glaz E, Papp Z. Low or high doses of spironolactone for treatment of maternal Bartter's syndrome. *Am J Obstet Gynecol* 1996; **174**: 297.

Sanson B-J, Lensing AWA, Prins MH *et al*. Safety of low-molecular-weight heparin in pregnancy. A systematic review. *Thromb Haemost* 1999; **81**: 668–72.

Turrentine MA, Braems G, Ramirez MM. Use of thrombolytics for the treatment of thromboembolic disease during pregnancy. *Obstet Gynecol Surv* 1995; **50**: 534.

Further references are available on the book's website at http://www.drugsandpregnancy.com

4

Endocrine disorders, contraception, and hormone therapy during pregnancy: embryotoxic versus fetal effects

Complex changes in maternal endocrine systems occur in normal women as a result of the altered metabolic demands of pregnancy. Disorders of endocrinologic systems may be associated with adverse maternal, embryonic, or fetal effects. These effects include increases in infertility, spontaneous abortion, fetal malformations, maternal and fetal metabolic derangements, and maternal and fetal death. Certain endocrine disorders, such as gestational diabetes mellitus, arise spontaneously during pregnancy, whereas preexisting endocrine disorders may be exacerbated, may improve, or may remain stable during gestation.

Abnormal fetal growth and development may occur as a result of the disease itself or from the medication(s) used to treat the disease. The teratogenic effects of certain drugs have long been considered a potential hazard for the embryo or fetus, particularly if such agents are administered during the first trimester of pregnancy. Pharmacokinetic behavior of hormones in pregnancy is not well documented.

The limited data available indicate that the volume of distribution (V_d) increases during pregnancy as does clearance for the drugs studied (Table 4.1).

This chapter is designed to address endocrine disorders, hormone therapy during pregnancy, and the possible teratogenic effects of medications. First, it describes briefly the pathogenesis of the major endocrine disorders of pregnancy and second, it enumerates the medications that may be used to treat such disorders and their potential embryotoxic and fetal effects.

Table 4.1 Pharmacokinetics of endocrine and hormone agents during pregnancy

Agent	n	EGA (weeks)	Route	AUC	V_d	C_{max}	C_{ss}	$t_{1/2}$	Cl	PPB	Control group[a]	Authors
Dexamethasone	6	33–40	IV		↑			=	↑		Yes (3)	Tsuei et al. (1980)
Dexamethasone	10	29	PO, IM		↑			=			Yes (1)	Elliot et al. (1996)
Methimazole	7	12–39	PO		=			→	↑		Yes (3)	Skellern et al. (1980)
Oxytocin	9	37–40	BU, IV			=	=	↑			Yes (4)	Dawood et al. (1980)

Source: Little BB. Obstet Gynecol 1999; **93**: 858.

EGA, estimated gestational age; AUC, area under the curve; V_d, volume of distribution; C_{max}, peak plasma concentration; C_{ss}, steady-state concentration; $t_{1/2}$, half-life; Cl, clearance; PPB, plasma protein binding; PO, by mouth; ↓ denotes a decrease during pregnancy compared to nonpregnant values; ↑ denotes an increase during pregnancy compared to nonpregnant values; = denotes no difference between pregnant and nonpregnant values; IV, intravenous; IM, intramuscular.

[a]Control groups: 1, nonpregnant women; 2, same individuals studied postpartum; 3, historic adult controls (sex not given); 4, adult male controls; 5, adult male and female controls combined.

MAJOR ENDOCRINE DISORDERS

Diabetes mellitus

Diabetes mellitus is a chronic disorder caused by a partial or total lack of insulin. It complicates 0.2–0.3 percent of all gestations (Connell *et al.*, 1985a; Cousins, 1991; Gabbe, 1980; Rodman *et al.*, 1976). Clinical manifestations vary with the severity of the disease, and range from an asymptomatic hyperglycemic state to severe diabetic ketoacidosis, coma, and death. Gestational diabetes mellitus is characterized by glucose intolerance arising in the second to third trimesters, and is found in approximately 2–3 percent of gestations.

Diabetic embryopathy

Children of women who have diabetes mellitus prior to pregnancy have a two- to fourfold increase in congenital anomalies compared to the general population (Cousins, 1983, 1987; Mills, 1982). Organ development occurs prior to the 8th week of gestation, and this is the critical window of time during which the teratogenic effect of overt maternal diabetes occurs (Mills *et al.*, 1979). Birth defects seen in infants of diabetic mothers involve cardiovascular, skeletal, and central nervous systems (Box 4.1). It is important to note, however, that infants of women who develop gestational diabetes mellitus are not at an increased risk for such defects because the exposure to the disease is outside the critical period of organogenesis (Mills, 1982).

FETAL COMPLICATIONS

Infants born to women who have diabetes prior to pregnancy and women who acquire gestational diabetes mellitus are at risk for significant neonatal morbidity. These neonates are at increased risk for respiratory distress syndrome, macrosomia, hypoglycemia, hyperbilirubinemia, and hypocalcemia. In addition, the risk of fetal death is

---

Box 4.1 Features of diabetic embryopathy

Cardiovascular	*Gastrointestinal*
Coarctation of the aorta	Bowel atresias
Situs inversus	Imperforate anus
Transposition of great vessels	Tracheoesophageal fistula
Ventricular septal defect	*Genitourinary*
Central nervous system	Absent kidneys
Hydrocephalus	Double ureters
Microcephaly	Polycystic kidneys
Neural tube defects	*Miscellaneous*
Skeletal	Cleft lip or palate
Caudal dysplasia syndrome	Polyhydramnios
Limb defects	Single umbilical artery

Adapted from Becerra *et al.*, 1990 and Dignan, 1981.

two- to three-fold greater than in the general population (O'Sullivan, 1980; Rust *et al.*, 1987). Although not conclusive, it is generally accepted that the frequency of these complications can be reduced with good maternal glucose control.

Medications

INSULIN

Insulin is a hormone produced by the beta cells in the pancreas that regulate glucose metabolism and other metabolic processes. Human insulin does not cross the placenta in physiologically significant amounts. Subcutaneous injection is the usual route of administration for insulin, but it can be administered intravenously in an emergency or during a stressful situation where a high degree of control is needed (e.g., labor), to lower the blood glucose rapidly.

Human insulin (semisynthetic or biosynthetic) is preferred over the animal insulins because it is much less antigenic. This is important because maternal insulin antibodies may alter insulin pharmacokinetics and cross the placenta, contributing to fetal hypoglycemia, beta-cell hyperplasia, and hyperinsulinemia (Knip *et al.*, 1983). Therefore, most diabetologists agree that immunogenic (animal) insulins should not be used in pregnant women.

Early studies suggested that the human placenta was impermeable to free insulin as well as insulin antibody complexes, but it appears that considerable amounts of antibody-bound animal insulin can cross the placenta. A nonoral drug available to treat diabetes is exenatide, but it has not been studied during pregnancy.

ORAL HYPOGLYCEMIC AGENTS

The classes of oral hypoglycemic drugs include: sulfonureas (acetohexamide, tolazamide, chlorpropamide, tolbutamide, glyburide, glipizide), biguanides (metformin), thiazolindinediones (rosiglitazone, pioglitazone), and alpha-glucosidase inhibitors (acarabose or Precose). Oral hypoglycemics are not recommended for use in pregnancy because they are known to cross the placenta and can stimulate fetal insulin secretion. These drugs have a very long half-life, and administration near term can result in a severely hypoglycemic neonate (Friend, 1981). No epidemiologic studies of birth defects among offspring of women treated with any of these oral hypoglycemic agents have been published.

ACETOHEXAMIDE

Acetohexamide administration throughout pregnancy has been associated with significant neonatal hypoglycemia (Kemball *et al.*, 1970). Pregnant rats, given acetohexamide at many times the usual human dose on days 9 and 10, had approximately 50 percent embryonic death, but no abnormalities (Bariljak, 1965). The frequency of congenital anomalies was not increased, other than those expected in diabetes mellitus. Chlorpropamide is a closely related drug.

CHLORPROPAMIDE

One out of 41 children born to women treated with chlorpropamide during the first trimester of pregnancy had congenital anomalies, but the malformations were consistent with diabetic embryopathy (Coetzee and Jackson, 1984). It is important to note that neonatal hypoglycemia may occur in infants of diabetic mothers treated with chlorpropamide late in pregnancy (Kemball *et al.*, 1970; Zucker and Simon, 1968). Rats treated during pregnancy with chlorpropamide in doses 200 to 300 times those usually employed in humans did not produce congenital anomalies in their offspring (Tuchmann-Duplessis and Mercier-Parot, 1959).

TOLBUTAMIDE

The frequency of congenital anomalies was not increased among 42 women who were treated with tolbutamide during pregnancy, but only 12 of these women had been treated during the first trimester. Several clinical series have suggested that the frequency of congenital anomalies among infants born to women who took tolbutamide in pregnancy is no greater than would be expected among infants of diabetic mothers (Coetzee and Jackson, 1984; Dolger *et al.*, 1969; Notelovitz, 1971). Rat and mouse studies show no increase in congenital anomalies with tolbutamide until the doses are maternally toxic. Tolbutamide does not seem likely to cause birth defects in exposed infants, but this is based on fewer than 50 exposed infants.

TOLAZAMIDE

There has been one case report of an ear malformation in an infant exposed to the oral hypoglycemic agent tolazamide during the first 12 weeks of gestation (Piacquadio *et al.*, 1991). It should be avoided in pregnancy since both tolazamide and tolbutamide will not provide good control in pregnant patients who cannot be controlled by diet alone (Friend, 1981). As with other sulfonylurea drugs, neonatal hypoglycemia is likely to occur with chronic use near the time of delivery.

GLYBURIDE

The transfer rate of glyburide through the human placenta was reported to be much lower than other oral hypoglycemics using *in vitro* techniques (Elliott *et al.*, 1991). Anencephaly and ventricular septal defect were reported in two infants exposed *in utero* to glyburide during the first 10 and 23 weeks of gestation, respectively (Piacquardio *et al.*, 1991). However, as with all of the agents in this class, prolonged neonatal hypoglycemia may be associated with maternal therapy (Coetzee and Jackson, 1984). Among more than 180 infants exposed to glyburide during the first trimester, the frequency of congenital anomalies was not increased (Towner *et al.*, 1995; Rosa, personal communication, cited in Briggs *et al.*, 2002). Given the high background risk for diabetic pregnancies (two- to four-fold higher than the general population), glyburide does not seem to pose a high risk for congenital anomalies.

GLIPIZIDE

Glipizide is a sulfonylurea drug used to treat noninsulin-dependent diabetes. In one study of 147 infants born to women who took glipizide during embryogenesis the frequency of congenital anomalies was not increased compared to infants born to women who took another sulfonylurea, used insulin, or controlled their diabetes with diet (Towner *et al.*, 1995).

THYROID GLAND

Maternal thyroid function changes during pregnancy

Thyroxine-binding globulin (TBG) concentrations increase to about twice normal values, resulting in significant elevations in serum L-thyroxine (T4) and liothyronine (T3) concentrations, coupled with a decrease in T3 resin uptake (T3RU) to values in the hypothyroid range (Glinoer et al., 1990; Harada et al., 1979; Osathanondh et al., 1976). Shortly after delivery, these values return to normal (Yamamoto et al., 1979). The concentrations of free T4, free T3, and the free thyroid index (FTI) in maternal serum remain normal throughout gestation (Glinoer et al., 1990). Mild diffuse thyromegaly occurs during gestation, probably due to an increased vascularity of the gland, and an increased thyroidal uptake of iodine secondary to elevated renal clearance (Dowling et al., 1961; Pochin, 1952). In addition, the placenta produces two hormones with thyroid-stimulating bioactivity. Human chorionic gonadotropin (hCG) and human chorionic thyrotropin (hCT) are secreted in variable amounts, yet are of questionable physiologic impact (Harada et al., 1979; Kennedy et al., 1992).

Maternal hyperthyroidism

Hyperthyroidism occurs in approximately two per 1000 pregnancies (Cheron et al., 1981; Mestman, 1980; Selenkow, 1975; Zakarija and McKenzie, 1983). Causes include Graves' disease, Plummer's disease, trophoblastic disease, and Hashimoto's thyroiditis. Symptoms include heat intolerance, tachycardia, tremulousness, palpitations, agitation, hyperreflexia, exophthalmos, lid lag, and weight loss, but many of these conditions are also seen during a normal pregnancy.

Thyroid hormones do not cross the placenta in significant amounts, but the maternal hyperthyroid state may be dangerous to the fetus and newborn. The incidence of prematurity, preeclampsia, and low birth weight is higher among hyperthyroid gravidas, and maternal weight loss can result in fetal undernutrition (Freedberg et al., 1957; Javert, 1940). Thyroid-stimulating immunoglobulins (TSI) can cross the placenta and produce fetal and/or neonatal thyrotoxicosis (McKenzie, 1964). This condition is typically transient and may last from 1 to 3 months in the neonate, until maternal TSI is finally cleared from the infant's serum. However, neonatal syndromes have been described for the transplacental passage of both blocking and stimulating antibodies (Zakarija et al., 1986).

Treatment of hyperthyroidism during pregnancy involves a choice between antithyroid drugs and subtotal thyroidectomy since maternal radioiodine treatment results in fetal thyroid ablation (Selenkow et al., 1975). Antithyroid drugs are commonly employed to control hyperthyroidism in pregnancy to avoid surgical intervention.

Medications for hyperthyroidism

PROPYLTHIOURACIL

Propylthiouracil (PTU), a thioamide, is the drug of choice in the therapy of thyrotoxicosis in pregnancy. Its antithyroid action blocks the synthesis but not the release of thyroid hormone and prevents the peripheral conversion of T4 to T3. Data suggest that pregnancy does not have a major effect on the pharmacokinetic disposition of PTU (Sitar *et al.*, 1982). PTU crosses the placenta (Marchant *et al.*, 1977). The fetus may attempt to compensate for the PTU-induced hypothyroidism, but this is infrequent (1–5 percent). The drug is not associated with an increased risk of congenital anomalies (Becks and Burrow, 1991; Davis *et al.*, 1989; Masiukiewicz and Burrow, 1999). Finally, maternal PTU administration has been used with some success to treat congenital fetal hyperthyroidism caused by increases in maternal thyroid-stimulating immunoglobulins (Check *et al.*, 1982; Serup and Petersen, 1977). Long-term follow-up of children exposed to PTU *in utero* revealed no difference in postnatal intellectual and physical development compared with nonexposed siblings (Burrow *et al.*, 1968, 1978). In summary, PTU is the drug of choice for treating hyperthyroidism in pregnancy, although it can lead to fetal goiter formation in a small number of cases (5 percent or fewer).

METHIMAZOLE AND CARBIMAZOLE

Methimazole (a thioamide) and carbimazole (a thioamide metabolized to methimazole) are not recommended for use during pregnancy, but should be considered if other medications are not efficacious. Their antithyroid action blocks the synthesis, but not the release, of thyroid hormone.

Methimazole crosses the placenta (Marchant *et al.*, 1977). Fourteen cases of aplasia cutis (scalp defect) among infants exposed to methimazole *in utero* are described in the literature (Bachrach and Burrow, 1984; Farine *et al.*, 1988; Kalb and Grossman, 1986; Milham, 1985; Milham and Elledge, 1972; Mujtaba and Burrow, 1975). The scalp, skull, and underlying cerebral cortex development is complete by the 3rd month of gestation, suggesting that first-trimester exposure to methimazole is critical for induction of the scalp defects (Kokich *et al.*, 1982). However, in the largest series of cases reported (243 infants) of methimazole use in pregnancy, no relationship was found between maternal methimazole therapy and scalp malformations (Momotani *et al.*, 1984). It is possible that the association of maternal use of methimazole and carbimazole during pregnancy with congenital skin defects in children is not as strong as originally thought (Van Dijke *et al.*, 1987). Two cases of fetal goiter development were reported in association with carbimazole use in pregnancy (Sugrue and Drury, 1980). Follow-up of children exposed to carbimazole *in utero* found no physical growth or development deficits (McCarroll *et al.*, 1976). Maternal carbimazole or methimazole therapy for hyperthyroidism is not recommended for use during pregnancy.

ETHIONAMIDE

Maternal ethionamide administration during pregnancy is known to suppress fetal thyroid hormone synthesis and to result in fetal hypothyroidism and goiter. Based on very limited information, ethionamide (thioamide) does appear to pose a high risk of congenital anomalies (Zierski, 1966).

PROPRANOLOL

Propranolol is a beta-adrenergic blocker medication that has been used in pregnancy for a variety of indications. The two most common disorders of pregnancy for which propranolol has been used are hypertension and hyperthyroidism. An extensive review of the use of propranolol in pregnancy can be found in Chapter 3.

IODIDE (POTASSIUM IODIDE)

Iodide compounds are contraindicated for use during pregnancy. Iodides cross the placenta, and the fetus is particularly sensitive to the inhibitory effects of excessive iodide (Wolff, 1969). More than 400 cases of neonatal goiter have been reported in infants of mothers treated with potassium iodide during pregnancy (Ayromlooi, 1972; Carswell *et al.*, 1970; Galina *et al.*, 1962; Mehta *et al.*, 1983; Miyagawa, 1973; Parmelee *et al.*, 1940). These goiters, due to fetal thyroid inhibition with secondary compensatory hypertrophy, can be very large and in some cases lead to tracheal compression and neonatal death.

Only in one scenario is potassium iodide not only useful, but is indicated during pregnancy – the case of 'thyroid storm.' Treatment of this entity is acute administration of 1 g of potassium iodide orally with 1 g of propylthiouracil.

RADIOIODINE (IODINE ^{131}I)

This isotope of iodine is contraindicated for use during pregnancy. One survey of 182 pregnancies inadvertently exposed to radioiodine therapy for hyperthyroidism in the first trimester revealed six infants with hypothyroidism; of these, four were mentally retarded (Stoffer and Hamburger, 1976). A number of case reports document children who developed either congenital or late-onset hypothyroidism after their mothers were treated with ^{131}I during various stages of pregnancy (Fisher *et al.*, 1963; Goh, 1981; Green *et al.*, 1971; Hamill *et al.*, 1961; Jafek *et al.*, 1974; Russel *et al.*, 1957).

Maternal hypothyroidism

Untreated hypothyroidism can impair fertility and increase the incidence of spontaneous abortion, stillbirth, and congenital anomalies (Davis *et al.*, 1988; Mestman, 1980; Montoro *et al.*, 1981; Pekonen *et al.*, 1984). Possible causes of hypothyroidism include iodine deficiency, iatrogenic (thyroidectomy or ^{131}I therapy) or thyroiditis. Symptoms include cold intolerance, irritability, difficulty with concentration, dry skin, coarse hair, and constipation. Clinical diagnosis may be difficult because many of these symptoms are commonly seen in normal pregnancy. The mechanism by which maternal hypothyroidism affects the fetus is unknown. Several reports suggest that it is not a major cause of concern (Kennedy and Montgomery, 1978; Montoro *et al.*, 1981), but others have reported a high prevalence of congenital malformations and impaired mental and somatic development among the offspring of hypothyroid women (Pharoah *et al.*, 1971; Potter, 1980).

Medications for hypothyroidism

LEVOTHYROXINE (L-THYROXINE)

L-Thyroxine (T4) is a hormone normally produced in the thyroid gland. It is used to treat thyroid deficiency and is suitable for use during pregnancy. The frequency of congenital anomalies was not increased among 537 pregnancies exposed to exogenous thyroxine or thyroid hormone during the first trimester, and 1605 pregnancies exposed at any time during pregnancy (Heinonen *et al.*, 1977a). Experimental studies agreed with the findings in humans. Thyroxine should be considered safe for use during pregnancy.

LIOTHYRONINE

Liothyronine (T3) is a hormone normally produced in the thyroid gland, which is used to treat thyroid deficiency states and is suitable for use during pregnancy. Evidence indicates no increased risk of congenital anomalies in infants whose mothers used liothyronine during pregnancy (Heinonen *et al.*, 1977a) (see Levothyroxine).

PARATHYROID GLAND

Maternal parathyroid function

Parathyroid glands, usually four in number, are located along the posterior border of the thyroid gland, and function primarily in the regulation of bone mineral metabolism. They secrete parathyroid hormone (PTH), which serves to maintain extracellular fluid calcium concentration. Pregnant women require three to four times the nonpregnant daily requirement for calcium, particularly during the latter half of gestation when most of the fetal bone mineral is deposited. Active transfer of calcium and phosphorus across the placenta results in lowering of maternal serum calcium concentration, an increase in PTH secretion, and a reduced calcitonin production (Schedewie and Fisher, 1980). Maternal 1,25 dihydroxy vitamin D levels and intestinal absorption of calcium increase markedly (Bouillon and Van Assche, 1982; Heany and Skillman, 1971; Kumar *et al.*, 1979).

Maternal hyperparathyroidism

Secretion of excess parathyroid hormone during pregnancy causes increased bone resorption and serum calcium, and other clinical manifestations similar to those in the nonpregnant state. Gravidas may seem asymptomatic; however, 80 percent present with generalized muscle weakness, nausea, vomiting, pain, renal colic, and/or polyuria. Primary hyperparathyroidism is most frequently caused by an adenoma in one of the inferior parathyroid glands. An unusually high frequency of hyperparathyroidism was reported among women with a history of irradiation to the head or neck in childhood (Gelister *et al.*, 1989; van der Spuy and Jacobs, 1984). Maternal effects include an increased incidence of renal stone formation caused by hypercalciuria, hyperphosphaturia, and thinning of bone trabeculae, secondary to increased bone resorption (Peacock., 1978; Stanbury *et al.*, 1972). Embryo and fetal effects include a high incidence of spontaneous abortion, stillbirth, neonatal death, and low birth weight (Delmonico *et al.*, 1976; Johnstone *et al.*, 1972; Kristofferson *et al.*, 1985; Ludwig, 1962; Mestman, 1980; Wagner *et al.*, 1964). The incidence of severe hypocalcemia and tetany in infants born to mothers with hyperparathyroidism approaches 50 percent (Butler *et al.*, 1973; Mestman, 1980; Pederon and Permin, 1975), and is caused by elevated maternal ionized calcium crossing the placenta (active transport) and blunting, ultimately suppressing the fetal parathyroid. Infants are usually unable to maintain normal serum calcium concentration in the perinatal period. Neonatal calcium supplementation is needed, but this effect is transient and usually resolves by 2 weeks of age without sequelae (Pederon and Permin, 1975).

Treatment of choice for primary hyperparathyroidism during the pregnant or nonpregnant state is surgery to avoid maternal, fetal, and perinatal complications.

Maternal hypoparathyroidism

Hypoparathyroidism is characterized by inadequate PTH, presenting as severe hypocalcemia. Symptoms are similar to the nonpregnant state, including weakness, fatigue, tetany (by Chvostek's and Trousseau's tests) and seizures. The etiology is usually idiopathic, autoimmune or iatrogenic (parathyroid glands removed or blood supply compromised during thyroid surgery). In contrast, pseudohypoparathyroidism is caused by deficient end-organ response to the endogenous PTH. Fetal effects of maternal hypoparathyroidism vary. Untreated maternal hypoparathyroidism is associated with neonatal hyperparathyroidism, hypercalcemia, and osteomalacia (Aceto et al., 1966; Bronsky et al., 1970; Goloboff and Ezrin, 1969; Landing and Kamoshita, 1970). Symptoms are transient and normally resolve over time (Landing and Kamoshita, 1970). Neonatal hyperparathyroidism secondary to low maternal calcium (Loughhead et al., 1990) is associated with neonatal skeletal disease and bone demineralization.

Medications for hypoparathyroidism

VITAMIN D

Vitamin D comes in a variety of commercially available forms which incur a similar metabolic fate, thus having a very similar effect on the mother and fetus. Along with calcium, vitamin D is used to treat hypoparathyroidism in both the pregnant and nonpregnant state. Pregnant patients treated for hypoparathyroidism with vitamin D apparently do not have an increased incidence of embryotoxic effects or fetal malformations (Goodenday and Gordon, 1971a,b; Sadeghi-Nejad et al., 1980; Wright et al., 1969), even high doses of 1,25 dihydroxy vitamin D were used (Marx et al., 1980).

PITUITARY GLAND

Maternal pituitary function

Adenohypophysis, or the anterior lobe of the pituitary gland, doubles or triples in size during normal pregnancy due to hypertrophy and hyperplasia of the lactotrophs (Goluboff and Ezrin, 1969). Physiologic changes that occur during pregnancy are outlined in Box 4.2.

Certain abnormalities in pituitary function are associated with infertility (e.g., hyperprolactinemia, Cushing's disease), but with proper therapy fertility may be restored. Pituitary disorders that may complicate pregnancy include: enlargement of a prolactinoma, acromegaly, Cushing's disease, and diabetes insipidus.

Prolactinoma

The pituitary gland enlarges during pregnancy and the presence of prolactinoma and its enlargement in pregnant women is a concern. A review of 16 investigations and 246 patients revealed a low incidence of symptomatic microadenoma (less than 10 mm in size) enlargement of 1.6 percent, and an incidence of symptomatic macroadenoma (more than 10 mm in size) enlargement of 15.5 percent during pregnancy (Gemzell and Wang, 1979).

Box 4.2 Pituitary gland function changes during pregnancy

- Low basal luteinizing hormone (LH) and follicle-stimulating hormone (FSH) levels, blunted gonadotropin response to gonadotrophin-releasing hormone (GnRH) infusion (Jeppsson *et al.*, 1977; Reyes *et al.*, 1976) secondary to a negative feedback inhibition from elevated levels of estrogen and progesterone.
- Low basal growth hormone (GH) levels and blunted response to insulin-induced hypoglycemia and arginine infusion (Spellacy *et al.*, 1970; Tyson *et al.*, 1969).
- Normal to low adrenocorticotropic hormone (ACTH) levels, that rise markedly during labor and delivery (Beck *et al.*, 1968; Carr *et al.*, 1981).
- Normal levels of thyroid-stimulating hormone (TSH) with a similar response to thyroid-releasing hormone (TRH) stimulation, as in the nonpregnant state (Fisher, 1983a).
- Ten- to 20-fold increase in serum prolactin levels (Rigg *et al.*, 1977; Tyson *et al.*, 1972), secondary to marked hypertrophy and hyperplasia of the lactotrophs.
- Neurophysins are intraneuronal protein carriers for oxytocin and vasopressin that are present in the neurohypophysis, and their plasma concentrations may be elevated during pregnancy (Robinson *et al.*, 1973). However, maternal plasma oxytocin and vasopressin levels are low and do not vary throughout gestation (Fisher, 1983b).

MEDICATIONS FOR PROLACTINOMAS – BROMOCRIPTINE (PARLODEL)

Bromocriptine is a dopamine agonist and ergot alkaloid known to have prolactin-lowering activity, and is commonly used to treat hyperprolactinemia associated with infertility.

Bromocriptine crosses the placenta and is associated with fetal hypoprolactinemia (del Pozo *et al.*, 1977, 1980). Effects on fetal neuroendocrine development are unknown. Outcomes of 1410 pregnancies in 1135 women who received bromocriptine in the early weeks of pregnancy was associated with a higher frequency of spontaneous abortion (11.1 percent), but a congenital anomaly rate (3.5 percent) similar to that observed in the general population (Turkalj *et al.*, 1982). Children (*n* = 212) from this study who were followed for up to 5 years were normal on mental and physical development assessments. Similar findings with fewer patients were reported by other investigators (Canales *et al.*, 1981; Hammond *et al.*, 1983; Konopka *et al.*, 1983). Evidence indicates that there is no increased risk to the fetuses of women treated with bromocriptine during pregnancy, and if symptomatic tumor enlargement should occur, bromocriptine therapy is preferred to surgical intervention (MacCagnan *et al.*, 1995).

Acromegaly

Acromegaly is caused by the overproduction of growth hormone (GH) resulting in the overgrowth and thickening of bones and soft tissues. The most common cause is a pituitary adenoma, and therapy often consists of surgery, radiation, medical therapy, or some combination. Menstrual irregularity (amenorrhea) is frequent and fecundity is low in acromegalic women. Acromegaly during pregnancy is extremely rare (van der Spuy and Jacobs, 1984). Symptomatic tumor expansion may arise during gestation as a result of increased maternal estrogen levels (Yap *et al.*, 1990). Optimal management is conservative and definitive therapy is preferably postponed until after delivery. The human placenta secretes its specific GH variant in increasing amounts up to delivery (Frankenne *et al.*, 1987). A recent study of GH secretory patterns in two pregnant acromegalic women suggests that the increased insulin-like growth factor (IGF-I) level present in late pregnancy is not pituitary-GH-dependent (Beckers *et al.*, 1990). In addition, there is no evidence that excessive maternal GH crosses the placenta to any significant degree. Bromocriptine is used to treat acromegaly.

Cushing's syndrome and Cushing's disease

Cushing's syndrome is characterized by increased cortisol secretion, whether the etiology is from overproduction of corticotropin-releasing factor (CRF), excessive pituitary adreno-corticotrophic hormone (ACTH) stimulating the adrenals (Cushing's disease), adrenal hyperplasia/adenoma, ectopic sources of ACTH or cortisol, or excessive glucocorticoid therapy. Hence, Cushing's disease refers simply to pituitary-dependent Cushing's syndrome. The etiology of Cushing's syndrome is usually a pituitary adenoma or hyperplasia, and during pregnancy the frequency of primary adrenal lesions is much higher (Gormley *et al.*, 1982). Pregnancy is very uncommon among women with Cushing's syndrome because most such patients are amenorrheic (Gormley *et al.*, 1982; Grimes *et al.*, 1973). The diagnosis may be difficult because many of the symptoms (hypertension, weight gain, fatigue, striae, and increased pigmentation) are common in normal pregnancies. Thinning of the skin, spontaneous bruising and muscle weakness are symptoms more specific of Cushing's syndrome. Hirsutism and acne are common in pregnant women with Cushing's syndrome because of increased adrenal androgens (Grimes *et al.*, 1973). Pregnancy outcome is extremely poor, with approximately 50 percent of gestations ending in spontaneous abortion, premature delivery or stillbirth (Aaron *et al.*, 1990; Gormley *et al.*, 1982; Grimes *et al.*, 1973). Treatment depends on the etiology of the disorder and the stage of pregnancy at diagnosis. Pituitary and adrenal adenomas should be removed surgically (van der Spuy and Jacobs, 1984). In the first trimester, pregnancy termination may be considered, especially if adrenal carcinoma is suspected. In late gestation, medical therapy with metyrapone may be considered until delivery of the infant, after which definitive surgery may be undertaken.

METYRAPONE FOR CUSHING'S DISEASE

Metyrapone is a 11-hydroxylase inhibitor that causes a decrease in cortisol production if given to normal subjects. This is followed by a subsequent rise of desoxycortisol, the immediate precursor of cortisol. Animal studies have shown that metyrapone does cross the placenta (Baram and Schultz, 1990). Metyrapone has been used infrequently during late pregnancy as medical therapy for Cushing's disease to delay surgical intervention until after delivery (Connell *et al.*, 1985b; Gormley *et al.*, 1982). In summary, the ideal therapy for Cushing's disease in pregnancy is surgical intervention. However, surgery should be postponed until fetal maturity.

Diabetes insipidus

Diabetes insipidus (DI) in pregnancy occurs in approximately three per 100 000 pregnancies (Hime and Richardson, 1978). Hypothalamic or neurogenic diabetes insipidus is a disorder caused by deficient arginine vasopressin (AVP) release from the posterior pituitary in response to normal physiologic stimuli. This results in low blood levels of AVP and impaired renal conservation of water. Clinical characteristics are polyuria, excessive thirst, polydipsia, and low urinary specific gravity. The etiology is idiopathic, inherited as autosomal dominant, or secondary to trauma or tumor. Patients with diabetes insipidus who are successfully treated do not have impaired fertility, and fetal outcome is not adversely affected by the disease (Hime and Richardson, 1978; Jouppila and Vuopala, 1971). Therapy consists of hormonal replacement, and the drug of choice in pregnancy is DDAVP (1-deamino-8-arginine vasopressin) administered as a nasal spray. Other modes of therapy in the patient with partial diabetes insipidus are not recommended for use during pregnancy (chlorpropamide, clofibrate, and carbamazepine). Note that DDAVP is not effective for the treatment of nephrogenic diabetes insipidus.

ADRENAL GLAND

Maternal adrenal function

A number of changes occur in maternal adrenal function during pregnancy. The rise in estrogen during gestation causes an increase in the liver production of cortisol-binding globulin (CBG), and thus a rise in plasma cortisol levels. Plasma ACTH concentrations are low (Carr et al., 1981). There is a two- to three-fold increase in plasma-unbound cortisol coupled with a two-fold increase in free cortisol excretion (Clerico et al., 1980; Nolten et al., 1980). In spite of the elevation of free cortisol in pregnancy, clinical evidence of cortisol hypersecretion is not seen (Gibson and Tulchinsky, 1980). Increased renin activity is associated with elevated aldosterone levels, although this does not appear to be clinically significant (Smeaton et al., 1977). Certain adrenal disorders that may complicate pregnancy include Addison's disease, Cushing's syndrome, and congenital adrenal hyperplasia. Cushing's syndrome was discussed in the previous section on the pituitary gland.

Maternal adrenal insufficiency (Addison's disease)

Adrenal corticosteroid insufficiency may be caused by insufficient ACTH secretion by the pituitary, insufficient adrenal secretion of corticosteroids, or inadequate steroid replacement. Atrophy of the adrenals secondary to autoimmune disease accounts for 75 percent of the cases. The diagnosis of Addison's disease in pregnancy can be difficult because the signs and symptoms (weakness, fatigue, anorexia, nervousness, increased skin pigmentation) are very similar to those occurring in a normal pregnancy. This disorder may take a chronic, indolent course or progress into a true medical emergency characterized by an 'Addisonian crisis' – severe nausea and vomiting, diarrhea, abdominal pain, and hypotension. Pregnancy may exacerbate the course of Addison's disease; however, the spontaneous abortion rate, prematurity rate, and neonatal outcome are apparently not affected by the disease (Brent, 1950; Satterfield and Williamson, 1976).

Chronic adrenal insufficiency requires adequate adrenal replacement in the form of cortisone acetate or prednisone and 9-alpha-fluoro-hydrocortisone. During labor, delivery, and the first few days postpartum, the mother should be monitored closely, ensuring a good state of hydration with normal saline and adequate cortisol hemisuccinate replacement. It is common for women with adrenal insufficiency to be diagnosed for the first time during the puerperium when they develop adrenal crisis (Brent, 1950). Treatment involves replacement steroids during an Addisonian crisis including cortisol hemisuccinate (Solu-Cortef), with fluid replacement as isotonic saline, and glucose administration.

Medications for Addison's disease

CORTISONE ACETATE

Cortisone is a glucocorticoid normally excreted by the adrenal gland. It is used for replacement therapy and to treat allergic and inflammatory diseases. The Collaborative Perinatal Project included 34 pregnancies exposed during the first trimester to cortisone, and the frequency of congenital anomalies among the exposed pregnancies was no greater than expected (Heinonen et al., 1977a).

Prednisone and prednisolone

Prednisone and prednisolone are synthetic glucocorticoids. Prednisone is biologically inert but is metabolized in the liver to prednisolone, a biologically active compound. Prednisone and prednisolone are used for replacement therapy and to treat a variety of allergic and inflammatory conditions. Among infants born to 43 and 204 women who had been treated with prednisone/prednisolone during the first trimester of pregnancy, the frequency of malformation was not increased (Heinonen et al., 1977b; Kallen, 1998). Perinatal death does not appear to be excessively frequent in most series of infants born to women treated with prednisone or prednisolone, but the incidence of fetal growth retardation may be increased (Reinisch et al., 1978). No such effect was apparent in two smaller studies, one of which also involved women treated throughout pregnancy (Lee et al., 1982; Walsh and Clark, 1967). Newborn infants of women who take prednisone throughout pregnancy usually have normal adrenocortical reserves and no symptoms of adrenal suppression (Arad and Landau, 1984). Dose-related fetal growth retardation, cleft palate, genital anomalies, and behavioral alterations occur in the offspring of mice treated in pregnancy with prednisone or prednisolone in doses within or above the human therapeutic range (Ballard et al., 1977; Gandelman and Rosenthal, 1981; Pinsky and DiGeorge, 1965; Reinisch et al., 1978). Increased frequencies of cleft palate are also observed among the offspring of pregnant hamsters treated during pregnancy with prednisolone in doses 80–240 times that used in humans (Shah and Kilistoff, 1976).

Corticosteroids in general

In one study of 631 whose mothers used therapeutic corticosteroids during the first trimester, the risk of non-syndromic cleft palate was increased more than sixfold (Rodriguez-Pinilla and Martinez-Frias, 1998). However, given the prevalence of the use of these drugs and of cleft palate, the absolute risk is probably less than 1 percent in pregnancies exposed to corticosteroids in the first trimester (Shepard et al., 2002), if the association is causal.

FLUDROCORTISONE

No epidemiologic studies have been reported regarding malformations in women treated with this drug during pregnancy.

CORTISOL HEMISUCCINATE

No epidemiologic studies have been reported regarding malformations in women treated with this drug during pregnancy.

CONGENITAL ADRENAL HYPERPLASIA

Five principal enzymatic steps are required for the conversion of cholesterol to cortisol in the adrenal gland. An inherited defect in any one of these enzymes may result in congenital adrenal hyperplasia (CAH). In over 90 percent of cases, the deficient enzyme is 21-hydroxylase (New *et al.*, 1983). This enzyme is necessary for the conversion of 17-hydroxyprogesterone to 11-desoxycortisol, and a deficiency results in a decrease in cortisol, and a compensatory rise in ACTH, followed by adrenal hyperplasia with elevated cortisol precursors and adrenal androgens. Classical CAH is the most severe form; it is characterized by a salt-wasting crisis soon after birth owing to impaired aldosterone production. Genital virilization is common in female infants, and both sexes manifest electrolyte imbalance and hypotension that can be life-threatening if not promptly treated by steroid hormone replacement. Simple virilizing CAH is a less severe form characterized by female virilization, but without the salt-wasting component. Adult-onset CAH may not manifest until adolescence, with (in females) oligomenorrhea, progressive hirsutism, and relatively short stature. Chorionic villus sampling, using DNA probes for HCA genes, when compared to parental chromosomes, will allow an earlier diagnosis. Currently, all known heterozygotes are treated with high-dose glucocorticoids until chorionic villus sampling occurs. If a male fetus is present, treatment stops. If a female fetus is present, treatment is continued because virilization of affected females can be prevented. Once DNA/HLA results are known, medication is discontinued only if the female fetus is unaffected.

Medications used to treat congenital adrenal hyperplasia include prednisone, fludrocortisone (see the section on Medications for Addison's disease), and dexamethasone.

CONTRACEPTION

Oral contraceptives

A wide variety of oral contraceptive formulations are available, including estrogen/progestin combinations and progestational agents that suppress ovulation and implantation. If exposure to oral contraceptives during embryogenesis increases the risk of birth defects, the increase is small compared to the risk of malformations in the general population (3.5–5 percent). Congenital anomalies were not increased in frequency among more than 500 infants born to women who took oral contraceptives during the first trimester (Harlap and Eldor, 1980; Heinonen *et al.*, 1977b; Nora *et al.*, 1978; Vessey *et al.*, 1979). A slight increase of congenital anomalies was associated with use of oral contraceptives in the first trimester in several studies, but it is generally accepted that the risk is not real, or extremely small.

Norplant

The Norplant system is a unique subdermal contraceptive system providing 5 years of continuous birth control.

No epidemiologic studies have been published regarding malformations in the off-spring of women who became pregnant with a Norplant system in place. Levonorgestrel is the progestin component in many oral contraceptive preparations.

Intrauterine device

Pregnancy with an intrauterine device (IUD) in place is associated with increased inci-dence of spontaneous abortion, approximately threefold greater than among women without an IUD (Lewit, 1970; Tatum et al., 1976; Vessey et al., 1974). When the device is removed or expelled spontaneously, spontaneous abortion is reduced to approximately 20–30 percent, which is much closer to the rates of miscarriage in the general population (Alvior, 1973; Tatum et al., 1976). Several studies of women who had copper-containing IUDs in place during pregnancy have found no increase in the rate of abnormalities over the expected rate in the general population (Guillebaud, 1981; Poland, 1970; Tatum et al., 1976). The frequency of congenital anomalies in the offspring of women who had progesterone-containing IUDs in place during pregnancy has not been published.

NEW INTRAUTERINE DEVICES

New IUD devices available ease insertion and removal, and reduce pain, bleeding, and expulsion rates. They include the intrauterine system (IUS) that gradually releases levono-gestrel (Mirena), or progesterone (Progesterasert). Rather than T-shaped copper IUDs of the 1980s and 1990s, the frameless IUD devices (e.g. GyneFix) are copper cylinders secured together with a string.

Spermicidal agents (nonoxynols)

Spermicidal intravaginal sponges, foams, creams, and suppositories contain nonoxynols, surfactants that are extremely toxic to sperm. The risk of congenital anomalies was not increased in frequency among more than 1200 infants whose mothers used nonoxynol spermicides during embryogenesis (Heinonen et al., 1977a; Mills et al., 1982). Similar results were found in large studies of the frequency of congenital anomalies among infants whose mothers used a multiagent spermicide that contained nonoxynol (Huggins et al., 1982; Polednak et al., 1982; Strobino et al., 1988). The frequency of heterogenous anomalies (chromosomal abnormalities, hypospadias, limb reduction defects, neoplasms) was statistically increased in more than 700 infants born to women who had used any vaginal spermicide within 10 months of conception (Jick et al., 1981). However, method-ological flaws in that study (Cordero and Layde, 1983), combined with simple data errors in classification of spermicidal exposures in the cases, cast doubt on the meaning of this study. It is now widely accepted that neither nonoxynols nor other spermicides are associated with an increased risk for chromosomal abnormalities and congenital anom-alies (Bracken, 1985). A case–control study of the use of topical contraceptives among mothers of infants with chromosomal abnormalities or limb reduction defects found no difference in the frequency of spermicide use around the time of conception between the case and the normal control groups (Cordero and Layde, 1983).

However, it was spermicides that spawned the term 'litogen.' Despite overwhelming scientific data that indicate spermicides are harmless, more than $3 million were awarded to parents of an infant born with multiple congenital anomalies whose mother had used nonoxynol during pregnancy.

Depo-Provera

This agent is discussed under Progestational agents (p. 93).

INFERTILITY

Ovulation induction agents

CLOMIPHENE CITRATE (CLOMID)

This drug has nonsteroidal estrogenic and antiestrogenic activity, and is given orally to stimulate ovulation. It is sometimes inadvertently given in an unrecognized early pregnancy. Women using clomiphene should be cautioned that pregnancy is to be excluded before each new course of the drug.

Malformations were not increased in frequency among 1500 infants of women who had clomiphene preconceptionally (Barrat and Leger, 1979; Harlap, 1976; Kurachi *et al.*, 1983). Multiple case–control studies of neural tube defects failed to find a significant association with artificial induction of ovulation and risk of a congenital anomaly (Cornel *et al.*, 1989; Cuckle and Wald, 1989; Czeizel, 1989). In a well-designed, case–control study, the frequency of clomiphene usage was not increased among more than 500 women who delivered children with a neural tube defect compared with a similar number of normal controls (Mills *et al.*, 1990). In summary, clomiphene is not associated with an increased risk of congenital anomalies.

HUMAN MENOPAUSAL GONADOTROPINS (PERGONAL, METRODIN)

Pergonal is an extract of urine from postmenopausal women; it contains follicle-stimulating hormone (FSH) and luteinizing hormone (LH). It is administered by intramuscular injection and is used to stimulate multiple ovarian follicular development in ovulation induction cycles. Metrodin is a purified extract of urine from postmenopausal women and primarily contains FSH. It is similar to Pergonal in its administration protocols. No epidemiologic studies have been reported regarding malformations in the offspring of women exposed to Pergonal or Metrodin before or during pregnancy. However, the risk does not appear to be high, although a very small risk cannot be excluded.

GONADOTROPIN-RELEASING HORMONE AGONISTS

Gonadotropin-releasing hormone (GnRH) agonists are widely used in clinical gynecologic practice for the treatment of endometriosis and uterine leiomyomas. Leuprolide acetate (Lupron) is an agent that is frequently used for these conditions. Although no epidemiological studies are published of infants born following Lupon therapy, it is unlikely that the risk of congenital anomalies is high following exposure to this drug during pregnancy (Friedman and Polifka, 2006). Chronic administration of the agonists downregulates the pituitary gonadotropin receptors, thereby suppressing release of LH and FSH and leading to a hypoestrogenic state. The likelihood of pregnancy occurring while a woman is given GnRH agonists is extremely low. However, GnRH agonists may also be used prior to HMG therapy in infertile women undergoing *in vitro* fertilization cycles. Typically, administration is begun in the luteal phase of the cycle, when a patient may be in the early stage of a pregnancy. No epidemiologic studies are published on the risk malformations in the offspring of women treated with this drug during pregnancy.

GENERAL HORMONAL THERAPY

Estrogens

ETHINYL ESTRADIOL

Ethinyl estradiol is a synthetic estrogen used to treat menopausal symptoms and menstrual disorders. This drug and progestin are common combinations in oral contraception. Congenital anomalies were not increased in frequency among infants born to women given ethinyl estradiol during embryogenesis or at any time during pregnancy (Heinonen *et al.*, 1977a). Results from two other studies of ethinyl estradiol use during pregnancy showed that it was not associated with an increased risk of congenital anomalies (Kullander and Kallen, 1976; Spira *et al.*, 1972). Congenital anomalies were not increased in frequency in teratology studies of three species of nonhuman primates given large doses of ethinyl estradiol during pregnancy (Hendrickx *et al.*, 1987). An increased frequency of intrauterine deaths was observed at doses that were also maternally lethal in one monkey species studied. Miscarriages occurred more frequently among monkeys given approximately 100 times the amount of ethinyl estradiol included in oral contraceptive dose regimens (Prahalada and Hendrickx, 1983). In rodent teratology studies, no increase in the frequency of congenital anomalies after embryonic treatment was found, but early intrauterine deaths were increased in frequency at the highest doses (Chemnitius *et al.*, 1979; Yasuda *et al.*, 1981).

CONJUGATED ESTROGENS

Conjugated estrogens are a mixture of estrogens obtained from natural sources, and are used to treat menopausal symptoms, osteoporosis, and hypothalamic amenorrhea. They are not indicated for use during pregnancy. Among 614 infants born to women who used estrogenic compounds during gestation, an increase in certain congenital anomalies was found – cardiovascular, eye and ear defects, and Down's syndrome (Heinonen *et al.*, 1977b). However, this association was reevaluated in another report, and the link between estrogens and cardiac malformations was not borne out (Wiseman and Dodds-Smith, 1984).

DIETHYLSTILBESTROL

This nonsteroidal synthetic estrogen, approved by the Food and Drug Administration in 1942 for use in pregnancy to prevent miscarriages, is strongly associated with an increased frequency of clear-cell adenocarcinoma of the vagina and cervix among daughters of women treated with diethylstilbestrol (DES) early in pregnancy. Between 500 000 and two million pregnant women took this drug. In a registry including more than 400 cases of clear-cell adenocarcinoma of the vagina and cervix diagnosed in the USA since 1971, no less than 65 percent of patients' mothers took DES in early pregnancy (Herbst, 1981). Of the women who took DES early in pregnancy, 80 percent had taken it during the 12 weeks prior to conception. The malignancy was diagnosed among females 7–30 years old, with a median age of 19 years. Estimates suggest that 0.14–1.4 per 1000 daughters of women treated with diethylstilbestrol during pregnancy will develop clear-cell adenocarcinoma of the vagina or cervix by the age of 24.

Nonmalignant abnormalities, especially adenosis, are common among the daughters of pregnant women who were treated with diethylstilbestrol. Gross structural abnormalities of the cervix or vagina are identified in about one quarter and abnormalities of the vaginal epithelium in one-third to one-half of women whose mothers took diethylstilbestrol during gestation (Bibbo, 1979; Herbst et al., 1978; Robboy et al., 1984; Stillman, 1982). T-shaped uterus, constricting bands of the uterine cavity, uterine hypoplasia or paraovarian cysts also occur with increased frequency among females exposed in utero (Kaufman et al., 1984). Among males exposed to DES in utero, epididymal cysts, hypoplastic testes, and cryptorchidism are reported with increased frequency (Stillman, 1982). Preterm delivery, spontaneous abortions, and ectopic pregnancy occurred with increased frequency in females whose mothers took diethylstilbestrol during gestation (Barnes et al., 1980; Herbst, 1981).

Progestational agents

PROGESTINS: ANALOGS OF PROGESTERONE

Progestins are a group of chemically related hormones with similar actions. Progesterone is the only natural progestin and is not well absorbed by the oral route unless given in micronized form. Synthetic progestins structurally related to progesterone are more commonly used. Low-dose progestins are used for contraception with an estrogen, and are used in the therapy of menstrual disorders at higher doses. In the 1960s and 1970s much higher doses of progesterones were used for oral contraception (Schardein, 1985), and are currently used to treat threatened abortion. In a review, female pseudohermaphroditism, including various degrees of clitoral hypertrophy with or without labioscrotal fusion, was reported in several-hundred children born to women treated with progesterone analogs in high doses during early pregnancy (Schardein, 1980, 1985). The frequency of occurrence of this anomaly varies with different progestins. Fewer than 100 cases of male pseudohermaphroditism have been reported, and the anomaly is usually isolated hypospadias (Aarskog, 1979; Mau, 1981; Schardein, 1985). Exposure to progestational agents during embryogenesis, therefore, seems not to increase substantially the risk for nongenital congenital anomalies in infants born to treated women.

NORETHINDRONE

Norethindrone is a synthetic progestational agent derived from 19-nortesterone, which is used as an oral contraceptive and to treat menstrual disorders. Among more than 100 infants born to women who took norethindrone during the first trimester, congenital anomalies were not increased in frequency, or in more than 100 infants whose mothers took this drug after the first trimester (Heinonen *et al.*, 1977a). Two case–control studies of 365 infants with congenital anomalies yielded similar results (Kullander and Kallen, 1976; Spira *et al.*, 1972). Several cases were reported in which use of norethindrone during pregnancy, at doses that were much greater than those used in contemporary practice, was associated with masculinization of the external female genitalia (clitoral hypertrophy with or without labioscrotal fusion), but internal genitalia and subsequent pubertal development were normal (Schardein, 1980, 1985). The genital anomalies observed include various degrees of masculinization (Wilkins *et al.*, 1958). Clitoral hypertrophy may occur in exposures any time after the 8th embryonic week, but labioscrotal fusion is limited to exposure during the 8th to 13th embryonic weeks. The risk for pseudohermaphroditism among female infants born to women who took norethindrone during pregnancy is probably less than 1 percent (Bongiovanni and McPadden, 1960; Ishizuka *et al.*, 1962). No increased risk of fetal sexual malformation was reported in a meta-analysis of published reports of women exposed to sex hormones after conception (Ramin-Wilms *et al.*, 1995). Masculinized external female genitalia were observed in several species of experimental animals, including nonhuman primates, following maternal treatment with high doses of norethindrone during pregnancy (Hendrickx *et al.*, 1983; Schardein, 1985). Nongenital malformations were not increased in frequency among three species of nonhuman primates given up to 100 times the oral contraceptive dose of norethindrone during pregnancy in combination with ethinyl estradiol (Hendrickx *et al.*, 1987; Prahalada and Hendrickx, 1983). Contemporary low-dose therapy with norethindrone is not a risk factor for genital malformations, and probably poses no increased risk for congenital anomalies in general.

NORETHYNODREL

Norethynodrel is a synthetic progestational agent that is a component of oral contraceptive preparations and is used to treat menstrual disorders. Congenital anomalies were not increased in frequency among more than 150 infants born to women who took norethynodrel during the first trimester, or among more than 150 women who took the drug after the first trimester (Heinonen *et al.*, 1977a). Virilization of female fetuses has not been reported in the human; however, female rat fetuses born to mothers that received several-hundred times the human contraceptive dose had masculinized external genitalia (Kawashima *et al.*, 1977). Treatment of human pregnancy within the low-dose range presently employed for contraception and for menstrual irregularity will not cause female virilization.

NORGESTREL

This synthetic progestational agent is used with estrogen compounds in oral contraceptives and for menstrual disorders. There are no controlled studies of congenital anomalies among infants born to women who used norgestrel during pregnancy. Although no human reports have associated the use of norgestrel during pregnancy with masculinization of external female genitalia, large doses administered in the latter two-thirds of pregnancy would be expected to produce virilization based upon clinical experience with other closely related compounds. The frequency of congenital anomalies was not increased among mouse and rabbit litters born to females treated with very large doses of norgestrel during pregnancy (Heinecke and Kohler, 1983; Klaus, 1983).

MEDROXYPROGESTERONE ACETATE

Medroxyprogesterone is the most widely used oral and parenteral progestational agent. It is used to treat menstrual disorders and as an injectable contraceptive. Major congenital anomalies were not increased in frequency among almost 500 infants born to women treated with medroxyprogesterone during the first trimester, or among 217 infants whose mothers took the drug after the first trimester of pregnancy (Heinonen *et al.*, 1977a; Yovich *et al.*, 1988).

Claimed associations between maternal use of high-dose progestins early in pregnancy and masculinization of the genitalia in female children, feminization of the genitalia in male children, a variety of malformations of other organ systems and certain behavioral alterations (Hines, 1982; Schardein, 1980, 1985; Wilson and Brent, 1981) are apparently not true. A large study that included 1274 cases where medroxyprogesterone was taken for first-trimester bleeding failed to reveal an increased rate of malformations when compared to 1146 control infants (Katz *et al.*, 1985).

Although ambiguous external genitalia occurred among both sons and daughters of women who were treated with high doses of medroxyprogesterone to prevent miscarriage during pregnancy, these abnormalities were isolated and very rare (Schardein, 1985; Yovich *et al.*, 1988). Growth, sexual maturation, and sexually dimorphic behavior were unaltered among 74 teenage boys and 98 teenage girls whose mothers had taken medroxyprogesterone during pregnancy (Jaffe *et al.*, 1989, 1990). Animal teratology studies in rats, rabbits, and monkeys demonstrated that nongenital anomalies were not increased in frequency, and genital ambiguity occurred only at very high doses of medroxyprogesterone during pregnancy (Andrew and Staples, 1977; Eibs *et al.*, 1982; Foote *et al.*, 1968; Kawashima *et al.*, 1977; Lerner *et al.*, 1962; Prahalada *et al.*, 1985a,b; Tarara, 1984).

MEGESTROL ACETATE

Megestrol is a synthetic oral progestational agent. The risk for virilization of female fetuses appears minimal with maternal use of large doses of this agent during pregnancy. No studies of congenital anomalies among infants whose mothers were treated with megestrol during pregnancy have been published. External genitalia of female rats born to mothers treated with very large doses of megestrol during pregnancy were virilized (Kawashima *et al.*, 1977).

Androgens

Androgen use during pregnancy is strictly contraindicated, primarily due to the risk of masculinization of a female fetus.

DANAZOL

Danazol is a synthetic steroid absorbed by the gastrointestinal tract, metabolized by the liver, and has a half-life of 4.5 h. The drug has moderate androgenic activity, and is used to treat endometriosis. Inadvertent use during early pregnancy results in virilization of female infants (Duck and Katayama, 1981; Kingsbury, 1985; Peress *et al.*, 1982; Quagliarello and Greco, 1985; Rosa, 1984; Shaw and Farquhar, 1984). A review of fetal exposure to danazol in 129 cases compiled from case reports revealed miscarriages in 12 cases and 23 elective abortions. There were 57 female fetuses whose mothers took dana-zol during the period of sensitivity to androgenic substances (8th week of embryogene-sis and thereafter), and 23 (40 percent) presented with virilization (clitoromegaly, par-tial fusion of labia majora) (Brunskill, 1992). The lowest daily dose that resulted in vir-ilization was 200 mg (Brunskill, 1992). Androgen influences on development of internal genitalia were present in only two cases (Quagliarello and Greco, 1985; Rosa, 1984). Therefore, the available data strongly indicate that virilization of the female fetus is a risk when there is exposure to danazol during the period of androgen receptor sensitiv-ity (beginning at the 8th week of embryogenesis and continuing through the fetal period). Virilization was not found among any infants exposed before the 8th week of embryogenesis (Rosa, 1984).

Danazol is usually prescribed for only a 3–6-month course. A patient who becomes pregnant while taking the medication may not be diagnosed until a considerable fetal exposure has occurred because the drug is expected to cause amenorrhea. Therefore, physicians should be aware of the risk of female genital ambiguity occurring in the off-spring of women who are prescribed this drug.

METHYLTESTOSTERONE

Methyltestosterone is a synthetic derivative of testosterone, the primary endogenous androgen. More than a dozen female infants were born to women treated with methyltestosterone during pregnancy, and they all had varying degrees of virilization of the external genitalia (clitoral enlargement and labioscrotal fusion) (Grumbach and Ducharme, 1960; Schardein, 1985). Paralleling other androgenic agents, clitoral enlargement may be induced by exposure to methyltestosterone throughout the postem-bryonic period, but labioscrotal fusion seems restricted to the period between the 8th and 13th weeks of gestation, and the degree of virilization appears dose related. Successful surgical correction of the defects associated with virilization is available. Sexual maturation seems normal, while menarche in virilized girls seems close to the median, following a healthy course.

Female rats, dogs, and rabbits born to mothers treated with methyltestosterone in doses similar to those used medically had a dose-dependent increased frequency of vir-ilization (Jost, 1947; Kawashima *et al*, 1975; Neumann and Junkmann, 1963; Shane *et al.*, 1969) similar to humans.

Methyltestosterone and testosterone proprionate were associated with clitoromegaly with or without fusion of the labia minora. Hoffman and colleagues (1955) reported a masculinized fetus following administration to the mother of testosterone enanthate from the 4th to the 9th months. Grumbach and Ducharme (1960) summarized the human reports and concluded that masculinization of the female fetus was a significant risk with the use of these drugs.

NANDROLONE

Nandrolone is an androgenic and anabolic steroid administered parenterally to treat metastatic breast cancer. Illicitly, it is used to increase muscle mass and enhance athletic

Table 4.2 Summary of endocrine drugs: TERIS and FDA risk estimates

Drug	Risk	Risk rating
Acetohexamide	Undetermined	C
Bromocriptine	Unlikely	C$_m$
Carbimazole	Unlikely	D
Clorpropamide	Undetermined	C$_m$
Conjugated estrogens	None	NA
Cortisone	Unlikely	C*
Danazol	Undetermined	X$_m$
Desmopressin	Unlikely	B$_m$
Dexamethasone	Minimal	C*
Diethylstillbestrol	Unknown	X$_m$
Ethinyl estradiol	Unlikely	X$_m$
Ethionamide	Undetermined	C$_m$
Fludrocortisone	None	NA
Glyburide	Unlikely	C$_m$
Hydrocortisone	Unlikely	C*
Insulin	Unlikely	B
Iodine	Unlikely	D
Levothyroxine	None	A$_m$
Liothyronine	Unlikely	C$_m$
Medroxyprogesterone	Unlikely	X$_m$
Megestrol	Undetermined	NA
Methimazole	Goiter: minimal to small	D
	Cuts aplasia of scalp: minimal to small	
	Embryopathy: minimal to small	
Methyltestosterone	Undetermined	NA
Metyrapone	Undetermined	NA
Nandrolone	Undetermined	NA
Norethindrone	None	X$_m$
Norethynodrel	None	X$_m$
Norgestrel	None	X$_m$
Oxymethalone	Undetermined	NA
Potassium iodide	Undetermined	D
Prednisone	Oral clefts: small	C*
	Other congenital anomalies: unlikely	
Propranolol	Undetermined	C$_m$*
Propylthiouracil	Malformations: none	D
	Goiter: small to moderate	
Stanozolol	Undetermined	NA
Tolazamide	Undetermined	C$_m$
Tolbutamide	Unlikely	C$_m$
Vitamin D	None	A*

NA, not available.

Compiled from: Friedman *et al.*, *Obstet Gynecol* 1990; **75**: 594; Briggs *et al.*, 2005; Friedman and Polifka, 2006.

performance. No studies have been published that have analyzed congenital anomalies among infants born to women treated with nandrolone during pregnancy. However, the strong androgenic action of this agent would be expected to cause virilization of the external genitalia in female fetuses. Intrauterine deaths were increased in frequency among rats born to mothers who were given up to twice the medically administered dose (Naqvi and Warren, 1971).

STANOZOLOL

No animal or human studies of the use of stanozolol, an anabolic steroid, during pregnancy have been published. As with other androgenic steroids, it is reasonable to expect virilization of the external genitalia of a female fetus with maternal use of stanozolol.

OXYMETHALONE

Another anabolic androgen is oxymethalone, which is used to treat anemia. Oxymethalone possesses significant androgenic action, and would be expected to cause virilization of the external genitalia of female fetuses.

No human studies are published of oxymethalone exposure during pregnancy. Embryonic loss occurred frequently after injection of about four times the usual human dose of oxymethalone in rats in early pregnancy (Naqvi and Warren, 1971). Significant virilization was found in female rats born to mothers given large doses of oxymethalone during pregnancy (Naqvi and Warren, 1971), and embryonic death was increased in frequency in pregnant rats given several times the medically administered dose (Kawashima *et al.*, 1977).

TIBOLONE

Tibolone is an antiandrogenic compound used primarily to treat menopausal symptoms and osteoporosis. It is contraindicated for use during pregnancy. No studies are published of its use during pregnancy.

SPECIAL CONSIDERATIONS

Morning after pill

The morning after pill, formerly RU-486, contains mifepristone. Other formulations may sometimes contain levonorgestrel. These drugs act by preventing implantation, rather than by preventing conception. The effects of either of these drugs on a post-implantation pregnancy are unknown. Friedman and Polifka (2006) state that the risk of congenital anomalies is unknown following a failed attempt at abortion but 'this risk may be substantial because the process of attempted abortion may disrupt normal embryogenesis or fetal development'.

Breast cancer

Aromatase inhibitors may be used to replace tamoxifen, because of fewer untoward effects, in the treatment of breast cancer. These agents include anastrozole (Arimidex), exemestane (Aromasin), and letrozole (Femara). These drugs are contraindicated for use during pregnancy.

Hyperprolactinemia

Excess pituitary prolactin secretion can lead to symptoms of galactorrhea, menstrual irregularities, and infertility. Menstrual cycle abnormalities caused by hyperprolactinemia include primary and secondary amenorrhea, oligomenorrhea, and luteal phase defects. Hyperprolactinemia may result from a variety of different causes (pituitary adenoma, hypothyroidism, various pharmacologic agents). Etiology should be established prior to beginning therapy. Primary therapy for idiopathic hyperprolactinemia, or a small pituitary adenoma, is an ergot alkaloid compound, such as bromocriptine. Many physicians prefer to use carbergone (Dostinex) to treat hyperprolactinoma instead of bromocriptine to avoid side effects. Dopamine agonist activity suppresses prolactin release from the pituitary. Surgical therapy is reserved for very large pituitary tumors or those unresponsive to medical treatment (see earlier sections on Prolactinoma and Bromocriptine).

Endometriosis

Endometriosis is the presence of endometrial implants (glands and stroma) outside the endometrial cavity. Most frequently implanted sites are the pelvic viscera and peritoneum. Various therapeutic regimens have been used to treat all stages of disease, including surgical ablation and extirpation, drug therapy, or both. Medical therapy for endometriosis includes hormonal regimens of oral contraceptives, danocrine, or gonadotropin-releasing hormone (GnRH) agonists. Pregnancy usually resolves endometriosis; therefore, treatment during pregnancy is probably not an issue.

SUMMARY

Hormonal agents should usually not be administered during pregnancy. Inadvertent oral contraceptive use during embryogenesis is not associated with an increased risk of congenital anomalies. Diethylstilbestrol, high doses of progestins derived from testosterone, and all androgens are strictly contraindicated during pregnancy A summary of endocrinedrugs and their risk estimates appears in Table 4.2.

Key references

Briggs GG, Freeman RK, Yaffe SJ. Drugs in pregnancy and lactation. *A Reference Guide to Fetal and Neonatal Risk*, 6th edn. Philadelphia: Lippincott Williams & Wilkins, 2005: 628.

Elliott CL, Read GF, Wallace EM. The pharmacokinetics of oral and intramuscular administration of dexamethasone in late pregnancy. *Acta Obstet Gynecol Scand* 1996; **75**: 213.

Kallen B. Drug treatment of rheumatic diseases during pregnancy. The teratogenicity of antirheumatic drugs – what is the evidence? *Scand J Rheumatol* 1998; **27** (Suppl. 107): 119.

Little BB. Pharmacokinetics during pregnancy. Evidence-based maternal dose formulation. *Obstet Gynecol* 1999; **93**: 858.

MacCagnan P, Macedo CL, Kayath MJ, Nogueira RG, Abucham J. Conservative management of pituitary apoplexy. A prospective study. *J Clin Endocrinol Metab* 1995; **80**: 2190.

Masiukiewicz US, Burrow GN. Hyperthyroidism in pregnancy. Diagnosis and treatment. *Thyroid* 1999; **9**: 647.

Ramin-Wilms L, Tseng AL, Wighardt S, Einarson TR, Koren G. Fetal genital effects of first trimester sex hormone exposure. A meta-analysis. *Obstet Gynecol* 1995; **85**: 141.

Rodriguez-Pinilla E, Martinez-Frias ML. Corticosteroids during pregnancy and oral clefts. A case–control study. *Teratology* 1998; **58**: 2.

Shepard TH, Brent RL, Friedman JM *et al.* Update on new developments in the study of human teratogens. *Teratology* 2002; **65**: 153.

Towner D, Kjos SL, Leung B *et al.* Congenital malformations in pregnancies complicated by NIDDM. *Diabetes Care* 1995; **18**: 1446.

Further references are available on the book's website at http://www.drugsandpregnancy.com

Antiasthma agents during pregnancy

Asthma is an obstructive pulmonary disease characterized by reversible airway hyperreactivity to a variety of stimuli (Box 5.1). During an acute asthmatic attack, resistance of the airways is increased while forced expiratory flow and volume rates are decreased. Asthma complicates approximately 1 percent of pregnancies (0.4–4 percent) pregnancy (deSwiet, 1977; Hernandez et al., 1980; National Asthma Education Program, 1993; Weinstein et al., 1979), and is increasing (ACOG, 1996). It is unclear whether or not pregnancy affects the severity of asthma. Among more than 1000 patients reported in nine investigations, 48 percent of gravid asthmatics experienced no change in clinical severity of their symptoms, 29 percent improved, and in 23 percent the disease worsened in severity (Gluck and Gluck, 1976). Other data indicate that approximately one-third of women with asthma experienced worsened disease severity during pregnancy (Cunningham, 1994; Schatz et al., 1988; Stenius-Aarniala et al., 1988). Most severe

Box 5.1 Stimuli that exacerbate asthma

Allergies
    Poison ivy, pollen
    Household pets, odors
Cold weather
Drugs
    Acetyl salicylic acid
    Indomethacin
    Beta-blockers (Inderal)
Emotional stress
Environmental pollutants (dust, smog, air pollution)
Exercise
Occupational factors (asbestos, plaster)
Respiratory tract infections (viral, bacterial)

asthma occurred among 0.1–0.2 percent of pregnancies (Hernandez *et al.*, 1980; Mabie *et al.*, 1992), implying that 10–20 percent of asthmatics have severe pregnancy-associated sequelae. Adverse effects of asthma on pregnancy include a doubling in the rate of preterm labor, low birth weight, and preeclampsia (ACOG, 1996; Clark, 1993; Gordon *et al.*, 1970; Kallen *et al.*, 2000; Lehrer *et al.*, 1993; Wendel *et al.*, 1996). In contrast, no differences in the frequency of prematurity, low birth weight, and perinatal mortality were found among 182 pregnancies complicated by asthma compared to 364 nonasthmatic controls. Importantly, complications were increased among gravidas with severe uncontrolled asthma (Jana *et al.*, 1995).

TREATMENT REGIMENS

Most medications to treat asthma can be used safely during pregnancy. The objectives of asthma treatment are: (1) to decrease the frequency and number of asthmatic exacerbations; (2) to prevent status asthmaticus – severe obstruction persisting for days or weeks; (3) to avoid respiratory failure; and (4) to prevent death (Greenberger and Patterson, 1983). Additional treatment objectives during pregnancy include: (1) maintenance of sufficient oxygenation to the fetus and (2) minimize fetal effects of the pharmacotherapy (ACOG, 1996).

These goals can be accomplished with available antiasthma agents at no added risk to either mother or fetus (Greenberger and Patterson, 1978; Turner *et al.*, 1980). There are several categories of treatment modalities for asthma (Box 5.2): methylxanthines, beta-adrenergic agonists, antiinflammatory agents and antihistamines, decongestants and antibiotics, glucocorticoids, chromones, anticholinergics, immunotherapy, and miscellaneous others. One medical authority has indicated that inhaled corticosteroids are the most efficacious of antiasthma agents (Dombrowski, 1997).

Box 5.2 Medications utilized for the treatment of asthma during pregnancy

Antiinflammatory agents	*Antihistamines*
Beclomethasone	Chlorpheniramine
Cromolyn sodium	Tripelennamine
Prednisone	
	Decongestants
Beta-adrenergic agonists	Oxymetazoline
Albuterol	Pseudoephedrine
Epinephrine	
Isoetharine	*Cough medications*
Isoproterenol	Dextramethorphan
Metaproterenol	Guaifenesin
Terbutaline	
	Other
Methylxanthines	Antibiotics
Aminophylline	Anticholinergics
Theophylline	

Adapted in part from the National Asthma Education Program, 1993; ACOG, 1996.

Table 5.1 Pharmacokinetics of xanthines and beta-agonists during pregnancy

Agent	n	EGA (weeks)	Route	AUC	V_d	C_{max}	C_{ss}	$t_{1/2}$	Cl	PPB	Control group[a]	Authors
Theophylline	10	13–39	PO	↑	↑			↑	↓	↓	Yes (2)	Gardner et al. (1987)
Theophylline	5	24–38	PO	↑	↑	=	=		↓	↓	Yes (2)	Frederiksen et al. (1986)
Theophylline	8	15–39	PO			↑	↑		↓		Yes (2)	Carter et al. (1986)
Caffeine	34	11–38	PO		=	↑		↑	↓		Yes (1)	Aldridge et al. (1981)
Caffeine	50	13–38	PO			↑	↑	↑			Yes (1, 2, 4)	Knutti et al. (1981)
Salbutamol	7	16–33	IV, PO	↓		=	=	=	=		Yes (3, 4)	Hutchings et al. (1987)
Terbutaline	8	27–35	IV			=	↓	↑	↑		Yes (4)	Berg et al. (1984)

Source: Little BB. Obstet Gynecol 1999; 93: 858.

EGA, estimated gestational age; AUC, area under the curve; V_d, volume of distribution; C_{max}, pleak plasma concentration; C_{ss}, steady-state concentration; $t_{1/2}$, half-life; Cl, clearance; PPB, plasma protein binding; PO, by mouth; ↓ denotes a decrease during pregnancy compared with nonpregnant values; ↑ denotes an increase during pregnancy compared with nonpregnant values; = denotes no difference between pregnant and nonpregnant values; IV, intravenous; IM, intramuscular.

[a]Control groups: 1, nonpregnant women; 2, same individuals studied postpartum; 3, historic adult controls (sex not given); 4, adult male controls; 5, adult male and female controls combined.

Table 5.2 Medication dosages for treatment of asthma during pregnancy

Drug	Dosage
Beclomethasone	2–5 puffs bid to qid (inhalation)
Cromolyn sodium	2 puffs qid
Epinephrine	0.3–0.5 mL of 1:1000 solution q 20 min
Prednisone	Burst for acute symptoms, 40 mg/day for 7 days, and then taper for 7 days
Theophylline	400–600 mg/day initial and increase to therapeutic level of 8–12 µg/mL
Terbutaline (inhaled)	2–3 puffs q 4–6 h prn
Terbutaline (subcutaneous)	250 µg q 15 min

Cunningham, 1994; National Asthma Education Program, 1993.

Methylxanthines

The xanthines and methylxanthines have a peculiar pharmacokinetic profile during pregnancy, and it important to note their unusual behavior. Xanthines tend to increase their steady-state concentration during pregnancy (Table 5.1), and this effect is magnified during the third trimester. Consequently, achieving the desired plasma concentrations will require different doses throughout pregnancy, and physicians should anticipate a decrease in doses required as the pregnancy advances (Table 5.2).

Theophylline

Theophylline is a xanthine derivative with potent diuretic effects commonly used for its bronchodilating actions. Theophylline is a competitive inhibitor of the enzyme phosphodiesterase which inactivates cyclic 3′ 5′-adenosine monophosphate (cAMP) (Feldman and McFadden, 1977). Increased in intracellular cAMP levels stimulates bronchodilation. For many years theophylline salts were the first line of therapy for control of asthma in the pregnant patient. The frequency of congenital anomalies was not increased among 606 infants whose mothers used theophylline during the first trimester, and among 1294 infants whose mothers used the drug any time during pregnancy (Heinonen et al., 1977; Schatz et al., 1997; Stenius-Aarniala et al., 1995).

Theophylline crosses the placenta readily and high maternal doses may result in toxicity in the neonate (Arwood et al., 1979; Horowitz et al., 1982; Labovitz and Spector, 1982; Omarini et al., 1993; Yeh and Pildes, 1977). Newborns may manifest tachycardia, jitteriness, vomiting, and occasional apneic episodes during theophylline withdrawal (Arwood et al., 1979; Horowitz et al., 1982; Spector, 1984; Turner et al., 1980; Yeh and Pildes, 1977).

Aminophylline

Aminophylline is the only salt preparation available for parenteral use, but there are numerous oral theophylline preparations. The range for therapeutic plasma concentrations of theophylline is between 10 and 20 mg/mL. Wide variation in the dosage necessary to achieve this plasma concentration in patients is apparent. Caution should be used because of the potential for toxicity. Parenteral aminophylline is given as a loading dose of 5–6 mg/kg body weight infused over 20–30 min followed by a continuous infusion of 0.2–0.9 mg/kg.h. The loading dose should be reduced by half or omitted for patients already taking oral theophylline preparations. Aminophylline was used in the past for initial therapy and as combination therapy with beta-adrenergic agonists. It has recently been replaced by corticosteroids (Dombrowski, 1997), but oral theophylline derivatives are still utilized by many clinicians (Cunningham, 1994; Weinberger and Hendeles, 1996). Intravenous aminophylline for the acute treatment of asthma in pregnant women 'offers no therapeutic advantages' and may be associated with toxicity (Wendel *et al.*, 1996).

Aminophylline is sometimes associated with uterine activity at higher dosages than those required to treat asthma, but it was not an effective agent for the treatment of premature labor (Lipshitz, 1978). Theophylline may have an additional benefit in the pregnant asthmatic because it may be associated with a decreased frequency of preeclampsia in these women (Dombrowski *et al.*, 1986). As noted by Hankins and Cunningham (1992) as well as Wendel *et al.* (1996), aminophylline should no longer be 'the mainstay of therapy for severe asthma,' and the primary role of theophylline derivatives is for chronic outpatient therapy (Hankins and Cunningham, 1992; Wendel *et al.*, 1996).

BETA-ADRENERGIC AGENTS

Epinephrine, isoetharine, isoproterenol, metaproterenol, and terbutaline are included in this class of drugs. These agents have beta$_2$ receptor activity; epinephrine has alpha, beta$_1$, and beta$_2$ receptor activity (Table 5.3).

Table 5.3 Adrenergic drugs used for the treatment of asthma

Drug	Receptor	Administration	Recommended dosages
Epinephrine	α, β_1, β_2	Subcutaneous	0.3–0.5 mL 1:1000 solution q 20 min
		Inhaled	200–300 μg/puff, 1–2 puffs q 4 h
Isoetharine	β_2	Inhaled metered dose	340 μg/puff, 3–7 puffs q 3–4 h
		Aerosolized	0.5 mL of 1% solution, diluted 1:3 with saline
Isoproterenol	β_1, β_2	Inhaled	1:100 solution, 3–7 inhalations q 4–6 h
			1:200 solution, 5–15 inhalations q 4–6 h
		Intravenous	0.5–5 μg/min by infusion
Metaproterenol	β_2	Inhaled metered dose	650 μg/puff, 2–3 puffs q 3–4 h
		Nebulizer	0.3 mL of 5% solution q 4 h
Terbutaline	β_2	Subcutaneous	250 μg q 15 min
		Oral	2.5 mg q 4–6 h

From Cunningham, 1994, with permission.

Epinephrine

Epinephrine has alpha and beta-adrenergic actions, and is used to alleviate bronchospasm and other allergic reactions. During an acute asthma attack, 0.3–0.5 mL of a 1:1000 dilution of epinephrine is given subcutaneously every 30 min and may be repeated up to three times (Table 5.3). Relative contraindications to epinephrine use include severe hypertension, cardiac arrhythmias, and a heart rate more than 140 beats per minute. No convincing evidence that epinephrine causes congenital anomalies or adverse fetal effects has been published. Congenital anomalies were increased in frequency among 189 women who used epinephrine during the first trimester, but not among 508 who used the drug only during the first and second trimesters (Heinonen et al., 1977). However, these were minor birth defects that were not of clinical significance, and probably not causally related to the drug exposure. Maternal epinephrine crosses the placenta readily. Epinephrine occurs naturally and is released from the adrenal medulla in response to stress. Therefore, it seems reasonable to conclude that it is unlikely that epinephrine is associated with an increased risk of malformations in the fetus when used in usual adult doses.

Epinephrine causes congenital anomalies in animal species, but only at doses hundreds to thousands of times greater than those administered to humans.

Isoproterenol

Isoproterenol stimulates beta-adrenergic receptors and is the most potent of the group. It is used in the treatment of asthma and cardiac arrhythmias. Isoproterenol is usually administered by inhalation although it has been used parenterally in the treatment of status asthmaticus (Table 5.3). There are no reports to date of an association between congenital anomalies and the use of isoproterenol. Congenital anomalies were not increased in frequency among 31 offspring exposed to this drug in the first trimester (Heinonen et al., 1977).

Isoetharine

Isoetharine is a sympathomimetic drug taken orally or as an aerosol (1 percent solution) to treat bronchospasms. Isoetharine is the most selective beta$_2$ agent of this class, but it has weak bronchodilating effects and does not stimulate the heart as much as other beta$_2$ agents. No published studies are available on congenital anomalies in infants of mothers exposed to isoetharine during pregnancy. No animal teratology studies in animals have been published. Isoproterenol is a closely related drug.

Metaproterenol and albuterol

Metaproterenol and albuterol are resorcinols, drugs that: (1) are acquired by manipulation of the catecholamine molecule; (2) confer more beta$_2$ selectivity; and (3) have somewhat longer duration of action than other agents in this class. They are administered orally, parenterally, or as inhalants. Any risk to the embryo or fetus that may be associated with these drugs is substantially reduced when the route of administration is inhalation.

Metaproterenol, albuterol, and terbutaline are the resorcinol agents available in the USA. Metaproterenol and albuterol are beta sympathomimetics used as bronchodilators and to arrest premature labor. In one series of 361 infants exposed to metaproterenol during the first trimester, the frequency of congenital anomalies was not increased in frequency (Rosa, personal communication, cited in Briggs *et al.*, 2002). Among 1090 infants exposed to albuterol during the first trimester, the frequency of congenital anomalies was not increased (Rosa, personal communication). Fetal tachycardia has been reported with maternal albuterol therapy in the third trimester, but has not been associated with any adverse neonatal effects (Hastwell *et al.*, 1978; Ryden, 1977).

Terbutaline

Terbutaline is a potent bronchodilator and has also been used to prevent or treat premature labor, although it does not have Food and Drug Administration (FDA) approval for this purpose. The oral dose of terbutaline is 2.5–5 mg three or four times daily. It can be administered subcutaneously (0.25–0.5 mg), but has less beta$_2$ selectivity. Congenital anomalies were not increased in frequency among 149 infants exposed to terbutaline during the first trimester (Rosa, personal communication, cited in Briggs *et al.*, 2005). Terbutaline crosses the placenta readily (Ingemarsson *et al.*, 1981) and has been associated with fetal tachycardia and transient hypoglycemia in the neonatal period when used as a tocolytic agent (Epstein *et al.*, 1979; Ingemarsson, 1976; Wallace *et al.*, 1978).

In summary, metaproterenol, albuterol, and terbutaline do not pose a substantial risk of birth defects at therapeutic doses, and it seems unlikely that these drugs are associated with an increased risk of congenital anomalies.

ANTIINFLAMMATORY AGENTS

Glucocorticoids

Glucocorticoids are a mainstay of asthma treatment. Several adrenal glucocorticoids are given to severely asthmatic pregnant women (Box 5.3). Steroids should be employed in acute exacerbations when severe airway obstruction persists or worsens despite optimal

---

Box 5.3 Steroid use in pregnancy

Patient unresponsive to bronchodilators
Hydrocortisone 4 mg/kg body weight IV loading dose followed by 3 mg/kg IV q 6 h for 2–3
  days. Switch to oral prednisone
Methylprednisolone 0.5–1 mg/kg (approximately 125 mg) IV bolus followed by 60 mg IV q 6 h
Prednisone 30–60 mg PO daily
Beclomethasone 2 puffs (100 µg) tid–qid
Patients on maintenance dose of steroids
Hydrocortisone 100 mg IM or IV q 6–8 h × 24 h
Methylprednisolone 125 mg IV bolus followed by 60 mg IV q 6 h

From ACOG, 1996.

bronchodilator therapy because severe asthma is dangerous to the mother. Chronic glucocorticoid use is of greatest benefit in patients with frequent recurrences and those with worsening disease despite a prior optimal regimen. Steroids act by inducing protein lipocortin production, thereby inhibiting phospholipase A_2 and decreasing arachidonic acid release (Townley and Suliaman, 1987). Enhancement of the bronchodilating effect of beta agonists occurs with steroid use, as well as a decrease in mucous gland secretions and an inflammatory response. In a prospective investigation of 503 pregnant patients with acute asthma, the risk of an attack when maintained on an inhaled steroid ($n = 257$) was reduced fivefold compared to those who did not receive an inhaled steroid (Stenius-Aarniala et al., 1996). Glucocorticoids effects are usually not felt until at least 6–8 h after initial administration. Therefore, it is of utmost importance to continue bronchodilator therapy.

Prednisone and prednisolone

Prednisone and prednisolone are synthetic glucocorticoids. Prednisone is biologically inert and is metabolized to prednisolone in the liver. The maternal-to-fetal gradient of prednisone/prednisolone is 10:1, and thus the fetus is exposed to only approximately 10 percent of the drug (Beitins et al., 1972; Levitz et al., 1978). Prednisone is the glucocorticoid of choice for asthma treatment.

Prednisone and prednisolone are discussed in Chapter 4. It is important to reiterate that it is unlikely that prednisone or prednisolone exposure during the first trimester is associated with an increased risk of congenital anomalies, particularly cleft palate.

Infants born to mothers who received prednisone throughout gestation usually had normal adrenocortical reserves and lacked symptoms of adrenal suppression (Arad and Landau, 1984). Additionally, in two other reports, no evidence of neonatal adrenal insufficiency was found in newborn infants of women who took prednisone daily (as much as 60 mg in one study) throughout pregnancy (Schatz et al., 1975; Weinberger et al., 1980).

Beclomethasone

Beclomethasone is a synthetic glucocorticoid administered by inhalation to treat bronchial asthma. Beclomethasone is now considered one of the key therapeutic agents for asthma. Readmissions decreased 55 percent in pregnant asthmatics receiving this inhaled steroid (Wendel et al., 1996). As with other steroids, beclomethasone has been reported to be teratogenic (i.e., cleft palate) in animals (Esaki et al., 1976; Furuhashi et al., 1977; Nomura et al., 1977; Tamagawa et al., 1982). However, beclomethasone was not associated with an increased frequency of congenital anomalies in 395 infants exposed to the drug during the first trimester (Rosa, personal communication, cited in Briggs et al., 2005; Schatz, 2001). In one prospective study of this agent in pregnancy, it was not associated with an increase in the frequency of malformations (Greenberger and Patterson, 1983).

In a prospective study of 503 gravid patients with acute asthma, risk of an attack when maintained on a beclomethasone ($n = 214$) was significantly reduced compared to those who did not receive an inhaled steroid. No reduction in birth weight or increase in the frequency of birth defects was found in the treated group compared to the untreated group (Stenius-Aarniala *et al.*, 1996).

Cortisone

Cortisone (hydrocortisone) is a glucocorticoid excreted by the adrenal cortex. Four of 27 newborns whose mothers were treated with cortisone had congenital anomalies, but no distinct patterns of malformations were found (Wells, 1953). No increase in the frequency of congenital anomalies was found among the small number of infants (*n* = 34) exposed to this steroid in the first trimester (Heinonen *et al.*, 1977).

Animal studies have demonstrated the teratogenic effects of cortisone in several species (Loevy and Roth, 1968). The pertinence of these findings to the clinical use of cortisone in human pregnancy remains unclear. It seems unlikely that cortisone therapy substantially increases the risk of cleft palate in infants born to women who used the drug during the first trimester.

Betamethasone

Betamethasone is a synthetic glucocorticoid that crosses the placenta readily (Ballard *et al.*, 1975). No epidemiological studies of congenital anomalies in newborns of pregnant women exposed to the drug during the first trimester have been published. Betamethasone has been used to accelerate fetal lung maturation in pregnant women with premature labor. In a 6-year follow-up evaluation of children exposed to betamethasone treatment, no consistent alterations in growth or intellectual function were noted (MacArthur *et al.*, 1982). Animal teratology studies with betamethasone have found effects similar to those of other corticosteroids, i.e., an increased frequency of cleft palate was observed among the offspring of pregnant rats, mice, and rabbits exposed to betamethasone during gestation (Ishimura *et al.*, 1975; Mosier *et al.*, 1982; Walker, 1971; Yamada *et al.*, 1981). The frequency of omphaloceles was increased in frequency among the offspring of betamethasone-exposed pregnant rats (Mosier *et al.*, 1982; Yamada *et al.*, 1981).

Dexamethasone

Dexamethasone has been used during pregnancy for the treatment of asthma and to stimulate fetal lung maturation. It crosses the placenta readily, resulting in therapeutic fetal serum levels (Osathanondh *et al.*, 1977). The use of dexamethasone, as well as other steroids, in treating the pregnant asthmatic was not associated with adverse maternal or fetal effects (Schatz *et al.*, 1975). There were no adverse effects of *in utero* exposure to dexamethasone observed in infants in a long-term follow-up by the Collaborative Group on Antenatal Steroid Therapy (1984). The teratogenic effects of dexamethasone in animal species are similar to those of cortisone. For example, neural tube defects were induced in rabbits (Buck *et al.*, 1962) and cleft palates in mice (Pinsky and DiGeorge, 1965). Also, Jerome and Hendrickx (1988) administered 10 mg/kg dexamethasone daily between days 22 and 50 in six pregnant rhesus monkeys and observed cranium bifidum and aplasia cutis congenita in one and three fetuses, respectively.

As discussed with prednisone previously, first trimester exposure may be associated with a very small risk of oral clefts (see Chapter 4).

CHROMONES

Cromolyn sodium

Cromolyn sodium inhibits degranulation of mast cells and thus the release of the chemical mediators of anaphylaxis. It is given by inhalation for asthma prophylaxis (Cunningham, 1994). Congenital anomalies were not increased in frequency among infants born to 151 and 191 women who used cromolyn sodium during the first trimester (Rosa, personal communication) (Schatz et al., 1997). Older reports of its use during pregnancy indicate no adverse fetal effects (Dykes, 1974; Wilson, 1982).

MISCELLANEOUS AGENTS

Anticholinergics

Anticholinergics, such as atropine, produce bronchodilation in asthmatics. Their systemic side effects limited their use (Van Arsdel and Paul, 1977). Atropine readily crosses the placenta to the fetal circulation and may cause fetal vagal blockade with subsequent fetal tachycardia (Hellman and Fillisti, 1965; Kanto et al., 1981; Kivalo and Saarikoski, 1977). No increase in congenital defects among 401 offspring of women with exposure to atropine during early pregnancy, or 1198 infants whose mothers used the drug anytime during pregnancy was found (Heinonen et al., 1977).

Antibiotics

Upper respiratory infections should be treated aggressively in the pregnant asthmatic patient, as in the nonpregnant patient (see Chapter 2). Penicillins are considered safe for use during pregnancy. Erythromycin is probably a safe alternative in the patient who is allergic to penicillin. However, hepatotoxicity has been observed in pregnant patients treated with the estolate salt of erythromycin (McCormack et al., 1977). Tetracyclines should be avoided during pregnancy (Table 5.4) because of their adverse effects on fetal teeth (permanent staining) and bones (abnormalities in bone formation) (Anthony, 1970; Cohlan et al., 1967; Harcourt et al., 1962; Rendle-Short, 1962; Swallow, 1964).

Table 5.4 Drugs that should be avoided in the treatment of asthma during pregnancy

Agent	Effects
Beta-blockers	Bronchospasm
Cyclopropane	Bronchoconstriction
Iodide-containing mixtures	Fetal goiter
	Congenital hypothyroidism
Opiates, sedatives, tranquilizers	Depress alveolar ventilation
Prostaglandin $F_{2\alpha}$	Bronchoconstriction
Tetracyclines	Stain fetal teeth
	Abnormalities in bone formation

Antihistamines and expectorants

Antihistamines and expectorant use during pregnancy during pregnancy is discussed in Chapter 11. Briefly, diphenhydramine, chlorpheniramine, pheniramine, and tripelennamine are generally considered safe for use during pregnancy. A few studies have shown that expectorants and mucolytics are efficacious in the treatment of asthma. It is of utmost importance that these agents, as well as theophylline mixtures containing iodides, not be used during pregnancy, because the iodine blocks the synthesis of thyroxine in the fetus, resulting in hypothyroidism or congenital goiter (Carswell *et al.*, 1970; Galina *et al.*, 1962). Other drugs used to treat asthma are also contraindicated for use during pregnancy (Table 5.4).

RISK SUMMARY

The FDA Pregnancy Risk Rating is compared to the Teratogen Information System (TERIS) risk rating in Table 5.5. Generally, the TERIS risk rating provides greater information than the FDA rating. However, the FDA rating is an aggregate risk of not only

Table 5.5 Summary of drugs used to treat asthma

Drug	TERIS risk	FDA risk rating
Albuterol	Undetermined	C_m
Atropine	Unlikely	C
Beclomethasone	Unlikely	C_m
Betamethasone	Undetermined	C*
Chlorpheniramine	Unlikely	B
Cortisone	Unlikely	C*
Cromolyn	Unlikely	B_m
Dexamethasone	Minimal	C*
Ephedrine	Unlikely	C
Epinephrine	Unlikely	C
Erythromycin	None	B_m
Hydrocortisone	Unlikely	C*
Isoetharine	Undetermined	C
Isoproterenol	Unlikely	C
Metaproterenol	Undetermined	C_m
Methylprednisolone	Unlikely	Not in book
Penicillin	None	B_m
Pheniramine	Unlikely	C
Prednisone	Oral clefts: small	C*
	Other congenital anomalies: unlikely	
Terbutaline	Unlikely	B_m
Tetracycline	Unlikely	D
Theophylline	None	C_m

NA, not available.

TERIS, Teratogen Information System; FDA, Food and Drug Administration.

Compiled from Friedman *et al., Obstet Gynecol* 1990; **75**: 594; Briggs *et al.*, 2005; Friedman and Polifka, 2006.

birth defects, but also of possible adverse events during the second and third trimester. The TERIS risk rating is directed toward the risk for birth defects (i.e., teratogenicity).

SPECIAL CONSIDERATIONS

Acute asthma

Patients with an acute asthma attack should have a clinical assessment, including evaluation for symptoms suggestive of complications such as pneumonia or pneumothorax and for the presence of agitation, pulse paradoxus, severe wheezing, or cyanosis. The beta-adrenergic agonists are a critical element of first-line pharmacological therapy (Cunningham, 1994). These include the medications listed in Table 5.3. During an acute asthma attack, 0.3–0.5 mL of epinephrine in a 1:1000 dilution is administered subcutaneously every 30 min. Alternatively, 0.25 mg of terbutaline in two to three doses can be given subcutaneously every 20–30 min. Some physicians advocate the use of inhaled beta agonists initially. Each dose should be followed by spirometry. Evaluation should include forced expiratory volume in 1 s (FEV_1) and peak expiratory flow rate (PEFR) (ACOG, 1996). Supplemental oxygen should be administered, as needed, to maintain a pO_2 greater than 60 mmHg. Intravenous hydration is also important, along with respiratory care to remove the tenacious secretions. If initial spirometry indicates severe obstruction, an intravenous bolus of 125 mg methylprednisolone should be considered. Methylprednisolone is indicated in patients who are on chronic corticosteroids. It has been recommended that corticosteroids should be part of the initial therapy for women with severe, acute asthma (Cunningham, 1994; National Heart, Lung and Blood Institute, 1991).

After two or three doses of epinephrine or inhaled beta-agonists, if the wheezing is not corrected, then intravenous aminophylline may be indicated. Dosing should be based on theophylline levels, if the patient has been receiving oral theophylline (it should be noted that theophylline requirements decrease as pregnancy advances; see Table 5.1). The patient should be admitted to the hospital if she demonstrates a poor spirometric response to therapy, has no symptom improvement, or has pneumonia or pneumothorax.

Endotracheal intubation and mechanical ventilation should be considered when signs of respiratory failure present. Specifically, $PaCO_2$ greater than 40 mmHg, PaO_2 less than 70 mmHg and pH less than 7.38 are indicators of impending respiratory failure. Immediate endotracheal intubation should be performed when (1) a $PaCO_2$ of greater than or equal to 55 mmHg or (2) a PaO_2 of less than or equal to 65 mmHg is obtained.

Patients who respond quickly to such therapy should be discharged on an intensified regimen. A tapering schedule of oral corticosteroids should be given if intravenous steroids were used. Close follow-up should be arranged to reassess their clinical condition and possible adjustments in medication. In addition, precipitating factors (Box 5.1) should be avoided.

Opiates, sedatives, and tranquilizers are contraindicated in asthmatics because they cause alveolar ventilatory depression, and are associated with respiratory arrest immediately after use (Table 5.4). Beta-adrenergic blockers and parasympathetic agents should also be avoided in asthmatics because they can cause bronchospasm. Additionally, if prostaglandins are needed for labor induction or termination of pregnancy, prostaglandin E_2 (PGE_2), a bronchodilator, should be administered, rather than prostaglandin $F_{2\alpha}$ ($PGF_{2\alpha}$), because it has potent bronchoconstricting effects and may precipitate status asthmaticus (Fishburne *et al.*, 1972a, 1972b; Hyman *et al.*, 1978; Smith, 1973).

Chronic asthma

Chronic asthma patients need additional steroid therapy for coverage during the stress of labor if they have received oral steroid therapy for more than 2 weeks within the previous year to prevent adrenal crisis. Hydrocortisone, 100 mg IM or IV every 6–8 h for 24 h, is usually given. Corticosteroids should be given in cases of severe or mild asthma with wheezing that is unresponsive to bronchodilators. Initially, prednisone, 30–60 mg daily is given to prevent status asthmaticus. Beclomethasone dipropionate is effective and safe when prolonged steroid use is necessary.

Beta-agonist by inhalation every 3–4 h as needed is used for outpatient management of chronic asthma, along with inhalation steroids such as beclomethasone (Cunningham, 1994).

Cromolyn sodium can be given chronically by inhalation, and is fairly effective in improving the symptoms of an asthmatic. An added benefit with cromolyn use is a decreased requirement for other antiasthma agents. Cromolyn therapy is best begun during remissions because it requires several days to reach an effective dosing regimen. Medications that cause bronchospasm or depress alveolar ventilation should be avoided in the pregnant woman with asthma (Table 5.4).

Key references

ACOG (American College of Obstetricians and Gynecologists). *Pulmonary Disease in Pregnancy.* Technical Bulletin No. 224, American College of Obstetricians and Gynecologists, Washington, DC, June 1996.

Briggs GG, Freeman RK, Yaffe SJ. *Drugs in Pregnancy and Lactation. A Reference Guide to Fetal and Neonatal Risk*, 6th edn. Philadelphia: Lippincott Williams & Wilkins, 2005: 873–4.

Dombrowski, M.P. Pharmacologic therapy of asthma during pregnancy. *Obstet Gynecol Clin North Am* 1997; **24**: 559–74.

Jana N, Vasishta K, Saha SC, Khunnu B. Effect of bronchial asthma on the course of pregnancy, labour and perinatal outcome. *J Obstet Gynaecol* 1995; **21**: 227.

Kallen B, Rydhstroem H, Aberg A. Asthma during pregnancy – a population-based study. *Eur J Epidemiol* 2000; **16**: 167–71.

Little BB. Pharmacokinetics during pregnancy. Evidence-based maternal dose formulation. *Obstet Gynecol* 1999; **93**: 858–68.

Schatz M. The efficacy and safety of asthma medications during pregnancy. *Semin Perinatol* 2001; **25**: 145–52.

Stenius-Aarniala B, Hedman J, Teramo KA. Acute asthma during pregnancy. *Thorax* 1996; **51**: 411.

Stenius-Aarniala B, Riikonen S, Teramo K. Slow-release theophylline in pregnant asthmatics. *Chest* 1995; **107**: 642.

Weinberger M, Hendeles L. Theophylline in asthma. *N Engl J Med* 1996; **334**: 1380.

Wendel PJ, Ramin SM, Barnett-Hamm C, Rowe TF, Cunningham FG. Asthma treatment in pregnancy. A randomized controlled study. *Am J Obstet Gynecol* 1996; **175**: 150.

Further references are available on the book's website at http://www.drugsandpregnancy.com

6

Anesthetic agents and surgery during pregnancy

Surgery during pregnancy is necessary among approximately 1–2 percent of gravidas in the USA (Brodsky, 1983; Friedman, 1988). Many surgeons are reluctant to perform operative procedures on women known to be pregnant, although emergency procedures are sometimes necessary. In addition, elective or indicated procedures may be carried out on women with an unrecognized pregnancy. Obstetrical surgery (i.e., Caesarean section) is increasingly common with a steady rise in the Caesarean section rate from 4–5 percent in the 1960s to rates exceeding 20 percent in contemporary practice (Gilstrap et al., 1984; Notzon et al., 1987).

General principles that the clinician should be aware of when surgery is anticipated in a pregnant woman are based on physiologic differences between the pregnant and non-pregnant state (Box 6.1). Most importantly, two patients are involved, the mother and her fetus. Virtually all anesthetic agents and 98 percent of medications cross the placenta, exposing the fetus to medically significant levels. In addition, mild changes in maternal cardiopulmonary status (i.e., changes in blood pressure or oxygen saturation) may have physiologically important sequelae for the fetus, but are of little consequence

Box 6.1 General principles regarding surgery and anesthesia during pregnancy

Two patients: Mother and embrofetus
Assume that all anesthetics and 98 percent of medications cross the placenta, resulting in fetal levels
Minor maternal cardiopulmonary status changes may have profound effects on the fetus
Numerous maternal physiological changes occur during pregnancy (Table 6.1)
Aspiration pneumonitis risk is increased during pregnancy
Laboratory and radiologic procedures should be performed as indicated
Indicated surgery during pregnancy showed be performed *statim* because delays increase risks of morbidity and mortality

to the mother. Even a minimal degree of hypotension and hypoxia is to be avoided because this may result in placental hypoperfusion and fetal hypoxemia. Pregnant women being prepared for surgery should be placed on their left side, adequately hydrated, and preoxygenated prior to induction of anesthesia.

Pharmacokinetics of anesthetic agents have been reported for only pancuronium, and its disposition was a pregnancy-associated decreased half-life, and this was probably due to significantly increased clearance (Little, 1999).

Table 6.1 *Physiologic changes in pregnancy*

System	
Cardiovascular	
Cardiac output	Increase
Blood volume	Increase
Heart rate	Increase
Blood pressure	Initial decrease[a]
Peripheral resistance	Decrease
Hematocrit	Decrease
Hematologic	
Leukocytes	Increase
Fibrinogen (I)	Increase
Factors VII–X	Increase
Factors II	Slow increase
Factors XI, XIII	Decrease
Platelets	Unchanged
Prothrombin time/ partial thromboplastin time	Slow decrease
Respiratory	
Tidal volume	Increase
Vital capacity	Unchanged
Functional residual capacity	Decrease
Compliance	Unchanged
Minute ventilation	Increase
pCO_2	Decrease
HCO_3	Decrease
Renal	
Serum creatinine	Decrease
Serum blood urea nitrogen	Decrease
Creatinine clearance	Increase
Gastrointestinal	
Gastric emptying	Decrease
Cardiac valve competency	Decrease
Regurgitation	Increase

[a]Returns to prepregnancy levels by term.
From Little, 1999; Gilstrap and Hankins, 1988.

Several maternal physiologic changes occur during pregnancy (Table 6.1), and the most marked is expansion of the maternal blood volume by up to 50 percent. Increased blood volume is caused by a plasma volume increase of approximately 1000 cc and a 300–500 cc increase in red cells. This usually results in lower hematocrit compared to the nonpregnant woman, and is commonly known as physiologic anemia of pregnancy. Increased renal blood flow is a result of the increase in blood volume. Accordingly, the glomerular filtration rate increases (as measured by the endogenous creatinine clearance) because of increased blood volume. Serum creatinine and blood urea nitrogen decrease because of dilution by increased plasma volume. Other changes in the renal system include dilatation of the ureters and a relative stasis of urine, resulting in a 'relative' hydronephrosis. The relative hydronephrosis is frequently more pronounced on the right than on the left side.

Other cardiopulmonary changes that occur during pregnancy include a slight increase in heart rate, and decreased systolic and diastolic blood pressures in the second trimester. Blood pressure gradually returns to prepregnancy levels by the third trimester. Most women have a systolic flow murmur by midpregnancy. Respiratory rate increases slightly during pregnancy with a decrease in physiologic 'dead space' as pregnancy progresses. Tidal volume is increased during pregnancy, but minute ventilation and compliance do not change during pregnancy. Blood pCO_2 and HCO_3 decrease during pregnancy, while pH is slightly increased during pregnancy. Hence, upper normal range pCO_2 for nonpregnant women probably indicates CO_2 retention.

Gastrointestinal system changes with pregnancy affect pregnant women that require anesthesia and/or surgery. The risk for aspiration pneumonitis in surgery on the gravid patient is increased because of pregnancy-associated decreases in intestinal motility and gastric emptying. Hepatic function is also altered during pregnancy. Maternal alkaline phosphatase levels are increased during gestation.

Liver cytochrome P-450 (CYP) 3A4 and CYP2D6 activities increase during pregnancy. Importantly, the enzyme responsible for metabolism of 50 percent of pharmacologic agents (CYP1A2) is downregulated. This has implications for anesthesia dose management of the pregnant patient; lower doses than in the nongravid patient may achieve the desired anesthetic effect. CYP2C19 activity is upregulated in pregnant compared to nonpregnant women, but even during pregnancy its activity is not higher than normal adult male levels. Extrahepatic enzymes (e.g., cholinesterase) that also metabolize some anesthetics have diminished activity during pregnancy.

Liver fibrinogen production is also increased during pregnancy. Serum levels as high as 400 mg percent are not unusual during the third trimester and cause increased red cell sedimentation rate in pregnant women. Hematocrit is decreased during pregnancy accompanied by a relative leukocytosis (white blood cell count greater than or equal to 10 000–12 000 or even higher during labor). Several hematologic measures are unchanged during pregnancy: for example, the relative percent of immature forms (i.e., 'bands'), lymphocytes, eosinophils, and platelet count. Whole blood clotting time, prothrombin time, and partial thromboplastin time remain in normal ranges during pregnancy.

Surgery should be performed without delay when it is indicated for life-threatening maternal conditions. Indicated laboratory tests and radiologic procedures should be performed without hesitation to properly guide life-saving surgical procedures.

ANESTHETIC AGENTS

Secondary effects of anesthetic agents (hypotension, hypoxia) are important to avoid in the gravid patient as these may cause adverse fetal effects. Anesthetic adjuncts, or other 'nonanesthetic' drugs and medications during the pre-, intra-, and post-operative periods may also adversely affect the fetus.

LOCAL ANESTHETICS

Local anesthetics may be injected in subdural or epidural spaces for regional anesthesia (Table 6.2). Topical application results in negligible fetal exposure and minimal risk. Regional techniques (spinal and epidural procedures, paracervical and pudendal blocks) result in physiologically important fetal exposure to clinically significant anesthetic levels.

Table 6.2 Frequently used anesthetic agents

Agent	Class	Principal use
Benzocaine	Ester	Topical
Bupivacaine	Amide	Local and epidural blocks
Chloroprocaine	Ester	Local and epidural blocks
Etidocaine	Amide	Epidural block
Lidocaine	Amide	Local, epidural, and spinal blocks
Mepivacaine	Amide	Local and epidural blocks
Procaine	Ester	Local block
Tetracaine	Ester	Spinal

Local anesthetics have an aromatic ring with an intermediate alkyl chain with (1) an amide or (2) ester linkage. Anesthetic potency is related to protein-bound fraction, and the amount of binding determines the duration of action. Highly protein bound anesthetics are lipid soluble and readily cross the placenta (Morishima *et al.*, 1966; Pedersen and Finster, 1987). Malformations were not increased in frequency among offspring of women who used procaine, lidocaine, benzocaine, or tetracaine during the first trimester, and there were no adverse fetal effects when these agents were utilized at any time during pregnancy (Heinonen *et al.*, 1977). No animal teratology studies of these agents have been published.

No investigations of bupivacaine, chloroprocaine or prilocaine have been published with regard to their teratogenic effects. Transient newborn neurobehavioral changes in infants whose mothers received local anesthetic agents have been reported, and vary from moderate for regional blocks (Rosenblatt *et al.*, 1981; Scanlon *et al.*, 1974; Standley *et al.*, 1974) to minimal for epidural anesthesia on newborn behavior (Tronick *et al.*, 1976).

Epinephrine

Epinephrine is added to local anesthetics to prolong their action. Following first trimester exposure there was a significantly increased frequency of inguinal hernias in the epinephrine-exposed group (Heinonen *et al.*, 1977). However, it is unlikely that epinephrine is a teratogen. Epinephrine is also used as a test agent to detect intravascular injection of local anesthetics.

Some local anesthetics (e.g., lidocaine), especially those used in combination with epinephrine, have been associated with fetal heart rate bradycardia when utilized for paracervical block anesthesia during labor. It has been suggested that bradycardia is secondary to vasoconstriction of uterine artery caused by the anesthetic agent (Fishburne *et al.*, 1979). Thus paracervical blocking techniques are not recommended in the presence of fetal heart rate abnormalities or compromised uterine blood flow (Carlsson *et al.*, 1987).

GENERAL ANESTHETICS

Regional anesthetic techniques are preferred for pregnant women undergoing obstetrical procedures, general anesthesia often used for nonobstetrical or emergency procedures in pregnant women. The fetus will be exposed to a variety of agents that include narcotics, paralyzing agents, and inhalational anesthetic agents.

Thiopental and ketamine

Thiopental and ketamine are narcotic anesthetics, and are given intravenously for rapid induction of anesthesia prior to the intubation and initiation of inhalational anesthetic agents. Thiopental is the most often used agent for this purpose. The frequency of congenital malformations was not increased in human or animal studies (Heinonen *et al.*, 1977; Friedman, 1988). Ketamine is rarely used in obstetrics, except for rapid anesthesia in emergency operative vaginal deliveries. Ketamine presents two problems: (1) clinically significant increase in blood pressure; and (2) significant maternal hallucinations. Ketamine was not teratogenic in one animal study (Friedman, 1988).

NEUROMUSCULAR BLOCKING AGENTS

The most commonly used agent for inducing paralysis prior to intubation and the initiation of actual surgical procedures is probably succinylcholine. Perhaps 20 percent of patients have lowered cholinesterase activity, and pregnancy reduces cholinesterase activity in general. Therefore, pregnant patients probably require a smaller dose of succinylcholine than nongravid women. Newborns may be exposed to enough drug to experience neuromuscular blockade that requires supportive therapy. Other common agents used for neuromuscular blockade are vecuronium bromide, pancuronium bromide, and atracurium besylate (Box 6.2). Unlike succinylcholine, which is a depolarizing agent, these three neuromuscular blocking agents are nonpolarizing in action.

Box 6.2 Neuromuscular blocking agents

Depolarizing agents
Succinylcholine (Anectine)
Nondepolarizing agents
Atracurium besylate (Tracrium)
Pancuronium bromide (Pavulen)
Vecuronium bromide (Norcuron)

As mentioned above, this class of neuromuscular agents may require a dose increase because of a reduced half-life and increased renal clearance (Little, 1999). No reports are published regarding these neuromuscular blocking agents. However, according to its manufacturer, atracurium is potentially teratogenic in animals.

INHALED ANESTHESIA AGENTS

Commonly utilized inhalation agents for general anesthesia include nitrous oxide, halothane, methoxyflurane, enflurane, and isoflurane. Neither ether nor cyclopropane is commonly used in present-day anesthetic techniques, and there have been no adequate human studies regarding potential teratogenicity of either of these agents (Friedman, 1988).

Halothane and other halogenated agents

Halogenated agents are often used to supplement the standard nitrous oxide, thiopental and muscle relaxant regimens for balanced general anesthesia. Use of halogenated agents decreases maternal awareness and recall, allows for a higher percentage of inspired oxygen, and results in higher fetal oxygen concentrations (Shnider and Levinson, 1979).

The prototype halogenated anesthetic agent was not found to be associated with an increased risk of congenital malformations in children whose mothers received this agent during the first 4 months (Heinonen et al., 1977), but there were only 26 infants exposed. Increased fetal loss, growth retardation, malformations, and behavioral abnormalities have been reported with the use of halothane in animal studies (Friedman, 1988). No epidemiologic studies of congenital anomalies with the use of the other halogenated agents (enflurane, methoxyflurane, isoflurane) have been published. These agents were reported to cause a variety of malformations in animal studies at doses many times those used in humans (Friedman, 1988).

Placental transfer of enflurane and halothane in women who were delivered via Caesarean section had no apparent adverse effects on Apgar scores, newborn acid–base status, and early neonatal neurobehavioral scores. Significant levels of both of these agents were achieved in the fetus at about 50–60 percent of maternal concentrations (Abboud et al., 1985).

Halogenated agents have also been reported to be associated with an increase in blood loss in the mother at the time of Caesarean section in some studies (Gilstrap et al., 1987), but others have found no association between blood loss and use of halogenated agents, especially when used in low doses for Caesarean section (Abboud et al., 1985; Lamont et al., 1988; Warren et al., 1983).

Increased blood loss from uterine relaxation may occur, especially in prolonged high-dose use. Otherwise, it seems apparent that halogenated agents are safe for both mother and fetus, although the data are not conclusive.

Nitrous oxide

Nitrous oxide is the most commonly used inhalation anesthetic agent in obstetrics, and is usually part of a balanced general anesthetic regimen that includes: a fast-acting barbiturate (e.g., thiopental), a muscle relaxant (e.g., succinylcholine), and a halogenated agent (e.g., isoflurane). The frequency of congenital anomalies was not increased among more than 500 infants exposed to nitrous oxide during the first trimester (Heinonen et al., 1977; Crawford and Lewis, 1986). As with many other agents, nitrous oxide has been reported to be associated with increased fetal resorption, growth retardation, and congenital anomalies in animal studies (Friedman, 1988; Mazze et al., 1984).

Some anesthetists have used high concentrations (e.g., 70 percent nitrous oxide, 30 percent oxygen). Lower nitrous oxide concentrations (50 percent) have been used with higher oxygen concentrations (50 percent), responding primarily to concerns that higher nitrous oxide concentrations may be associated with neurobehavioral alterations. Altered neonatal neurobehavioral effects are associated with nitrous oxide and halothane and have been demonstrated in animal studies (Koeter and Rodier, 1986; Mullenix et al., 1986). Current recommendations are to use lower concentrations of nitrous oxide, higher concentrations of oxygen, and to add a halogenated agent to the regimen.

SYSTEMIC ANALGESICS

Systemic analgesics (meperidine, morphine, pentazocine, butorphanel, alphaprodine) are used for analgesia for women in labor and are discussed in the chapter on analgesics (Chapter 8). Three very potent synthetic opioid analgesics (fentanyl, sufentanil, and alfetanil) (Box 6.3) are often used as: (1) premedication prior to surgery; (2) an adjunct for induction of anesthesia; and (3) an adjunct in maintaining general anesthesia. Fentanyl is also used in combination with a neuroleptic agent (droperidol) for the same indications. None of these narcotic agents has been shown to be teratogenic in a variety of animal studies. First trimester exposure to meperidine was not associated with an increased frequency of congenital anomalies among 268 infants (Heinonen et al., 1977). Similarly, morphine was not teratogenic in humans (Table 6.3). Intravenous fentanyl was not associated with low Apgar scores or neonatal respiratory depression compared to controls (Rayburn et al., 1989).

Three synthetic narcotic analgesics (fentanyl, sufentanil, and alfetanil) have been used as an adjunct to epidural analgesia during labor (Ross and Hughes, 1987). However, neonatal respiratory depression is a risk with use of these agents during labor.

Box 6.3 Agents utilized for or as adjuncts for general anesthesia

Inhalational agents	Narcotic
Enflurane (Ethrane)	Alfentanil (Alfenta)
Halothane (Fluothane)	Fentanyl (Sublimaze)
Isoflurane (Forane)	Fentanyl + Droperidol (Innovar)
Methoxyflurane (Penthrane)	Sufentanil (Sufenta)
	Other
	Ketamine (Ketalar)
	Thiopental

Table 6.3 Summary of cardiovascular anaesthetics drugs: Teratogen Information System (TERIS) and Food and Drug Administration (FDA) risk estimates

Drug	Risk	Risk rating
Atracurium	Undetermined	C_m
Benzocaine	Unlikely	NA
Bupivacaine	Undetermined	NA
Cyclopropane	Undetermined	NA
Diazepam	Minimal	D
Droperidol	Undetermined	C_m
Enflurane	Undetermined	NA
Epinephrine	Unlikely	C
Ether	Undetermined	NA
Fentanyl	Undetermined	C_m^*
Halothane	Undetermined	NA
Isoflurane	Undetermined	NA
Ketamine	Undetermined	B
Lidocaine	Local administration: none	B_m
	Intravenous administration: undetermined	
Meperidine	Unlikely	B^*
Methoxyflurane	Undetermined	NA
Morphine	Congenital anomalies: unlikely	C_m^*
	Neonatal neurobehavioral effects: moderate	
Nitrous oxide	Occupational exposure: unlikely	NA
	Anesthesia: unlikely	
Pancuronium	Undetermined	C_m
Prilocaine	Undetermined	NA
Procaine	None	NA
Succinylcholine	Unlikely	C_m
Tetracaine	Undetermined	NA
Thiopental	Unlikely	NA
Vecuronium	Undetermined	NA

NA, not available.

Compiled from: Friedman *et al., Obstet Gynecol* 1990; **75**: 594; Briggs *et al.*, 2005; Friedman and Polifka, 2006.

SPECIAL CONSIDERATIONS

Nonobstetric surgery

Nonobstetric surgery is sometimes necessary during pregnancy, and ranges from 1 in 500 to 1 in 635 (Affleck *et al.*, 1999). Maternal mortality nonobstetric surgery is no greater than mortality in the nonpregnant patient. Risks to the fetus from surgery are probably related more to the specific condition requiring the surgery than to the surgery itself. Among 2565 women who underwent surgery during the first or second trimester compared to controls, the frequency of spontaneous abortion in women undergoing surgery with general anesthesia was greater for gynecologic procedures compared to surgery in other anatomic regions (risk ratio of 2 versus 1.54). The frequency of congenital anomalies was not different (Duncan *et al.*, 1986).

Appendicitis is the most common nontrauma indication for nonobstetric surgery during pregnancy, at approximately 1 in 3000 (Affleck *et al.*, 1999), and occurs with equal frequency in all three trimesters (Black, 1960).

Cholecystitis and biliary tract disease are the most common surgical conditions following appendicitis and occur in approximately 1–10 per 10 000 pregnancies (Affleck *et al.*, 1999; Hill *et al.*, 1975). Laparoscopic surgery morbidity and mortality was no different from the open cholecystectomy (Affleck *et al.*, 1999; Barone *et al.*, 1999).

Surgical procedures for intestinal obstruction, inflammatory bowel disease, breast disease, and diseases of the ovary are also relatively common. Surgery for cardiovascular disease during pregnancy is less common, but procedures such as mitral valvotomy (el-Maraghy *et al.*, 1983) valve replacement, and cardiopulmonary bypass (Bernal and Miralles, 1986) have been performed in pregnant women with reasonably good results.

Anesthesia for nonobstetrical surgery may be delivered via either general endotracheal or regional techniques. The choice depends on: (1) procedure to be performed; (2) emergent nature of the procedure; (3) length of time the patient has been fasting; and (4) preferences of the surgeon and the patient. General anesthesia should be accomplished through a balanced technique using nitrous oxide, oxygen, thiopental, succinylcholine, and a halogenated agent. As surgical patients, pregnant women should receive antacid prophylaxis to prevent aspiration pneumonia. The patient should also fast for 10–12 h prior to anticipated surgery, but this may not be possible in all cases (e.g., emergency procedures). Endotracheal intubation with timely extubation when reflexes have returned will help prevent aspiration complications. High-concentration oxygen should be used and hypotension should be avoided in the pregnant surgical patient.

Choice of anesthetic depends on length of the procedure and preference of the anesthesiologist. To prevent maternal hypotension and decreased uteroplacental blood flow, adequate preload with a balanced salt solution is recommended prior to initiation of the actual block. Regional anesthetic techniques have some complications (Box 6.4), but they can be minimized using preventative techniques to decrease the incidence and severity of hypotension from regional blocks (Box 6.5).

Anesthesia for Caesarean section: the uncomplicated patient

Regional anesthesia is the preferred method of anesthesia for the uncomplicated patient undergoing Caesarean section. Subarachnoid (spinal) or epidural block, or a combination, are suitable anesthetic techniques for these patients. The various agents which can

Box 6.4 Complications of regional anesthesia

Subarachnoid block	Total spinal block
Arachnoiditis	
Bladder dysfunction	*Epidural block*
Headaches	Hematoma or infection
Hypotension	Hypotension
Meningitis	Subarachnoid or intravascular injection

From Gilstrap and Hankins, 1988.

Box 6.5 Prevention and treatment of hypotension from regional anesthesia

Positioning
Left lateral position
Left uterine displacement

Preanesthetic hydration
500–1000 cc balanced salt solution

Ephedrine
25–50 mg IM prophylactically
10–15 mg IV for hypotension

From Gilstrap and Hankins, 1988.

Box 6.6 Anesthetic agents for regional anesthesia for Caesarean section

Subarachnoid block
Bupivacaine (Marcaine, spinal), 7.5–10.5 mg
Lidocaine (Xylocaine) 5% in 7.5% glucose, 60–75 mg
Tetracaine (Pontocaine) 1%, 8–10 mg

Epidural block
Bupivacaine (Marcaine) 0.5%
Chloroprocaine (Nesacaine) 2–3%
Lidocaine (Xylocaine) 1–2%

be utilized in these patients are listed in Box 6.6. Hypotension is the most common complication of these techniques and the one that has the greatest impact on the fetus (Box 6.5).

A potentially serious complication resulting from the inadvertent intravascular injection of local anesthetic is central nervous system (CNS) toxicity. Epidural veins are engorged and large during pregnancy, and may be punctured with a needle or catheter. Symptoms of CNS toxicity include: slurred speech, dizziness, metallic taste in the mouth, ringing in the ears, paresthesias of the face, seizures, and syncope. Epinephrine to detect intravascular injection has been discussed. Treatment of CNS toxicity is primarily supportive care: airway and ventilation support, oxygen, prevention and treatment of seizures (thiopental, diazepam), and treatment for hypotension (fluid, ephedrine, and lateral uterine displacement) (Gilstrap and Hankins, 1988).

General anesthesia is used even for uncomplicated Caesarean section. The estimated rate of general anesthesia is 21–26 percent (Shroff *et al.*, 2004). The previously described balanced general technique of nitrous oxide, oxygen, thiopental, succinylcholine and a halogenated agent provides satisfactory anesthesia for uncomplicated Caesarean sections. Patients should be preoxygenated and placed in the lateral position with left lateral uterine displacement. While avoiding hypotension, general anesthesia provides reliable and expeditious anesthesia. Aspiration pneumonitis is the major maternal risk and neonatal cardiorespiratory depression is the major fetal risk. As a precautionary rule, all pregnant women undergoing Caesarean section should be treated as if they have 'full stomachs,' hence the importance of endotracheal intubation.

Anesthesia for Caesarean section: The complicated patient

Many women who require Caesarean section have other medical complications, such as hypertension, diabetes, or heart disease. It is, therefore, imperative for the obstetrician and anesthesiologist to communicate. Importantly, this is the critical path where communication frequently breaks down (Shroff *et al.*, 2004).

Pregnancy-induced hypertension (PIH) occurs among about 5 percent of pregnancies and presents a significant challenge with regard to anesthesia when Caesarean section is required (Lopez-Jaramillo *et al.*, 2005). Severe PIH, blood pressure $\geq 160/110$ mmHg, is associated with several cardiovascular changes, the most important of which is changes in blood volume. Blood volume in women with severe PIH generally does not expand much above the nonpregnant state, unlike the normotensive pregnant woman. Severe PIH patients typically have low colloidal osmotic pressures and 'leaky vessels.' Hence, they are more likely to develop pulmonary edema following the intravenous infusion of crystalloid solutions. A small percentage of women with PIH may also have hematologic abnormalities (thrombocytopenia, hemolytic anemia). Anesthetic choice for Caesarean section in women with severe PIH is controversial. General anesthesia, preferred by some, is not without risk. Significant hypertension may develop during intubation or extubation, with increased risk of cerebral hemorrhage or cardiac failure. Hypertensive response to endotracheal intubation for general anesthesia may be dampened through antihypertensives such as nitroglycerin (Hodgkinson *et al.*, 1980; Snyder *et al.*, 1979). The efficacy and safety of general anesthesia in these patients is shown in one study of 245 cases of eclampsia in which no cases of cerebral hemorrhage, pulmonary edema, or mortality were observed (Pritchard *et al.*, 1984).

Hypotension is a major problem with conduction anesthesia (spinal or epidural), secondary to sympathetic blockade. Hypotension is difficult to treat in women with severe PIH because they may be overly sensitive to pressor agents. Preloading with crystalloid solutions must be done with great caution, being careful to prevent fluid overload in a vasoconstricted but not underfilled vascular tree. The general consensus is that spinal block is contraindicated in women with severe PIH, but many clinicians do advocate epidural anesthesia for these women (Jouppila *et al.*, 1982; Marx, 1974; Moir *et al.*, 1972; Newsome and Branwell, 1984). Careful attention to fluid preload, prevention of hypotension, and test of coagulation status are of paramount importance if epidurals are to be used in these gravidas. Epidural or general anesthesia is effective for women with mild PIH.

Diabetes mellitus complicates approximately 2 percent of pregnancies and many of these women require Caesarean section. When necessary among pregnant diabetics, Caesarean section should be scheduled as the first case in the morning with blood glucose well controlled prior to surgery. General anesthesia or regional techniques (including spinal) may be used. If preload is required for regional techniques, a nondextrose solution should be used to prevent neonatal hypoglycemia.

No single anesthetic technique is ideal for women with heart disease during pregnancy. Anesthetic technique choice will depend on the specific type of heart lesion present and the patient's functional cardiac status (New York Heart Association Classification; Dunselman *et al.*, 1988). Epidural anesthesia is preferred in pregnant women requiring surgery with most varieties of heart disease, and close attention must be paid to preload and hypotension.

General anesthesia is indicated for certain cardiac lesions. Pregnant women with aortic stenosis are at significant risk for hypotension and hypovolemia, and are better served by general anesthesia when Caesarean section is required. Women who have pulmonary hypertension and diminished venous return to the heart are especially at risk for hypotension and hypovolemia. Hence, they do not receive regional anesthesia when surgery is required. For women with recent myocardial infarctions, epidural or general anesthesia is efficacious.

Key references

Affleck DG, Handrahan DL, Egger MJ, Price RR. The laparoscopic management of appendicitis and cholelithiasis during pregnancy. *Am J Surg* 1999; **178**: 523.

Barone JE, Bears S, Chen S *et al.* Outcome study of cholecystectomy during pregnancy. *Am J Surg* 1999; **177**: 232.

Little BB. Pharmacokinetics during pregnancy. Evidence-based maternal dose formulation. *Obstet Gynecol* 1999; **93**: 858–68.

Lopez-Jaramillo P, Garcia RG, Lopez M. Preventing pregnancy-induced hypertension. Are there regional differences for this global problem? *J Hypertens* 2005; **23**: 1121.

Shroff R, Thompson ACD, McCrum A, Rees SGO. Prospective multidisciplinary general anesthesia in a district general hospital. *J Obstet Gynaecol* 2004; **24**: 641.

Further references are available on the book's website at http://www.drugsandpregnancy.com

7

Antineoplastic drugs during pregnancy

Cancer is uncommon during pregnancy and occurs in approximately one in 1000–6000 pregnant women (Haas, 1984; Kennedy *et al.*, 1993; Pepe *et al.*, 1989). It can be estimated that one in 118 women with cancer will be pregnant, because 12.8 percent of all cancers in women occur in the 15–44 age group (Third National Cancer Survey, 1975). Population- and hospital-based studies show that the most frequently occurring cancers that present during pregnancy are cervix, breast, and ovary (Haas, 1984; Pepe *et al.*, 1989). The frequencies of nongenital-type cancers during pregnancy are shown in Table 7.1. The frequencies of the various forms of genital cancers in pregnancy are shown in Table 7.2, with cervical cancer being the most common.

Table 7.1 Frequencies of nongenital cancers in pregnancy

Malignancy type	Incidence (per number of gestations)	Source
Malignant melanoma	1:1000–10 000	Pavlidis (2002)
Breast carcinoma	1:3000–1:10 000	
Lymphoma	1:1000–1:6000	
Leukemia	1:75 000–1:100 000	
Colon cancer	1:13 000	
Hodgkin's lymphoma	1 in 6000	Others, see below
Non-Hodgkin's lymphomas	Extremely rare (< 1 in 100 000)	
Acute leukemia	1 in 75 000 to 1 in 100 000	
Gastrointestinal (colon, gastric, pancreatic, carcinoid, hepatic)		Up to 1 in 10 000
Renal cell	Rare	
Thyroid	Rare	

Compiled from Pavlidis, 2002 and others (Donegan, 1983, 1986; Koren *et al.*, 1990; McLain, 1974; Orr and Shingleton, 1983; Parente *et al.*, 1988; Smith and Randal, 1969; Yazigi and Cunningham, 1990).

Table 7.2 Frequency of genital cancers in pregnancy

Type	Frequency	
Cervix		
Carcinoma *in situ*	1.3 in 1000 to 1 in 770	Others
Carcinoma of the cervix	1:2000–10 000	Pavlidis, 2002
Invasive carcinoma	0.5 in 1000 to 1 in 2200	Others
Ovarian	1 in 18 000 to 1 in 25 000	Others
Ovarian carcinoma	1:10 000–1:100 000	Pavlidis, 2002

Data compiled from Pavlidis, 2002 and Others (Chung and Birnbaum, 1973; Hacker *et al.*, 1982; Munnell, 1963; Yazigi and Cunningham, 1990).

When cancer is present during pregnancy, several dilemmas arise. Perhaps most important is whether the pregnancy should be continued or terminated. Several factors must be considered in this discussion: (1) the gestational age of the pregnancy; (2) the patient's desire to continue the pregnancy; (3) whether pregnancy *per se* affects the cancerous progression; and (4) the ultimate prognosis for the mother and infant. In general, pregnancies close to viability (i.e., 24–28 weeks gestation) may be continued with mild to moderate adverse effects on the fetus. Of the various therapeutic modalities available, none are known to be safe for use during pregnancy. Some patients with pregnancies less than 24 weeks gestational age may best be managed by pregnancy termination. Decisions regarding pregnancy termination between 24 and 28 weeks are more difficult. Management is most often dependent upon the patient's wishes, as well as the type and stage of the woman's cancer.

Available data suggest that pregnancy affects neither the progression nor prognosis for most cancers; the exception to this is the critical period of neural plate development (10–18 days postconception). However, pregnancy may interfere with the diagnostic procedures for some types of malignancies.

The pharmacokinetics of neoplastics is poorly studied, with only sufficient information to speculate on the effects of pregnancy on metabolism and clearance of cyclophosphamide. Of the five cytochrome P-450 enzymes that metabolize cyclophosphamide (Matalon *et al.*, 2004), the activity of one, CYP3A4 (Little, 1999), is significantly increased during pregnancy. This implies that dose size or dose frequency should be adjusted for pregnant women by monitoring levels, and adjusting these parameters to maintain therapeutic levels.

A major consideration in treating cancer during pregnancy is finding the optimal regimen. This must include consideration of: (1) the effects of diagnostic tests; (2) surgical procedures; (3) radiotherapy; and (4) chemotherapy (Gilstrap and Cunningham, 1996; Koren *et al.*, 1990; Yazigi and Cunningham, 1990). It is important to minimize the amount of fetal exposure to ionizing radiation. Many diagnostic tests can be performed safely during pregnancy because most diagnostic X-ray procedures expose the fetus to low doses of radiation, i.e., less than 1 rad per procedure; this holds true even for pelvic neoplasms. General 'rule of thumb' suggests that a fetal or embryonic radiation exposure of less than 5 'skin' rads is associated with little to no risk – the exception to this is the critical period of neural plate development (days 10–18 postconception) – with the threshold for significant risk being as high as 15–20 'skin' rads (Brent, 1987). Skin rads are the amount of radiation delivered to the mother's skin surface. Thus, procedures such as barium enemas, pyelography, chest films, and nonpelvic computerized tomography can be safely performed if deemed necessary during the initial diagnosis of malignancies during pregnancy. Other diagnostic modalities, such as magnetic resonance imaging and ultrasonography, can often provide the same diagnostic information as X-ray studies and carry no known risk to the fetus or embryo. Until the end of the second trimester, diagnostic techniques such as cystoscopy and sigmoidoscopy may be performed safely (Pentheroudakis and Pavlidis, 2006).

Most surgical oncology techniques can be used during pregnancy to treat life-threatening disease, especially if they do not involve the pelvis or pelvic organs (Miller and Bloss, 1995). Ovaries can generally be removed after 10 weeks gestational age (8 weeks postconception) without apparent adverse effects on pregnancy. However, progestational agents should be utilized if oophorectomy is necessary prior to this time (Gilstrap and Cunningham, 1996; Pentheroudakis and Pavlidis, 2006; Yazigi and Cunningham, 1990).

Most antineoplastic agents employed in chemotherapy have the capability to interfere with normal cell growth (hyperplasia, hypertrophy, and migration) in the embryo. Thus they are potentially teratogenic and may cause fetal growth retardation and congenital abnormalities. In one review of 163 pregnancies exposed to antineoplastic drugs in the first trimester, the frequency of congenital anomalies was 25 percent for polytherapy chemotherapeutic regimens and 17 percent for single-agent exposure (Doll *et al.*, 1989) (Table 7.3).

Table 7.3 Frequency of congenital anomalies associated with first-trimester use of chemotherapy

Class	Congenital anomalies (%)
Alkylating agents	6 in 44 (14)
Antimetabolites[a]	15 in 77 (19)
Plant alkaloids	1 in 14 (7)
Other	
Amsacrine	
Cisplatin	
Daunorubicin	
Procarbazine	
Total	24 in 139 (17%)

[a]13 (24%) exposed to aminopterin or methotrexate.
Compiled from Doll *et al.*, 1989.

The frequency of malformations in 131 pregnancies with second-trimester exposure was 1.5 percent, below the background risk for the human population (Doll *et al.*, 1988). Hence it would be expected that exposures to antineoplastic agents after the period of embryogenesis (second and third trimesters of pregnancy) carry little risk to the fetus other than fetal growth retardation (Gilstrap and Cunningham, 1996; Yazigi and Cunningham, 1990). Potential immediate fetal and neonatal effects are summarized in Box 7.1.

Box 7.1 Potential immediate effects of chemotherapeutic agents on the fetus and newborn

Spontaneous abortion

Teratogenic effects

Organ toxicity

Premature birth

Growth retardation

Adapted from Doll et al., 1989.

Box 7.2 Potential long-term or delayed effects of antineoplastic agents on the neonate

Carcinogenesis

Sterility

Growth retardation

Developmental retardation

Mutation

Teratogenic in future offspring

Adapted from Doll et al., 1989.

Antineoplastic agents may also have long-term or delayed effects, such as sterility or carcinogenesis for the child exposed prenatally (Box 7.2). For the benefit of the patient, some treatments (for example, for acute leukemia) should begin as soon as the diagnosis is made, including the first trimester (Koren et al., 1990).

Finally, there is a risk to the fetus from spread of the maternal cancer by transplacental metastasis. It is well documented that certain cancers may spread to the developing fetus, yielding a grave fetal prognosis (Read and Platzer, 1981). Malignant melanoma is the most common cancer to metastasize to the fetus and placenta (Anderson et al., 1989; Eltorky et al., 1995; Read and Platzer, 1981).

Management and treatment of specific types of cancers are discussed under Special Considerations below. Specific chemotherapeutic agents, considered below, can be divided into several classes: alkylating agents, antibiotics, antimetabolites, plant alkaloids, and miscellaneous (Boice, 1986). Antineoplastic agents can also be classified as cycle-specific and cycle-nonspecific agents. Cycle-specific agents (antimetabolites, antibiotics, and plant alkaloids) arrest cell division only during specific phases of the replication cycle. In contrast, cycle-nonspecific agents (alkylating agents) are cytotoxic during all phases of cell replication (Caliguri and Mayer, 1989).

ALKYLATING AGENTS

A number of alkylating agents are available (Box 7.3). These agents act by transferring alkyl groups to such biological substrates as nucleic acids and proteins. Alkyl groups

Box 7.3 The alkylating agents

Busulfan (Myleran)

Cyclophosphamide (Cytoxan, Neosar)

Chlorambucil (Leukeran)

Mechlorethamine (Mustargen)

Melphalan (Alkeran)

Triethylene thiophosphoramide (Thiotepa)

Carmustine (BCNU)

block replication of DNA via the cross-linking bioactive molecules (i.e., polymerases) needed for cell division.

Busulfan

Busulfan (Myleran) is Food and Drug Administration (FDA)-approved for the palliative treatment of chronic myelogenous leukemia, and is the primary treatment for acute non-lymphacytic leukemia. Summary of 16 different reports of 22 infants born to busulfan-exposed patients found two infants with major congenital anomalies (2/22, 9.1 percent) (Doll *et al.*, 1989). Subsequent reports of two exposed pregnancies resulted in normal neonates (Norhaya *et al.*, 1994; Shalev *et al.*, 1987). They also reported that six (14 percent) of 44 infants born to women who received an alkylating agent (30 different reports) had major congenital anomalies. Experimental animal studies also report an increased frequency of congenital anomalies with exposure to busulfan during gestation.

Cyclophosphamide

Cyclophosphamide (Cytoxan and Neosar) is biotransformed principally in the liver to active alkylating metabolites that cause crosslinking of tumor cell DNA. It is FDA-approved for treatment of a variety of cancers: (1) certain forms of acute and chronic leukemia; (2) ovarian; (3) multiple myeloma; (4) mycosis fungoides; and (5) breast carcinoma. This drug is also used to treat cancers of the bladder, cervix, colorectum, endometrium, Ewing's sarcoma, head and neck, lymphomas, kidney, lung, osteosarcoma, pancreas, and trophoblastic tumors. In addition, cyclophosphamide is efficacious in combination with other agents for the treatment of Ewing's sarcoma, lymphomas, osteosarcoma, and trophoblastic tumors. Several studies of cyclophosphamide metabolism in *in vitro* cultures with rat embryos showed that the compound must be bioactivated by a monofunctional liver oxygenase system in order to be teratogenic (Fantel *et al.*, 1979; Kitchen *et al.*, 1981; Mirkes *et al.*, 1981, 1985). The morphologic changes found *in vitro* were very similar to those seen *in vivo* (Greenway *et al.*, 1982), suggesting cyclophosphamide metabolites are the teratogenic agents (Mirkes *et al.*, 1985).

According to Mirkes *et al.* (1985), cyclophosphamide is 'one of the best studied teratogens'. There is no doubt that this agent produces skeletal and central nervous system anomalies in rats (Chaube *et al.*, 1968), mice (Gibson and Becker, 1968), rabbits (Fritz and Hess, 1971), and monkeys (McClure *et al.*, 1979). Available human data are minimal and include three case reports and one case series. A set of twins comprising one normal infant and one malformed twin exposed *in utero* was reported. The malformed twin had multiple congenital abnormalities and subsequently developed thyroid cancer and neuroblastoma (Zemlickis *et al.*, 1993). In another case report, a fetus with multiple anomalies (cleft palate, absent thumbs, and multiple eye defects) was born to a mother who was treated with cyclophosphamide in the first trimester (Kirshon *et al.*, 1988). A growth-retarded infant with bilateral absence of the big toe, cleft palate, and hypoplasia of the fifth digit was born to a mother who received cyclophosphamide throughout pregnancy (Greenberg and Tanaka, 1964). No ill effects have been reported in association with second and third trimester exposure to cyclophosphamide (Matalon *et al.*, 2004). Ten normal infants were reported following cyclophosphamide therapy during the first trimester (Blatt *et al.*, 1980).

Hematologic abnormalities, such as pancytopenia, were reported in infants whose mothers were treated with cyclophosphamide and other agents during pregnancy (Pizzuto *et al.*, 1980), but not all neonates exhibited such effects, even when their mothers developed severe pancytopenia (Meador *et al.*, 1987). The use of multiple agents seems more likely to be associated with pancytopenia in the fetus and newborn than does monotherapy.

Chlorambucil

Chlorambucil (Leukeran) is an oral bifunctional alkylating agent, nitrogen mustard type, FDA-approved to treat chronic leukemia and lymphomas. It is also used to treat breast, trophoblastic, and ovarian carcinomas. Several case reports of possible association of this agent with unilateral renal agenesis in the human have been published (Shotton and Monie, 1963; Steege and Caldwell, 1980), but no causal inference can be made. No epidemiological studies have been published. One of five fetuses exposed in the first trimester had a congenital anomaly (Doll *et al.*, 1989). Central nervous system anomalies, postcranial skeleton, and palatal closure were increased in frequency among rodents whose mothers were given large doses of chlorambucil during pregnancy (Chaube and Murphy, 1968; Mirkes and Greenaway, 1982; Monie, 1961).

Ifosfamide

Ifosfamide (Ifex) is a chemotherapeutic agent, chemically related to nitrogen mustards and a synthetic analog of cyclophosphamide, which requires metabolic activation by microsomal liver enzymes to produce biologically active metabolites. The mechanism of action is typical for alkylating agents and is mediated by formation of DNA adducts. Ifosfamide is particularly toxic to the urinary epithelium and must be given with mesna (Mesnex, Uromitexan). It is FDA-approved as third-line chemotherapy of germ cell testicular cancer. It is also used to treat acute leukemias and lung, pancreas, breast, cervix and endometrium cancers, as well as Ewing's sarcomas, lymphomas, osteosarcoma, soft tissue sarcoma, and ovarian cancer. No epidemiologic studies have been published of congenital anomalies in fetuses whose mothers used this agent during pregnancy. To date there are two case reports of fetuses exposed *in utero* to ifosfamide-containing combination chemotherapy, of which one developed oligohydramnios (Barrenetexa *et al.*, 1995; Fernandez *et al.*, 1989). The manufacturer reports that embryotoxic and teratogenic effects have been observed in mice, rats, and rabbits.

Mechlorethamine

Another alkylating agent, mechlorethamine (Mustargen), is an FDA-approved treatment for Hodgkin's disease, polycythema vera, mycosis fungoides, chronic leukemia, lymphomas, and carcinoma of the lung. It is also used to treat brain, breast, and ovarian cancers. Two case reports of congenital anomalies after first-trimester combination chemotherapy (Garrett, 1974; Mennuti *et al.*, 1975) are published, but no epidemiological studies of the use of this agent during pregnancy have been published. Chemotherapy with mechlorethamine and other drugs that were discontinued prior to conception did not increase the frequency of congenital anomalies among more than 40 infants above the 3.5–5 percent background rate expected in the general population (Andrieu and Ochoa-Molina, 1983; Schilsky *et al.*, 1981; Whitehead *et al.*, 1983). However, this is probably unrelated to use of this drug during pregnancy. No birth defects were reported among the children of 12 women treated with mechlorethamine and other antineoplastic agents during pregnancy in one series (Aviles *et al.*, 1991; Aviles and Neri, 2001), but the significance of these findings is unknown because most exposures were outside the first trimester.

Increased frequencies of congenital anomalies were found among the offspring of pregnant rodents that were given mechlorethamine in doses several times those normally used in humans (Beck *et al.*, 1976; Gottschewski, 1964; Murphy *et al.*, 1957; Nishimura and Takagaki, 1959).

Somatic chromosome breaks have been observed among embryos of pregnant animals who received this agent during gestation (Soukup *et al.*, 1967). The relevance of this finding to human reproduction is unknown because gonadal cell lines were not analyzed.

Melphalan

Melphalan (Alkeran) is a phenylalanine derivative of nitrogen mustard. It is a bifunctional alkylating agent, FDA-approved to treat multiple myeloma, ovarian, and breast carcinomas. It is also used for treatment of chronic myelocytic leukemia, melanoma, osteosarcoma, soft tissue sarcoma, and thyroid cancers. The manufacturer reports that oral melphalan is teratogenic and embryolethal in animals. Although there are no studies of the use of this drug during pregnancy in humans, its strong mutagenic and cytotoxic actions suggest that it is a likely human teratogen and should be avoided during pregnancy.

Triethylene thiophosphoramide

The alkylating agent triethylene (Thiotepa) is FDA-approved for the treatment of ovarian, bladder and breast carcinomas, and malignant effusions. As with most antineoplastics, no epidemiological studies have been published of pregnancy outcome after the use of this agent during human pregnancy. None of four fetuses exposed in the first trimester developed malformations (Doll *et al.*, 1989). One case was reported of fetal growth retardation associated with use of the drug in the latter half of pregnancy (Stevens and Fisher, 1965). An increased frequency of congenital anomalies and growth stunting was reported among the offspring of pregnant rodents that received this agent during pregnancy (Korogodina and Kaurov, 1984; Murphy *et al.*, 1958; Tanimura, 1968).

Carmustine

Carmustine (BCNU) is an alkylating agent, FDA-approved for chemotherapy of a variety of neoplasms including multiple myeloma, lymphomas, and brain tumors. A patient received carmustine throughout pregnancy and delivered a normal neonate (Schapira and Chudley, 1984). Carmustine must be suspected of being teratogenic because of its biochemical action (an alkylating agent). Rodents exposed to carmustine at several times the usual human dose during embryogenesis had increased frequency of birth defects (Wong and Wells, 1989). Otherwise, little information is published about the use of this agent during pregnancy in humans or animals.

Antimetabolites

Antimetabolites can be divided into three groups: folate antagonists, purine antagonists, and pyrimidine antagonists (Box 7.4). One of the original antimetabolites is the folate antagonist aminopterin. This antineoplastic agent was previously used as an abortifacient, but is no longer widely used as an antineoplastic or abortifacient. It is a well-known teratogen, causing the fetal aminopterin syndrome. This finding is relevant to other folate antagonist antineoplastics that are commonly used.

Box 7.4 The antimetabolites

Folate antagonist
Methotrexate (Folex, Mexate)

Purine antagonist
Mercaptopurine (Purinethol)
Thioguanine (Thioguanine)

Pyrimidine antagonist
Cytarabine (Cytosar)
Fluorouracil (Efudex, Fluoroplex)

Aminopterin/methylaminopterin

A variety of congenital anomalies was observed among infants and children whose mothers used aminopterin or methylaminopterin throughout pregnancy, including short stature, craniosynostosis, hydrocephalus, micrognathia, hypertelorism, limb anomalies, and neural tube defects (Char, 1979; Reich *et al.*, 1977; Thiersch, 1952; Thiersch and Phillips, 1950; Warkany, 1978). The precise risk of congenital anomalies following maternal exposure to this agent is unknown but is likely high (Warkany, 1978).

Malformations of the skull, face, eye, and abdominal wall were described among rodents born to mothers that were administered large doses of the aminopterin during pregnancy (Baranov, 1966; Puchkov, 1967). Even at doses lower than those used in humans, malformations were observed in rabbits (Goeringer and DeSesso, 1990). Fetal death occurred in another rat study (Thiersch and Phillips, 1950). As a group, folate antagonists appear to carry a substantially higher risk of congenital anomalies than other antineoplastic agents. Therefore, folate antagonists are uniformly contraindicated for use during pregnancy (Doll *et al.*, 1989).

Methotrexate

The folate antagonist methotrexate (Folex, Mexate) inhibits dihydrofolic acid reductase, interrupting DNA synthesis, repair, and cellular replication, including trophoblastic cells. It is used to treat a number of neoplasms, including acute leukemia, lymphoma, trophoblastic tumors, and carcinomas of the breast, cervix, ovary, bladder, kidney, prostate, lung, and testicles. It is also used to treat nonneoplastic diseases: rheumatoid arthritis, psoriasis, and ectopic pregnancy. Methotrexate is particularly toxic to trophoblastic cells and is used frequently as an abortifacient. It has been used successfully to treat ectopic pregnancies (Grainger and Seifer, 1995; Schink, 1995) and to induce abortion (Hausknecht, 1995).

Methotrexate is associated with a pattern of malformations similar to those in the aminopterin syndrome (Warkany, 1978). Congenital anomalies among more than a dozen children with first-trimester exposure to this agent included skeletal defects, ocular hypertelorism, and craniosynostosis (Adam *et al.*, 2003; Chapa *et al.*, 2003; Diniz *et al.*, 1978; Milunsky *et al.*, 1968; Nguyen *et al.*, 2002; Powell and Ekert, 1971; Sosa-Munoz *et al.*, 1983; Wheeler *et al.*, 2002; Zand *et al.*, 2003). The frequency of malformations seems to be dose-related, but some investigators speculate that the risk of congenital anomalies is lower than for aminopterin (Kozlowski *et al.*, 1990; Roubenoff *et al.*, 1988). The frequency of birth defects was not increased among the offspring of over 350 women who received methotrexate prior to conception (Rustin *et al.*, 1984; Van Thiel *et al.*, 1970). However, this finding is entirely irrelevant to exposure during embryogenesis or other times in pregnancy. Congenital anomalies were increased in frequency among the offspring of rodents given this folate antagonist during pregnancy (Darab *et al.*, 1987; Jordan *et al.*, 1977; Skalko and Gold, 1974; Wilson *et al.*, 1979).

Mercaptopurine

Mercaptopurine (Purinethol, 6-MP), a purine antagonist, is FDA-approved primarily for the treatment of acute leukemias. It is also used in the treatment of lymphomas. Although there are two published case reports of a possible association of congenital anomalies with the use of this agent during early pregnancy (Diamond *et al.*, 1960; Sosa-Munoz *et al.*, 1983), no controlled studies involving human pregnancies have been published. In a review of 12 case reports (Doll *et al.*, 1989) of 20 infants born to women given this agent during pregnancy, none had congenital anomalies (Perucca *et al.*, 1995). Among 34 infants born to women who were treated with mercaptopurine early in pregnancy, one infant had a birth defect (1/34, 2.9 percent), which does not seem unusually high compared to background risk (3.5 percent) (Francella *et al.*, 2003). In addition, the one birth defect was probably not related to the drug as the neonate had a chromosomal aberration. Infants of eight women treated with mercaptopurine and other antineoplastic agents during pregnancy had no congenital anomalies (Aviles *et al.*, 1991). Mercaptopurine is often a component of polydrug regimens, making it impossible to assess the teratogenic potential of an individual agent. This agent was associated with neonatal pancytopenia in several case reports (McConnell and Bhoola, 1973; Okun *et al.*, 1979; Pizzuto *et al.*, 1980), but most instances involved a polydrug regimen. Congenital anomalies (limb, facial, and central nervous system) were increased in frequency among rodents whose mothers were given up to several times the usual human dose of mercaptopurine during gestation (Mercier-Parot and Tuchmann-Duplessis, 1967; Puget *et al.*, 1975; Shah and Burdett, 1976).

Thioguanine

Another purine antagonist, thioguanine (Tabloid), is FDA-approved for the treatment of acute nonlymphocytic leukemia. It was part of a multiple drug regimen to which a fetus was exposed in the first trimester and it had multiple abnormalities similar to Baller–Gerald syndrome (Artlich *et al.*, 1994). An increased frequency of malformations was found in offspring of pregnant rats that were given thioguanine during embryogenesis (Thiersch, 1957).

Cytarabine

Cytarabine (cytosine arabinoside) (Cytosar-U, Ara-C, Tarabine) is a pyrimidine antagonist antimetabolite that inhibits DNA polymerase. It is approved for the treatment of leukemia (acute and chronic). It is also used against lymphomas. A few reports of monotherapy with this agent during early pregnancy have been published. Wagner and associates (1980) reported a newborn with limb and ear anomalies whose mother received this agent alone. In a review of leukemia treatment during pregnancy, 46 infants (summarized from 24 case reports) were born to mothers who received cytosine arabinoside (Ara-C) at some point during pregnancy, and several had received it during the first trimester (Caliguri and Mayer, 1989). Among exposed pregnancies, there were two spontaneous and six therapeutic abortions. Of the remaining 38 pregnancies, there were four intrauterine deaths (apparently grossly normal), one infant with polydactyly and one with adherence of the iris to the cornea; one newborn presented with neonatal pancytopenia (Caliguri and Mayer, 1989). Anecdotal reports seem to indicate an increased risk of birth defects following first trimester exposure to cytarabine, this kind of information cannot be used to attribute risk. However, this suspicion is bolstered by findings in experimental animal studies parallel to those in humans. In addition, it seems that treatment of leukemia during pregnancy given after the first trimester is not associated with a high frequency of congenital abnormalities. It is important to note that the folate antagonist methotrexate was a component of the polydrug therapy in several of these gravidas.

When given during embryogenesis, cytarabine was associated with an increased frequency of congenital anomalies in two rodent teratology studies (Chaube and Murphy, 1965; Percy, 1975).

Fluorouracil

Fluorouracil (Adrucil, 5-FU, Efudex, Fluoroplex) is a fluorinated pyrimidine analog that inhibits thymidine formation and blocks DNA and protein synthesis. Its FDA-approved indications are colon, rectum, breast, stomach, and pancreas neoplasms. Other uses include bladder, cervix, endometrium, esophagus, head and neck, liver, lung, ovary, prostate, and skin cancers.

Among 24 infants whose mothers were treated with intravenous fluorouracil in combination with doxorubicin and cyclophosphamide for breast cancer during the second and third trimesters of pregnancy, no congenital anomalies occurred (Berry *et al.*, 1999). However, it must be noted that these exposures occurred outside the period of embryogenesis, and do not indicate anything about the risk of birth defects that may be related to first trimester exposure to the drug. Multiple congenital anomalies in an abortus of a mother with colon malignancy who had received 5-fluorouracil during 11 and 12 weeks of gestation (9–10 weeks postconception) (600 mg IV five times weekly) has been reported (Stephens *et al.*, 1980). However, the patient had also undergone bowel resection and multiple diagnostic X-ray procedures during late embryogenesis. Malformations included bilateral radial aplasia, absent thumbs, abnormal fingers, a single umbilical artery, hypoplastic aorta, and esophageal atresia, imperforate anus, and renal dysplasia. These anomalies were probably not related to fluorouracil because of the gestational timing of the exposure (i.e., exposure occurred outside the period of morphogenesis of these organs).

Two normal infants were born following first-trimester maternal treatment with intravaginal 5-fluorouracil (Odom *et al.*, 1990), which is known to be absorbed systemically by this route (Markman, 1985). Skeletal and other major anomalies (cleft palate, central nervous system) were increased in frequency among offspring of several species of pregnant nonprimate animals born to mothers exposed to this antineoplastic during pregnancy (Chaube and Murphy, 1968; Dagg, 1960; Shah and Mackay, 1978; Wilson *et al.*, 1979).

ANTIBIOTICS

These agents work through a variety of mechanisms, including alkylation and induction of DNA breakage to prevent DNA replication in neoplasias and other cells (Box 7.5).

Box 7.5 The antibiotic antineoplastic agents

Anthracyclines	*Other*
Daunorubicin (Cerubidine)	Bleomycin (Blenoxane)
Doxorubicin (Adriamycin)	Dactinomycin[a] (Cosmegen)
	Mitomycin (Mutamycin)

[a]Also known as actinomycin-D.

Bleomycin

Bleomycin (Blenoxane) inhibits DNA and, to a lesser extent, RNA and other protein synthesis. The drug is FDA-approved to treat a variety of carcinomas (renal, cervical, penile, testicular, vulvar, and neck), lymphomas, and sarcomas. No reports regarding the use of bleomycin monotherapy during organogenesis have been published. Reports of bleomycin polytherapy (Christman *et al.*, 1990; Kim *et al.*, 1989) reported two normal infants following maternal therapy for a malignant ovarian germ cell tumor during the second trimester with bleomycin in combination with cisplatin and vinblastine. Other reports are of second-trimester exposure (Nantel *et al.*, 1990; Rodriguez and Haggag, 1995) to bleomycin-containing combinations for maternal lymphoma with normal infants. One newborn infant had profound but transient neonatal leukopenia (resolved by day of life 13) following maternal therapy for metastatic adenocarcinoma that was initiated very early in the third trimester with bleomycin in combination with etoposide and cisplatin (Raffles *et al.*, 1989). Limb and tail anomalies were reported in nine rat teratology studies involving bleomycin (Nishimura and Tanimura, 1976).

Dactinomycin

Dactinomycin (Cosmegen), also known as actinomycin-D, is one of a group of antibiotics produced by various species of streptomyces called the actinomycins. It is FDA-approved to treat choriocarcinoma, Ewing's and Wilms' tumors, rhabdomyosarcoma, and cancers of the testis and uterus. Primary indication for dactinomycin in obstetrics is to treat gestational trophoblastic tumors.

No studies are available regarding dactinomycin use during pregnancy, but it is an FDA category C drug. Four normal infants (one set of twins) were born to mothers who received dactinomycin in the second and/or third trimesters of pregnancy as part of combination therapy in two pregnancies (Gililland and Weinstein, 1983), but there was no exposure during embryogenesis. The manufacturer of dactinomycin reported that malformations were increased in frequency in various animals whose mothers were given doses of the drug several times those normally used in humans, but the information is unpublished and no details were provided.

Mitomycin

Mitomycin (Mitomycin-C) is an antibiotic with antitumor activity that acts by blocking DNA synthesis. It is isolated from the broth of *Streptomyces caespitosus*, similar to dactinomycin. It is FDA-approved as part of combination therapy for pancreatic and stomach cancers. Occasionally, it is used to treat hypercalcemia secondary to malignancy.

No reports have been published regarding the use of mitomycin during pregnancy and infant outcome. Congenital anomalies were increased in several mouse teratology studies that employed several times the usual human therapeutic dose of the drug during pregnancy (Friji and Nahatsuka, 1983; Gregg and Snow, 1983; Snow and Tam, 1979). In an experimental animal model, approximately 6 percent of mitomycin crossed the placenta in pregnant rats (Boike *et al.*, 1989). One investigator conducted embryo studies in mice that suggest that as early as the four-cell embryo stage, mitomycin has a genetic imprinting effect acting at the proliferative DNA level (Snow, personal communication).

Anthracycline antibiotics

Anthracycline antibiotic antineoplastics (daunorubicin or Cerubidine; doxorubicin or Adriamycin, Rubex) are potent inhibitors of nucleic acid synthesis and are nonspecific cell cycle-phase agents. Daunorubicin is FDA-approved for neuroblastoma and acute leukemias. Doxorubicin is FDA-approved for acute leukemias, lymphomas, Wilms' tumor, and sarcomas, as well as a variety of carcinomas (bladder, breast, ovary, gastric, thyroid, and small-cell cancers).

No studies are available of either of these agents during pregnancy, but there are a number of case reports. In reviews from 18 reports of 28 pregnancies that were exposed to one of the anthracyclines at various stages of gestation, eight of the pregnancies were at 16 weeks' gestational age or less at exposure. All but one received polytherapy chemotherapy. There were 24 normal infants (one set of twins), two spontaneous abortions, one therapeutic abortion, and two fetal deaths (Turchi and Villasis, 1988; Wiebe and Sipila, 1994). Fetal deaths were secondary to maternal deaths. One infant was reported with multiple abnormalities, similar to Baller–Gerold syndrome; was exposed *in utero* at conception to combination therapy containing doxorubicin and daunorubicin (Artlich *et al.*, 1994). Among 43 infants published in 26 reports, the frequency of birth defects was not increased, with two malformed infants (Friedman and Polifka, 2006).

The cytotoxic nature of these drugs suggests that embryonic exposure may not be without risk, depending upon the timing of the exposure. Adverse fetal effects do appear to be appreciably increased. The manufacturer of daunorubicin reported multiple defects in rabbits; prematurity and low birth weight was found in mice exposed to the drug *in utero*, but this information has not been published. Published data indicate increased frequencies of birth defects (heart, digestive system, eye, genitourinary (GU) defects) in rats, but not rabbits.

PLANT ALKALOIDS

Vinblastine (Velban) and vincristine (Oncovin) are antimitotic *Vinca* alkaloids and they act through inhibition of microtubule formation, and this produces arrest of the cell cycle in metaphase (Box 7.6). The mechanism of action of etoposide is probably similar.

Box 7.6 The plant alkaloid antineoplastics

Vinblastine (Velban, Velsar)
Vincristine (Oncovin, Vincasar, Vincrex)
Etoposide (VePesid)

Vinblastine

Vinblastine (Velban, Velsar) is FDA-approved to treat lymphoma, Hodgkin's disease, chronic myelocytic leukemia, and several carcinomas: breast, bladder, lung, and testis (Jacobs *et al.*, 1981). A review from five separate reports of pregnant women with Hodgkin's disease gave details of 13 normal infants following maternal vinblastine therapy. Eleven of these infants had first-trimester exposure and two had second-trimester exposure. Among the offspring of five pregnant women who used vinblastine during the first trimester, congenital anomalies were observed in two infants, there was one spontaneous abortion and two normal neonates (Metz *et al.*, 1989). No anomalies were reported in 27 infants, 17 of whom were exposed during the first trimester (Aviles and Neri, 2001; Wiebe and Sipila, 1994). One normal infant was reported who was exposed following maternal vinblastine, bleomycin, and cisplatin therapy for a malignant teratoma during the second trimester (Christman *et al.*, 1990). It should be noted that there is considerable overlap in the published reports included in the different reviews. Vinblastine was associated with an increased frequency of congenital anomalies in rats, mice, hamsters, and rabbits exposed during embryogenesis.

Vincristine (Oncovin)

Vincristine is FDA-approved to treat leukemia (acute and chronic), lymphomas, Hodgkin's disease, neuroblastoma, rhabdomyosarcoma, and Wilms' tumor. It is also used to treat melanoma, trophoblastic tumors, and some carcinomas (breast, cervical, ovarian, and lung). The cytotoxic nature of vincristine suggests high potential to cause birth defects in exposed embryos, although no published studies document this. Among 35 infants born to women who received vincristine as part of polydrug antineoplastic regimens at various stages of gestation, there were two spontaneous and three therapeutic abortions, two intrauterine deaths (without anomalies), and 29 live-born infants with no gross anomalies (Caliguri and Mayer, 1989). It is important to note that only 11 of 29 infants were exposed to vincristine in the first trimester, and none were malformed. However, all vincristine-polytherapy-exposed newborns had significant transient pancytopenia, and one infant had polydactyly (most probably not drug-related). Among 31 infants exposed to antineoplastic agents during gestation in another review, two major birth defects occurred among those exposed to vincristine polytherapy regimens (Wiebe and Sipila, 1994). Of five infants born to women who sustained exposure to the drug during the first trimester, one had a major congenital anomaly (Metz et al., 1989). Vincristine and vinblastine were associated with an increased frequency of congenital anomalies in nonhuman primates and in rat studies (Courtney and Valenio, 1968; Demeyer, 1964, 1965).

Etoposide

Etoposide (VePesid, VP-16VPP) is a semisynthetic derivative of podophyllotoxin that inhibits DNA synthesis. Its related sister molecule, podophyllum, is used to treat condylomas. It is approved for use against testicular and small-cell lung cancer. Acute leukemia, lymphomas, gestational trophoblastic tumors, and a variety of carcinomas are also treated with etoposide. No anomalies were reported in one infant exposed whose mother was treated with an etoposide-containing polytherapy during pregnancy (Rodriguez and Haggag, 1995). One infant was born with cerebral atrophy following first trimester exposure to etoposide (Elit et al., 1999), but 16 infants in other case reports were found to have no congenital anomalies. According to the manufacturer of the drug, this agent was teratogenic in animals, but these studies have not been subjected to peer review.

MISCELLANEOUS AGENTS

Other antineoplastic agents that do not belong to the categories previously discussed are classified as miscellaneous in this text (Box 7.7).

Asparaginase

Asparaginase (Elspar) contains the enzyme L-asparagine amidohydrolase (derived from *Escherichia coli*), and is FDA-approved to treat acute lymphocytic leukemia. Occasionally, this agent is used to treat chronic leukemias and lymphomas. The mode of action is thought

---

Box 7.7 Miscellaneous antineoplastic agents

Asparaginase (Elspar)	Hydroxyurea (Hydrea)
Altretamine (Hexalen)	Paclitaxel (Taxol)
Cisplatin (Platinol)	Procarbazine (Matulane)

to be asparagine catabolism. No studies have been published regarding use of this drug during the first trimester of pregnancy. Treatment during the second and third trimesters was associated with pancytopenia. It is classified as FDA fetal risk category C. In a review of seven infants whose mothers were given L-asparaginase as part of polydrug therapy for leukemia, all were live-born and none had congenital anomalies (Caliguri and Mayer, 1989). Importantly, only one of these infants was exposed to the drug during the first trimester.

Asparaginase was associated with an increased frequency of congenital anomalies in the offspring of pregnant rats, rabbits, and mice (Adamson and Fabro, 1970; Lorke and Tettenborn, 1970; Ohguro et al., 1969).

Cisplatin

Cisplatin (Platinol) is a heavy-metal complex that inhibits growth of cancer cells by inducing interstrand crosslinks in DNA. It is FDA-approved for the treatment of testicular, ovarian, and bladder cancers. Cisplatin is also used to treat a number of carcinomas: adrenal, head and neck, lung, neuroblastoma, osteosarcoma, prostate, stomach, cervical, endometrial, and breast.

No studies of this agent have been published, but there are case reports. A review of case reports suggested that cisplatin has been administered in the second and third trimesters without untoward fetal effects (Christman et al., 1990; King et al., 1991), but case reports cannot adequately address safety. Caution is recommended for its use in the first trimester because platinol interferes with neurolation (complete development of the neural tube) in experimental animals. This corresponds to the 3rd to 4th weeks postconception in humans (Wiebe and Sipila, 1994). In animal teratology studies, investigators found growth retardation but no malformations following exposure during embryogenesis to cisplatin in mice, rats, and rabbits (Anabuki et al., 1982; Kopf-Maier et al., 1985; Nagaoka et al., 1981).

Carboplatin

Carboplatin (Paraplatin) is a platinum compound whose action is similar to cisplatin, producing predominantly interstrand DNA crosslinks rather than DNA protein crosslinks. Its FDA-approved indications are for the primary and secondary treatment of advanced ovarian cancer. It is also used to treat other types of cancer: bladder, brain, breast, endometrium, head and neck, lung, neuroblastoma, testis, and Wilms' tumor. No studies have been published of use of this agent during pregnancy in humans. One case report of carboplatin treatment during the second trimester stated that subsequent fetal and neonatal development was normal (Henderson et al., 1993). Manufacturer package inserts report that carboplatin is embryotoxic and teratogenic in rats. In one study, in offspring of rats exposed to carboplatin during embryogenesis, fetal weight was reduced, but there were no congenital anomalies (Kai et al., 1988).

Procarbazine

Procarbazine (Matulane) is a hydrazine derivative that inhibits RNA, DNA, and other protein synthesis. It is FDA-approved for treatment of Hodgkin's disease.

Procarbazine is also used to treat lymphomas, lung and brain carcinoma, and melanoma.

No studies have been published of infants born to women who were exposed to this drug during embryogenesis. A clinical series of six pregnancies were published following exposure to procarbazine in the first trimester (four in combination with other agents). Among these infants two were normal, one infant had hemangiomas on its extremities, one elective abortion occurred, and two miscarriages were reported. Of the miscarriages, one had malpositioned, hypoplastic kidneys and the other had four toes on each foot, with bilateral webbing (Gililland and Weinstein, 1983). In a review of collected cases, the authors summarized their findings, stating that procarbazine use 'in early pregnancy, particularly during the period of fetal neurolization and morphogenesis (3rd to 12th weeks menstrual in humans) *does* appear to be associated with the risk of teratologic effects' (Wiebe and Sipila, 1994) (emphasis added). Congenital anomalies were increased in frequency among rats whose mothers were treated with procarbazine during embryogenesis (Chaube and Murphy, 1968; Tuchmann-Duplessis and Mercier-Parot, 1967). Notably, both animal studies found an increased frequency of eye defects.

Hydroxyurea

Hydroxyurea (Hydrea) inhibits DNA synthesis and is FDA-approved for chronic myelocytic leukemia, ovarian carcinoma, head and neck cancers, and melanoma. No studies have been published on the use of hydroxyurea during pregnancy in humans. A case report of two infants exposed to hydroxyurea during the second and third trimesters as part of polydrug therapy had no congenital anomalies in the fetus (therapeutic abortion) or the live born infant (Caliguri and Mayer, 1989). Three subsequent case reports of fetuses exposed in the first and second trimesters revealed no anomalies (Fitzgerald and McCann, 1993; Jackson *et al.*; 1993; Patel, 1991). Among seven women treated from conception to delivery, one stillborn premature infant and one fetal death occurred (Koh *et al.*, 2002). Five apparently normal infants were born after exposure to hydroxyurea throughout gestation. Importantly, hydroxyurea is suspected to be a human teratogen based upon its mechanism of inhibitory action on DNA and essential proteins.

Altretamine

Altretamine (hexamethylmelamine, Hexalen) was used early (1964) as an antineoplastic and is FDA-approved to treat epithelial ovarian cancer (Moore *et al.*, 1991). The mechanism of action is unknown. No studies of congenital anomalies in infants whose mothers used this agent during pregnancy have been published. Offspring of rats and rabbits exposed to hexamethylmelamine during embryogenesis had an increased frequency of congenital anomalies (Thompson *et al.*, 1984).

Paclitaxel

Paclitaxel (Taxol) is a natural plant product derived from the bark of the Pacific yew tree. It promotes assembly and stabilization of microtubules by preventing depolymerization, and subsequently halting mitosis. It is FDA-approved for the treatment of ovarian and breast cancer. It is also used against endometrial and non-small-cell lung cancer. No studies of paclitaxel in pregnant women have been published. Unpublished data from the manufacturer states that paclitaxel has been shown to be embryo- and feto-toxic in rats and rabbits.

SPECIAL CONSIDERATIONS

Nongenital cancers

Breast carcinomas and melanoma appear to be the most frequently occurring of several forms of nongenital cancers that may occur in the pregnant patient (Table 7.1).

Breast carcinoma

Breast carcinoma is the most common malignancy that occurs in women, and affects approximately 10 percent of all women at some time during their lives. Breast carcinoma occurs in approximately one to seven per 10 000 pregnancies (3 percent of all breast carcinomas) (Parente et al., 1988).

Apparently, pregnancy per se has little, if any, adverse effect on the course or prognosis of breast cancer when analyzed stage for stage (Marchant, 1994). Pregnant women seem to be more likely to have: (1) advanced lesions when diagnosed, and (2) estrogen-receptor-negative tumors (Ishida et al., 1992; Elledge et al., 1993). Both of these factors are associated with a worse prognosis than less advanced lesions and estrogen-receptor-positive tumors. The average delay in the diagnosis of breast carcinoma in pregnancy is from 1.5–6 months longer than diagnosis in nonpregnant women (Barnavon and Wallack, 1990). Delays in diagnosis of 3–6 months significantly diminish the chances of survival in both pregnant and nonpregnant patients. As part of family history collected, any genetic relative of the patient who has had breast cancer should trigger a simple screening for breast carcinoma.

Treatment strategy depends upon (1) stage of the carcinoma and (2) gestational age of the pregnancy. Surgery can generally be performed throughout gestation (see Chapter 6). If the procedure is done close to term, risk to the fetus can be eliminated if the infant is delivered first (Bloss and Miller, 1995). The usual accepted surgical technique for breast carcinoma in the pregnant patient is modified radical mastectomy with axillary node dissection (Marchant, 1994). 'Lumpectomy' and sampling of axillary nodes followed by radiotherapy has not been satisfactorily evaluated in the pregnant patient. Moreover, radiotherapy may present a significant risk to the fetus (Petrek, 1994). These guidelines are consistent with the recommendations made in 2005 (Pentheroudakis and Pavlidis, 2006).

Chemotherapy is frequently recommended for either adjunctive therapy or treatment in advanced cases. Women with axillary lymph node metastases appear to be the best candidates for adjunctive chemotherapy (Barnavon and Wallack, 1990). As detailed previously in this chapter, chemotherapy with currently available antineoplastic agents carries an increased risk of congenital anomalies with first-trimester exposure, and fetal growth retardation is the major risk in the latter two-thirds of pregnancy, although long-term effects are unknown.

The efficacy of breast carcinoma treatment during pregnancy appears to be enhanced little, if at all, by therapeutic abortion and prophylactic oophorectomy (Donegan, 1986). Therapeutic abortion might be a consideration if radiotherapy is deemed necessary or if chemotherapy is necessary during the first trimester. However, with proper shielding and focused radiotherapy above the maternal diaphram, it may be possible to minimize the adverse effects of radiation on the fetus (Pentheroudakis and Pavlidis, 2006).

Leukemia

Acute leukemia is extremely rare during pregnancy, occurring in approximately one in 100 000 pregnancies. However, it is among the most common neoplasms in young women (Caliguri and Mayer, 1989; Catanzarite and Ferguson, 1984; Koren *et al.*, 1990). Review of 72 cases of leukemia during pregnancy (13 separate reports), 64 (89 percent) women had acute leukemia and eight (11 percent) had chronic or other forms of leukemia (Caliguri and Mayer, 1989). Acute myelocytic leukemia (AML) was the most common malignancy encountered, and most cases were recognized in the latter half of pregnancy (see Table 7.4). The survival rate was approximately 75 percent in one report of 45 pregnant women with acute leukemia (Reynoso *et al.*, 1987), which is similar to the rate among nonpregnant patients with acute leukemia (Caliguri and Mayer, 1989). Therefore, pregnancy *per se* does not affect the course of leukemia.

Antineoplastic drugs most commonly used to treat chronic leukemia include antimetabolites (methotrexate, thioguanine, mercaptopurine, and cytarabine), anthracycline antibiotics (daunorubicin and doxorubicin), and plant alkaloids (vincristine). Alkylating agents are also used as antileukemic drugs. Notably, all of these drugs are cytostatic, although their methods of accomplishing this differs (cyotoxicity, DNA, and protein synthesis suppression). Therefore, all antineoplastics have a very high potential for production of birth defects during embryogenesis because this period is characterized by the highest rate of cell division (hyperplasia) in a human's life.

The prognosis for survival in the untreated woman is extremely poor, with life expectancy of less than 3 months (Catanzarite and Ferguson, 1984; Hou and Song,

Table 7.4 Cases (*n* = 72) of leukemia in pregnancy, 1975–1988

	n	%
Trimesters		
First	16	22
Second	26	36
Third	30	42
Types of leukemia		
Acute lymphoblastic	20	28
Acute myelocytic	44	61
Chronic myelocytic	5	7
Hairy cell	1	1.3
Not specified	2	2.7

Adapted from Caliguri and Mayer, 1989.

1995; Kawamura *et al.*, 1994; Koren *et al.*, 1990). Therefore, chemotherapy should be initiated immediately (even during the first trimester) once the diagnosis of acute leukemia is made. However, folate antagonists (e.g., methotrexate) should be avoided in the first trimester, if possible.

Among a series of 58 infants born to pregnant women who had either acute myelocytic or lymphoblastic leukemia, there were 31 (53 percent) premature births (including five stillbirths), and 23 (43 percent) full-term infants (two of whom were of low birth weight) (Caliguri and Mayer, 1989). No studies have been published of congenital anomalies among the infants born to women with leukemia during pregnancy. No congenital anomalies have been reported among the 13 fetuses exposed to chemotherapy for leukemia during the first trimester (Caliguri and Mayer, 1989).

Lymphomas and Hodgkin's disease

An estimated 40 percent of malignant lymphomas are of the Hodgkin's variety and are the most commonly encountered lymphoma among pregnant women, and occur among approximately one in 6000 pregnancies. Non-Hodgkin's lymphoma is 'very rare' in pregnancy (Lishner *et al.*, 1994). As with breast carcinoma, pregnancy does not seem to affect the prognosis for Hodgkin's disease (Lishner *et al.*, 1992). Both leukemias and lymphomas are known to metastasize to the placenta, but the empirical risk is unknown.

Treatment of Hodgkin's lymphoma, like that of most other malignancies, depends on the stage of the disease and the gestational age at which the disease is diagnosed. Staging is of paramount importance, and pregnancy may interfere with the types of diagnostic studies that can be performed. Most diagnostic radiographic procedures not involving the abdomen or fetus can be accomplished, if necessary, with minimal risk to the conceptus. Moreover, an abdominal X-ray and computed tomography (CT) scan usually expose the fetus to less than 1 rad of actual radiation. Magnetic resonance imaging (MRI) may also prove useful in early to mid-pregnancy as an alternative to x-ray. Staging laparotomy lymphomas is somewhat controversial and difficult, if not impossible, to accomplish in the latter half of pregnancy because the large uterus obstructs the operating field (Bloss and Miller, 1995).

For early stages of lymphomas in the first half of pregnancy, several options are available. Obviously, therapeutic abortion is one consideration, although it is not always necessary. Modified radiotherapy can be utilized if done at a significant distance from the shielded pelvis, i.e., in supradiaphragmatic disease, head and neck, etc. (Woo *et al.*, 1992). If chemotherapy is deemed necessary, it is best to wait until after the first trimester.

For patients with early-stage disease during the latter half of pregnancy, one reasonable option is simply to wait until after delivery to initiate therapy, especially if the patient is asymptomatic. Chemotherapy after the first trimester causes little known risk to the fetus except for pancytopenia and mild to moderate growth retardation. For patients with advanced disease, early treatment is obviously much more of a concern. Some physicians recommend therapeutic abortion if the advanced-stage lymphoma is diagnosed early in pregnancy (Jacobs *et al.*, 1980). For advanced disease after the first trimester, chemotherapy should be initiated. If the patient is near term, early delivery is usually indicated.

In a review of 15 pregnancies among women with Hodgkin's disease (Jacobs *et al.*, 1981), outcomes observed were six normal pregnancies (radiation in five, bleomycin in one), six therapeutic abortions, one spontaneous abortion, and one preterm delivery. One patient developed a subdiaphragmatic relapse, and her treatment was delayed until after delivery. These data suggest that the prognosis for Hodgkin's disease during pregnancy is reasonably good for the mother.

Nineteen pregnancies (reported in 15 publications) are published with first-trimester exposure to chemotherapeutic agents for treatment of lymphomas. Of these 19 pregnancies, 15 (79 percent) resulted in normal infants (three were exposed to mechlorethamine, two to thiotepa, and 10 to vinblastine). One patient who received mechlorethamine had a therapeutic abortion. Another patient who received chlorambucil delivered an infant with unilateral renal agenesis. One patient who received procarbazine gave birth to an infant with multiple hemangiomas. Another patient who received polydrug therapy during pregnancy had an infant with an atrial septal defect (Jacobs *et al.*, 1981).

Melanomas

Melanomas are one of the more common cancers that occur during pregnancy, with approximately three per 1000 deliveries (Gilstrap and Cunningham, 1996; Smith and Randal, 1969; Yazigi and Cunningham, 1990). It is important to note that melanoma is the tumor type with the highest risk to metastasize to the placenta and fetus (Anderson *et al.*, 1989; Read and Platzer, 1981). Pregnancy does not seem to affect the growth or prognosis of melanoma, although pregnancy is associated with an increased level of melanocyte-stimulating hormone (Gilstrap and Cunningham, 1996; Holly, 1986; Yazigi and Cunningham, 1990). There was no difference in survival of 58 pregnant women with melanoma compared to nonpregnant controls with melanoma (Reintgen *et al.*, 1985). Treatment usually comprises surgical resection, with or without lymph node dissection. A variety of chemotherapeutic agents are used, but their success rate is poor, with little success whether chemotherapy is given as adjuvant or primary therapy in metastatic disease.

Other nongenital cancers

Other nongenital types of cancer, such as colorectal carcinoma, gastric carcinoma, pancreatic or hepatic cancer, and sarcoma, are rare during pregnancy (Gilstrap and Cunningham, 1996; Yazigi and Cunningham, 1990). Treatment during pregnancy is similar to that of nonpregnant women, with certain chemotherapeutic and radiation limitations as consideration for the pregnancy (as mentioned above). If the patient is in the first trimester, therapeutic abortion should be considered an option. In the latter half of pregnancy, early delivery followed by treatment is a prudent option. As previously mentioned, chemotherapy carries little known risk, other than fetal growth retardation, when used in the second and third trimester. If chemotherapy is given in the first trimester, folic acid antagonists should be avoided.

Pregnancy following nongenital cancer

No data support the misconception that women with breast cancer should not become pregnant following initial therapy. Similarly, no scientific data support the misconception that pregnancy after mastectomy for breast cancer adversely affects survival of the mother (Donegan, 1983; Gilstrap and Cunningham, 1996; Yazigi and Cunningham 1990). Among 227 consecutive breast cancer patients 35 years of age or younger who received doxorubicin as adjuvant chemotherapy, 33 pregnancies occurred in 25 patients. Twelve abortions (10 therapeutic) and 19 full-term pregnancies with normal outcomes occurred following treatment before conception for nongenital cancer, leading the authors to conclude that subsequent pregnancy 'did not affect the disease-free or overall survival of the patient' (Sutton *et al.*, 1990).

In general, it seems prudent to delay subsequent pregnancy for 2–3 years following successful treatment of any cancer, allowing an appropriate period of time for observation and retreatment, if necessary. More than 90 percent of recurrences occur during the 3 years following remission of nongenital cancer (Yazigi and Cunningham, 1990).

Fertility and outcome in subsequent pregnancies

In one of the largest reviews (*n* = 2283 patients) of survivors of childhood cancers, cancer survivors of reproductive age were less likely to become pregnant than their siblings. In addition, radiation below the diaphragm resulted in a decrease in fertility of both sexes by approximately 25 percent (Byrne *et al.*, 1987). Alkylating agent therapy is associated with an estimated two-thirds reduction in male fertility, but had no effect on female fertility. Green *et al.* (1989) found that '... Pregnancy outcome is not adversely affected by treatment received during childhood or adolescence for acute lymphoblastic leukemia'.

Among 34 women of reproductive age treated with combined radiation therapy and polydrug chemotherapy (vincristine, vinblastin, thiotepa, and procarbazine) for stage II and III Hodgkin's disease, the ability to become pregnant was comparable to the patient's pretreatment history (Lacher and Toner, 1986).

Genital cancers

Both cervical and ovarian cancer occur during pregnancy, although cervical cancer is much more frequent than ovarian.

Cervical cancer

The incidence of cervical carcinoma in pregnancy is approximately 1.3 per 1000 pregnancies (Hacker *et al.*, 1982; Yazigi and Cunningham, 1990), ranging from 1:1000 to 1:10 000. One of the major problems associated with this neoplasm is determining the stage of the lesion and the treatment plan. The extent of the tumor in the pregnant patient tends to be underestimated (Pentheroudakis and Pavlidis, 2006; Yazigi and Cunningham, 1990).

The treatment depends upon the stage of the cancer and gestational age of the pregnancy. In the first half of pregnancy, treatment consists basically of radical hysterectomy and lymphadenectomy for small lesions and radiotherapy for more extensive lesions (Yazigi and Cunningham, 1990). Radiotherapy will generally result in spontaneous abortion, and therapeutic abortion should be offered as an option.

In pregnancies close to viability (i.e., 24 weeks gestation and beyond), it is appropriate to follow these patients conservatively and to deliver them when fetal pulmonary maturity is reached (ACOG, 1989). Chemotherapy is generally utilized for advanced or metastatic disease, and the best prognosis for the infant is probably associated with treatment initiated after the first trimester if possible. Patients with microinvasion or preinvasive lesions can generally be treated with cone biopsy or conservative therapy until after pregnancy (Pentheroudakis and Pavlidis, 2006).

Ovarian cancer

Approximately 6 percent of adnexal masses in pregnancy are malignant compared to 15–20 percent in the nonpregnant patient, and the incidence of ovarian cancer during pregnancy is approximately one in 18 000–25 000 deliveries (Beischer *et al.*, 1971; Chung and Birnbaum, 1973; Jubb, 1963; Munnell, 1963; Yazigi and Cunningham, 1990). The most recent estimate for ovarian cancer is 1:10 000 to 1:100 000 (Pavlidis, 2002).

Epithelial cell, germ cell, gonadal stromal cell, and endodermal sinus tumors have all been reported during pregnancy. Therapy depends on the stage of the disease and gestational age of the pregnancy. For stage IA disease, unilateral oophorectomy may be satisfactory, with appropriate surgical staging (Yazigi and Cunningham, 1990).

Depending on the stage of pregnancy, more advanced disease may require hysterectomy or radical surgery. Chemotherapy may be indicated as adjuvant therapy, and the same principle applies as with other cancers (with the exception of acute leukemia); i.e., therapy should be started after the first trimester (Pentheroudakis and Pavlidis, 2006).

In a recent survey of 23 cases of ovarian carcinoma during pregnancy, Dgani and colleagues (1989) reported that 35 percent were borderline grade and that overall survival was much better than expected for ovarian cancer because more of the cases in pregnancy are of an earlier stage. The types of ovarian tumors encountered in this review are summarized in Table 7.5. Fourteen of the 23 women gave birth to normal live-born infants. The overall 5-year survival for women in this series was 61 percent and 92 percent for stage I lesions.

Table 7.5 Type and trimester of occurrence in 23 cases of ovarian cancer during pregnancy

Ovarian cancer	Stage of pregnancy	Percentage
	First trimester	44
	Second trimester	17
	Third trimester	9
	Delivery or postpartum	30
Type of cancer		
	Borderline	35
	Epithelial	30
	Dysgerminoma	17
	Granulosa cell	13
	Undifferentiated	5

Adapted from Dgani *et al.*, 1989.

Occupational exposure

There may be an increased frequency of fetal loss from occupational exposure to various chemotherapeutic agents (Selevan *et al.*, 1985).

SUMMARY

All antineoplastic agents are devoted to the purpose of suppressing cell replication. The conflict arises because the predominant cellular event that occurs during *in utero* development is replication. Cell differentiation and replication dominate embryonic development; increases in cell number (hyperplastic growth) are the major occurrences during fetal growth and development. Hence, the greatest risk of antineoplastic agents during the first trimester is for birth defects, and the greatest risk during the fetal period is for intrauterine/fetal growth retardation.

Key references

Adam MP, Manning MA, Beck AE *et al*. Methotrexate/misoprostol embryopathy. Report of four cases resulting from failed medical abortion. *Am J Med Genet* 2003; **123**: 72.

Aviles A, Neri N. Hematological malignancies and pregnancy. A final report of 84 children who received chemotherapy *in utero*. *Clin Lymphoma* 2001; **2**: 173.

Berry DL, Theriault RL, Holmes FA *et al*. Management of breast cancer during pregnancy using a standardized protocol. *J Clin Oncol* 1999; **17**: 855.

Chapa JB, Hibbard JU, Weber EM, Abramowicz JS, Verp MS. Prenatal diagnosis of methotrexate embryopathy. *Obstet Gynecol* 2003; **101** (5 Pt 2): 1104.

Francella A, Dyan A, Bodian C, Rubin P, Chapman M, Present DH. The safety of 6-mercaptopurine for childbearing patients with inflammatory bowel disease. A retrospective cohort study. *Gastroenterology* 2003; **124** (1): 9.

Grainger DA, Seifer DB. Laparoscopic management of ectopic pregnancy. *Curr Opin Obstet Gynecol* 1995; **7**: 277.

Hausknecht RU. Methotrexate and misoprostol to terminate early pregnancy. *N Engl J Med* 1995; **333**: 537.

Pavlidis NA. Coexistence of pregnancy and malignancy. *Oncologist* 2002; **7**: 279–87.

Pentheroudakis G, Pavlidis N. Cancer and pregnancy. Poena magna, not anymore. *Eur J Cancer* 2006; **49**: 126–40.

Zand DJ, Blanco C, Coleman B, Huff D, Zackai E. *In utero* methotrexate exposure resulting in long bone aplasia. *Am J Hum Genet* 2003; **73** (Suppl. 5): 591.

Further references are available on the book's website at http://www.drugsandpregnancy.com

8

Analgesics during pregnancy

Pregnant women experience a variety of aches and pains and most do not require analgesic therapy. Headaches or pain secondary to dental procedures are common during pregnancy. Many nonnarcotic analgesics are commercially available (many of them over-the-counter medications) and fortunately, with few exceptions, can be utilized safely for the treatment of minor pain during pregnancy.

Limited data are available on the pharmacokinetics of analgesics during pregnancy, and the findings are not entirely consistent. For example, acetaminophen has a decreased half-life and increased clearance in one study, but it is unchanged in another at about the same gestational age (Table 8.1). The pharmacokinetics of meperidine in pregnancy are unchanged compared to nonpregnant controls, and the same is true of the kinetics of meptazinol. In contrast, morphine has a decreased half-life and increased clearance, implying the need for increased frequency or dose regimen to maintain adequate analgesia. Indomethacin has a decreased half-life, C_{max}, and C_{ss}, which also implies dose or frequency regimen adjustment. In contrast, sodium salicylate has an increased half-life during late pregnancy. Low-dose aspirin does not appear to significantly affect umbilical artery circulation (Owen *et al.*, 1993; Veille *et al.*, 1993). Notably, the half-life for aspirin increases during pregnancy, implying that a dose decrease in amount and/or frequency may be needed (Table 8.1).

NONSTEROIDAL ANTIINFLAMMATORY AGENTS

Most of the agents in this group are relatively new analgesics and all are prostaglandin synthetase inhibitors. Some of the commonly used agents in this class are listed in Box 8.1. Phenylbutazone and indomethacin are two of the 'oldest' agents in this group.

Box 8.1 Nonsteroidal antiinflammatory agents

Phenylbutazone	Diflunisal
Indomethacin	Ketorulac
Ibuprofen	Piroxicam
Fenoprofen	Diclofenac
Meclofenamate	Rofecoxib
Naproxen	Celecoxib
Tolmentin	Etodolac
Sulindac	

Table 8.1 Pharmacokinetics analgesic agents during pregnancy: pregnant compared with nonpregnant

Agent	n	EGA (weeks)	Route	AUC	V_d	C_{max}	C_{SS}	$t_{1/2}$	Cl	PPB	Control group[a]	Authors
Acetaminophen	8	3rd trimester	PO					↓	↑		Yes (1)	Miners et al. (1986)
Acetaminophen	6	36	PO	↑		=	=	=	=		Yes (2)	Rayburn et al. (1986)
Indomethacin	5	36–38	IV			↓	↓	↓			Yes (1)	Traeger et al. (1973)
Meperidine	18	Term	IV		=	=	=	=			Yes (1)	Kuhnert et al. (1980)
Meptazinol	5	36–38	IV	=	=	=	=	=			Yes (1)	Murray et al. (1989)
Morphine	13	Term	IM, IV	↑	=			↓	↑		Yes (1)	Gerdin et al. (1990)
Sodium salicylate	20	40	IV	↑				↑	↑		No	Noeschel et al. (1972)

Source: Little BB. Obstet Gynecol 1999; **93**: 858.

EGA, estimated gestational age; AUC, area under the curve; V_d, volume of distribution; C_{max}, peak plasma concentration; C_{SS}, steady-state concentration; $t_{1/2}$, half-life; Cl, clearance; PPB, plasma protein binding; PO, by mouth; ↓ denotes a decrease during pregnancy compared with nonpregnant values; = denotes no difference between pregnant and nonpregnant values; IV, intravenous, IM, intramuscular. ↑ denotes an increase during pregnancy compared with nonpregnant values.

[a]Control groups: 1, nonpregnant women; 2, same individuals studied postpartum; 3, historic adult controls (sex not given); 4, adult male controls; 5, adult male and female controls combined.

Nonnarcotic analgesics

SALICYLATES (ASPIRIN)

Aspirin has been used for a variety of therapeutic reasons, but is used primarily as an analgesic, antipyretic, or antiinflammatory agent. Salicylates have been used clinically use for over 100 years and are one of the most commonly used nonnarcotic analgesics. Aspirin is one of the drugs most used by pregnant women (Corby, 1978; Sibai and Amon, 1988; Streissguth et al., 1987). In one prospective study of 1529 pregnant women in 1974 and 1975 (Streissguth et al., 1987), almost 50 percent of the women reported taking aspirin, and about 3 percent took it daily. Salicylates are prostaglandin synthetase inhibitors, and act primarily via inactivation of the enzyme cyclo-oxygenase (COX) (Sibai et al., 1989), and are well known for inhibiting COX-1 and COX-2 enzymes. Suppression of COX-1 inhibits production of protective esophageal and gastric mucosa, increasing the risk for gastrointestinal bleeds and associated complications. Suppression of COX-1 also inhibits synthesis of vasoactive prostaglandins (prostacyclin and thromboxane A_2). Prostacyclin, a potent vasodilator, also inhibits platelet aggregation, while thromboxane A_2, a potent vasoconstrictor, stimulates platelet aggregation (Bhagwat et al., 1985; Ellis et al., 1976). Prostaglandin E and prostaglandin $F_{2\alpha}$ are also inhibited. In usual human therapeutic doses, aspirin results in 'nonselective inhibition of prostaglandin synthetase in various tissues' (Sibai and Amon, 1988), thus suppressing COX-2. Suppression of COX-2 has an analgesic effect by blocking prostaglandins associated with inflammation.

High or normal doses (>325 mg) block production of prostacyclin and thromboxane, and low-dose aspirin (60–83 mg) results in selective block of thromboxane production, and favors the prostacyclin (vasodilation) pathway (Beaufils et al., 1985; Masotti et al., 1979; Schiff et al., 1989; Sibai et al., 1989; Spitz et al., 1988; Wallenberg, 1995; Wallenberg et al., 1986). This provides the basis for the use of low-dose aspirin to forestall or prevent pregnancy-induced hypertension (Gant and Gilstrap, 1990) (see Special considerations). Importantly, low-dose aspirin does not completely inhibit thromboxane and does not completely 'spare' prostacyclin. One group of investigators found that 81 mg of aspirin inhibited thromboxane by 75 percent, but also inhibited prostacyclin by approximately 20 percent (Spitz et al., 1988).

There have been several large studies regarding the effect of aspirin on preeclampsia (Hauth et al., 1993; Sibai et al., 1993), as well as a meta-analysis, Collaborative Low-Dose Aspirin Study in Pregnancy (CLASP, 1994). These results indicate that low-dose aspirin does decrease the incidence of preeclampsia (Hauth and Cunningham, 1995). Review of four large controlled trials that included over 13 000 pregnant women led to the conclusion that daily low-dose aspirin significantly reduced the risk of preeclampsia (Wallenberg, 1995). In a follow-up study, compared to untreated women, aspirin-treated women had: (1) a greater than twofold longitudinal reduction in serum thromboxane B_2 levels; (2) a significantly decreased frequency of preeclampsia; and (3) fewer premature and growth-stunted newborns (Hauth et al., 1995a).

Aspirin readily crosses the placenta and results in physiologically significant fetal levels (Levy et al., 1975; Palminsano and Cassudy, 1969; Turner and Collins, 1975). Aspirin has been reported to be teratogenic in various laboratory animals when given at several times the human adult dose (Wilson et al., 1977), and there have been anecdotal case reports of congenital anomalies in humans (Agapitos *et al.*, 1986). However, the risk of congenital anomalies in infants of mothers exposed to aspirin in the first 16 weeks of pregnancy was not increased when compared to unexposed infants (Slone *et al.*, 1976). The major malformation rate in a large national study in the USA was 6.7 percent for heavy aspirin use, 6.8 percent for intermediate use, and 6.3 percent for women who did not use aspirin (Heinonen *et al.*, 1977). Among 144 pregnant women who were 'heavy aspirin' users, the frequency of major birth defects in offspring was 4.2 percent – not significantly different from that in the general population (3.5–5 percent; Turner and Collins, 1975). Similarly, among 62 women who used aspirin in the first trimester, the rate was not significantly higher than that expected in the general population (Aselton *et al.*, 1985).

High-dose aspirin taken late in the third trimester may be associated with (1) closure of the ductus arteriosus, (2) persistent pulmonary hypertension (Levin *et al.*, 1978; Sibai and Amon, 1988), (3) decreased fetal renal function, and (4) oligohydramnios (Witter and Niebyl, 1986). Lower IQs in offspring of mothers who took aspirin in the first trimester of pregnancy have been reported by some investigators (Streissguth *et al.*, 1987), but not others (Klebanoff and Berendes, 1988). Maternal use of high-dose aspirin is associated with increased frequency of post-term pregnancies (Collins and Turner, 1975), low birth weight (Lewis and Schulman, 1973), neonatal bleeding disorders, and intracranial hemorrhage in premature infants (Rumack *et al.*, 1981; Stuart *et al.*, 1982), and premature closure of the ductus arteriosus in the fetus (Levin *et al.*, 1978). However, these complications are not associated with aspirin use when pharmacologically controlled doses of salicylates were used (Sibai and Amon, 1988). This implies that gravidas may be self-adjusting their doses and/or frequency regimens upward, increasing the risk of untoward outcomes.

There were no significant differences in the frequency of congenital anomalies, motor or developmental delay, or height or weight between those exposed to low-dose aspirin and controls at 12- and 18-month follow-up (CLASP, 1995).

In one study, a significantly increased frequency of placental abruption was found among women taking low-dose aspirin therapy compared to controls (Sibai *et al.*, 1993). However, meta-analysis of 11 clinical trials found no significant difference in the incidence of placental abruption among women taking aspirin compared to controls (Hauth *et al.*, 1995b).

In summary, aspirin at therapeutic or low doses is not associated with a significant risk of birth defects, although in very large, chronic doses close to the time of delivery, aspirin may be associated with an increase in bleeding disorders in the mother and fetus.

ACETAMINOPHEN

Acetaminophen is also commonly used during pregnancy, second only to aspirin. Forty-one percent of pregnant women reported acetaminophen use during pregnancy in a large longitudinal study (Streissguth *et al.*, 1987). The frequency of congenital birth defects in several studies was not increased above background among more than 1200 offspring whose mothers used acetaminophen during the first trimester (Aselton *et al.*, 1985; Heinonen *et al.*, 1977; Jick *et al.*, 1981). The IQs of offspring at 4 years of age whose mothers had ingested acetaminophen during pregnancy were no different than controls (Streissguth *et al.*, 1987).

The potential association of maternal acetaminophen use and polyhydramnios is unclear, but is based upon one case report of one single infant (Char *et al.*, 1975). Ingestion of large doses of acetaminophen or the protracted use of this drug may result in renal and hepatic failure in the adult and could result in the same complications in the fetus (see Chapter 14).

In summary, acetaminophen is one of the safest nonnarcotic analgesics available for use in the pregnant woman when doses are kept in the therapeutic range.

PHENACETIN

Phenacetin is an analgesic and antipyretic with poor antiinflammatory activity. It is often used in combination with other analgesics, and one of its major metabolites is acetaminophen. The frequency of malformations was not increased among more than 18 000 offspring of mothers who utilized this analgesic either alone or in combination with other agents (Heinonen *et al.*, 1977; Jick *et al.*, 1981). There are also no reports of this analgesic being teratogenic in animals.

PHENYLBUTAZONE

Phenylbutazone is a nonsteroidal antiinflammatory agent (NSAID) with analgesic, antipyretic, and antiinflammatory actions. It is commonly used to treat women with arthritic conditions (rheumatoid arthritis, degenerative joint disease). No scientific studies are published regarding the safety and efficacy of this medication in pregnant women. Two major congenital anomalies were among 27 infants exposed to phenylbutazone, but these data were not peer reviewed (Rosa, personal communication, cited in Briggs *et al.*, 2005). Some of the prostaglandin synthetase inhibitors are associated with premature closure of the ductus arteriosus in the newborn (Csaba *et al.*, 1978; Levin *et al.*, 1978), and theoretically phenylbutazone could also be associated with this complication. However, there are no reports of this to date.

INDOMETHACIN

Indomethacin has antipyretic action in addition to analgesic and antiinflammatory effects. It is used for the treatment of rheumatoid arthritis and osteoarthritis, bursitis, and tendonitis. It has also been used to treat premature labor in the second and third trimesters of pregnancy (Niebyl *et al.*, 1980; Sibony *et al.*, 1994; Zuckerman *et al.*, 1974, 1984). In addition, intravenous indomethacin has been used to close a hemodynamically significant patent ductus arteriosus in premature infants. Indomethacin has also been used for the treatment of symptomatic leiomyomata during pregnancy (Dildy *et al.*, 1992).

The frequency of congenital anomalies among more than 400 infants following exposure to indomethacin during the first trimester is no different from the population background rate (Aselton *et al.*, 1985; Kallen, 1998). Congenital anomalies have also not been found to be increased in several reports in which animals received several times the adult human dose of indomethacin (Kalter, 1973; Klein *et al.*, 1981; Randall *et al.*, 1987).

Indomethacin is associated with premature closure of the ductus arteriosus and pulmonary hypertension in the fetus and newborn in several reports (DeWit *et al.*, 1988; Levin *et al.*, 1978; Manchester *et al.*, 1976; Moise *et al.*, 1988). Ductal constriction was found by echocardiography in seven of 14 fetuses in 13 pregnant women who received indomethacin for premature labor at 25–31 weeks gestation (Moise *et al.*, 1988). Ductal constriction was transient and resolved within 24 h after discontinuation of the indomethacin. Fetal ductus arteriosus closure in the fetus was also associated with indomethacin exposure in several animal models (Harker *et al.*, 1981; Harris, 1980; Levin *et al.*, 1979). No evidence was reported of either premature closure of the ductus arteriosus or pulmonary hypertension in 15 fetuses whose mothers had received indomethacin in a randomized trial (Niebyl *et al.*, 1980). A review of 167 newborns [<35 weeks estimated gestational age (EGA)] whose mothers received indomethacin for tocolysis found no cases of premature closure of the ductus arteriosus or persistent fetal circulation (Dudley *et al.*, 1985).

Among 818 women who received indomethacin during pregnancy near the time of delivery, perinatal complications occurred in 13 percent compared to 1.8 percent for controls (Marpeau *et al.*, 1994). A study of 57 infants born at 30 weeks EGA reported an increase in necrotizing enterocolitis, intracranial hemorrhage, and patent ductus arteriosus compared to 57 infants not exposed to indomethacin (Norton *et al.*, 1993), paralleling adverse neonatal outcomes shown in numerous other studies (Eronen *et al.*, 1994; Major *et al.*, 1994; Rasenen and Jouppila, 1995; van der Heijden *et al.*, 1994). In contrast, among 15 infants exposed to indomethacin chronically during gestation, no instances of patent ductus occurred (Al-Alaiyan *et al.*, 1996).

IBUPROFEN

Ibuprofen is another commonly used NSAID analgesic. The frequency of congenital anomalies was no greater than expected among 51 infants whose mothers took ibuprofen during the first trimester of pregnancy (Aselton *et al.*, 1985). In a case series, five infants were reported with abnormalities at birth, but no distinct anomaly syndrome (Barry *et al.*, 1984). Ibuprofen was also associated with decreased amniotic fluid volume (Hickok *et al.*, 1989).

MECLOFENAMATE

Among 166 infants exposed to meclofenamate during the first trimester, the frequency of congenital anomalies (3.6 percent) was not greater than expected in the general population (3.5–5 percent), but the study was neither peer reviewed nor controlled (Rosa, personal communication, cited in Briggs *et al.*, 2005).

NAPROXEN

In a series of children born to 23 women who took naproxen throughout pregnancy for rheumatic disease, no congenital anomalies were found (Ostensen and Ostensen, 1996).

SULINDAC

The frequency of major congenital anomalies was 4.3 percent among 69 infants born to women who used sulindac during the first trimester, and is within the range of that expected in the general population, i.e., 3.5–5 percent (Rosa, personal communication, cited in Briggs *et al.*, 2005). However, this study is neither peer reviewed nor controlled.

Sulindac is another NSAID that has been used as a tocolytic. In comparisons of sulindac to indomethacin for tocolysis, two studies found that sulindac was as effective as indomethacin but had fewer side effects (Carlan *et al.*, 1992; Rasenen and Jouppila, 1995).

Miscellaneous NSAIDS

No reports have been published regarding the other NSAID analgesics sometimes used during pregnancy: fenoprofen, tolmentin, rofecoxib, celecoxib, and etodolac. However, all of these drugs are prostaglandin synthetase inhibitors and could theoretically cause premature closure of the ductus arteriosus and/or oligohydramnios.

ROFECOXIB

Rofecoxib is a cyclooxygenase-2 (COX-2) selective analgesic. No studies of congenital anomalies in offspring exposed to rofecoxib during embryogenesis have been published. Premature closure of the ductus arteriosus is a theoretical risk of maternal therapy with rofecoxib because of the pharmacologic action of the drug. Rofecoxib (Vioxx) was withdrawn from the market in September 2004 because an increased risk of myocardial infarction or stroke was found.

CELECOXIB

Celecoxib is a COX-2 selective analgesic. No studies of congenital anomalies in infants exposed to celecoxib during organogenesis have been published. Premature closure of the ductus arteriosus is a theoretical risk because of the pharmacologic action of celecoxib. Ductus closure has been demonstrated in animal models, but not reported in humans.

ETODOLAC

Etodolac is a COX-2 selective analgesic. No studies of congenital anomalies in offspring exposed to etodolac during the first trimester have been published. Premature closure of the ductus arteriosus is a theoretical risk because of the pharmacologic action of etodolac. Etodolac was found to be safer for the gastrointestinal tract (i.e., fewer bleeding ulcers than naproxen) with chronic therapy (Weideman *et al.*, 2004). The frequency of congenital anomalies was increased among rats or rabbits exposed to etodolac during embryogenesis (Ninomiya *et al.*, 1990a, 1990b).

Narcotic analgesics

Some of the more commonly used analgesics are listed in Box 8.2. All of the opioid narcotic analgesics cross the placenta and have the potential to cause dependence and withdrawal symptoms in the fetus and newborn if regularly used or abused (see Chapter 16 regarding substance abuse). Many of these agents are commonly used for the relief of

Box 8.2 Narcotic analgesics

Alphaprodine	Morphine
Butorphanol	Nalbuphine
Codeine	Oxycodone
Fentanyl	Oxymorphone
Hydrocodone	Pentazocine
Hydromorphone	Propoxyphene
Meperidine	Sufentanil

pain during labor and as such are associated with few, if any, adverse fetal effects, with the possible exception of respiratory depression if used in sufficiently large doses close to delivery.

MEPERIDINE

Meperidine is one of the most commonly used analgesics during labor. Within 7 min of maternal injection, fetal levels are about equal to maternal levels (Fishburne, 1982; Spielman, 1987). The half-life in the newborn may be up to 23 h (Spielman, 1987). Meperidine is metabolized predominantly in the liver, and its major metabolite, normeperidine, is more potent and potentially more toxic than the parent compound itself.

The frequency of congenital anomalies was not increased among more than 300 infants born to women who took this analgesic in the first trimester (Heinonen *et al.*, 1977; Jick *et al.*, 1981). Neonates may manifest respiratory depression and behavioral changes because of the long half-life of this drug in the fetus and newborn (Belsey *et al.*, 1981; Busacca *et al.*, 1982; Koch and Wendel, 1968; Morrison *et al.*, 1973; Schnider and Moya, 1964). The neonatal behavioral changes are, however, transient as shown in a 5- to 10-year follow-up of 70 children born to mothers who received meperidine during labor. There were no significant persisting physical or psychological effects as a result of this medication (Buck, 1975). The frequency of central nervous system anomalies was increased in the offspring of hamsters who received meperidine in doses several times that used in humans (Geber and Schramm, 1975).

Meperidine is apparently a safe drug for use during pregnancy when taken within the therapeutic dose range, especially during labor. The dose needs extra consideration because of the long half-life of this drug in the neonate.

MORPHINE

Morphine is no longer commonly used as an analgesic during labor because neonatal respiratory depression occurs with a significantly greater frequency than with meperidine (Spielman, 1987). Nonetheless, pregnant women may be exposed to this narcotic analgesic for other indications (e.g., postoperative pain). The frequency of birth defects was no greater than expected among the offspring of 70 women who received this drug during the first trimester of pregnancy (Heinonen *et al.*, 1977). Two animal studies found that morphine exposure during embryogenesis did not increase the frequency of congenital anomalies (Fujinaga and Mazze, 1988; Yamamoto *et al.*, 1972). Three other experimental animal studies did find an increase in the central nervous system and other abnormalities in the offspring of animals treated with morphine in doses several times larger than those used in humans (Geber, 1977; Geber and Schramm, 1975; Harpel and Gautierie, 1968).

Newborns of addicted mothers may experience withdrawal symptoms, and this is discussed in more detail in the chapter on substance abuse (Chapter 16).

PENTAZOCINE

Pentazocine is a narcotic analgesic used for the relief of moderate to severe pain and is associated with a risk of respiratory depression similar to other narcotics. It crosses the placenta readily, but evidently not to the same extent as meperidine (Spielman, 1987).

The frequency of congenital anomalies was not increased in two studies encompassing 63 infants born to mothers who utilized pentazocine in association with tripelennamine, i.e., Ts and blues (see Chapter 16) (Chasnoff et al., 1983; Senay, 1985). In another study, the frequency of congenital anomalies was increased but concomitant heavy alcohol use in the study cohort was probably the proximate cause of the birth defects observed (Little et al., 1990). The authors concluded that it was very unlikely that the anomalies found were associated with the abuse of pentazocine.

An increased frequency of low birth weight infants was associated with the use of pentazocine and tripelennamine during pregnancy (Chasnoff et al., 1983; Dunn and Reynolds, 1982; Little et al., 1990; von Almen and Miller, 1986). No epidemiologic studies are published regarding the possible association of congenital anomalies with the therapeutic use of pentazocine.

There was an increased frequency of central nervous system defects in the offspring of hamsters which had received large doses of pentazocine, but not with smaller doses (Geber and Schramm, 1975).

As with all narcotics, fetal addiction and severe neonatal withdrawal symptoms occur with habitual maternal use of pentazocine (Goetz and Bain, 1974; Kopelman, 1975; Little et al., 1990; Scanlon, 1974).

BUTORPHANOL

Butorphanol is a parenterally administered labor analgesic with agonist and antagonist actions (Spielman, 1987). The main advantage of butorphanel is that it has the efficacy of other narcotic analgesics, but respiratory depressive effects are less of a risk than with other narcotics. The butorphanol metabolite has no analgesic or toxic effect, unlike meperidine, which is an advantage in the management of maternal dose and untoward neonatal effects (Spielman, 1987), because this agent readily crosses the placenta (Pittman et al., 1980). Importantly, it may cause fetal and neonatal cardiorespiratory depression at high and frequent dose regimens. Chronic use/abuse of this agent during pregnancy may lead to fetal dependence and severe neonatal withdrawal symptoms.

No studies regarding the use of this agent during pregnancy and the frequency of congenital anomalies have been published. However, butorphanel is not considered to increase the risk of birth defects substantially (Friedman and Polifka, 2006). The frequency of congenital anomalies among offspring exposed to butorphanol during embryogenesis was not increased above that observed in offspring of sham controls (Takahashi et al., 1982).

Butorphanol is compatible with breastfeeding (American Academy of Pediatrics, 1994).

HYDROCODONE

Hydrocodone is a synthetic narcotic used to treat moderate pain but it is not often used during labor and delivery. It is also used as a cough suppressant. The frequency of congenital anomalies (7.2 percent) was slightly increased above that expected in the general population (5 percent) in an unpublished study of 332 women who received prescriptions for this drug in the first trimester (Rosa, personal communication, cited in Briggs et al., 2005). No pattern of anomalies was observed in a clinical case series of 40 infants whose mothers used hydrocodone during the first trimester (Schick et al., 1996). An increased frequency of malformations was found in the offspring of animals that received extremely large doses of this agent (Geber and Schramm, 1975).

OXYMORPHONE

Oxymorphone is another narcotic analgesic, and no published reports are available regarding potential teratogenic effects in humans. Several early studies regarding the use of this analgesic during labor associate it with newborn respiratory depression (Sentnor et al., 1962; Simeckova et al., 1960).

An increased frequency of malformations was observed in offspring of animals given oxymorphone during embryogenesis, but a dose 5000 times that normally used in humans was used (Geber and Schramm, 1975).

OXYCODONE

Among 78 infants exposed to oxycodone during the first trimester, the frequency of birth defects was not increased above population background levels (3.5–5 percent) (Schick et al., 1996). In an unpublished study, the frequency of birth defects among 281 infants born to women who were prescribed oxycodone during the first trimester was not increased (Rosa, 1993). There are no published animal reproduction studies.

Pharmacologically, this analgesic is expected to result in neonatal respiratory depression and possibly withdrawal symptoms. Although there is a paucity of information regarding the last three drugs (hydrocodone, oxymorphone, and oxycodone), they are listed as FDA category B drugs by their manufacturers.

ALPHAPRODINE

Although this narcotic analgesic has been available since the 1940s (Hapke and Barnes, 1949), there are no available large human reproduction studies. Alphaprodine crosses the placenta readily and may result in newborn respiratory depression. This agent is no longer commonly used during pregnancy because of the potential for causing a sinusoidal heart rate pattern in the fetus (Gray et al., 1978).

FENTANYL

Fentanyl is a synthetic narcotic that is 1000 times more potent than meperidine (Spielman, 1987). No studies have been published on the use of fentanyl during the first trimester. It may, however, cause respiratory depression with chronic maternal use in the third trimester (Regan et al., 2000). No birth defects were found among rats given high doses of this drug throughout gestation (Fujinaga et al., 1986).

Alfentanil and sufentanil are discussed in Chapter 6.

PROPOXYPHENE

Propoxyphene is a commonly used analgesic agent similar in structure to methadone. It has neither an antipyretic nor antiinflammatory action. In epidemiological investigations, the frequency of congenital anomalies was not increased among the offspring of almost 800 women who used this agent during early pregnancy (Heinonen et al., 1977; Jick et al., 1981). A few case reports of malformations in the offspring of mothers who utilized propoxyphene during pregnancy have been published (Golden et al., 1982; Williams et al., 1983), but no causal links can be established. Propoxyphene is not teratogenic in rabbit, hamster, rat, or mouse animal models at doses 40-fold greater than the usual human dose (Buttar and Moffatt, 1983; Emmerson et al., 1971).

A neonatal withdrawal syndrome (irritability, hyperactivity, tremors, high-pitched cry) was reported among newborns of mothers who used propoxyphene chronically during late pregnancy (Ente and Mehra, 1978; Klein *et al.*, 1975; Quillian and Dunn, 1976; Tyson, 1974). Propoxyphene is opined to be safe for breastfeeding mothers (American Academy of Pediatrics, 1994).

NALBUPHINE

Nalbuphine is an opiate analgesic given parenterally for moderate to severe pain, or as an adjunct to balanced general anesthesia or regional techniques. This narcotic crosses the placenta readily. Nalbuphine, as other narcotics, has the potential to result in neonatal respiratory depression, fetal and neonatal addiction, fetal cardiac function alterations, and withdrawal symptoms in the newborn. For example, this agent was associated with a sinusoidal fetal heart rate pattern, similar to that produced by alphaprodine (Feinstein *et al.*, 1986).

No studies have been published regarding use of this agent during pregnancy during the first trimester. However, according to the manufacturer, this agent was not teratogenic in animal studies.

Narcotic antagonists

These are agents used primarily for the treatment of central nervous system and cardiorespiratory depression secondary to narcotic agonists.

NALOXONE

Naloxone (Narcan), a synthetic congener of oxymorphone, is the most commonly used antagonist agent for reversal of narcotic depression in the newborn. No studies have been published regarding congenital anomalies among the offspring of women who took this drug in the first trimester.

In experimental animal studies (hamsters, mice), the frequency of congenital anomalies was not increased among offspring exposed to naloxone at many times the usual human dose (Geber and Schramm, 1975; Jurand, 1985). It is well known that naloxone may precipitate withdrawal symptoms in newborns whose mothers are addicted to narcotics, and who used very high doses of narcotics near the time of delivery.

NALTREXONE

Another narcotic antagonist, naltrexone (Trexan), is also a congener of oxymorphone. No studies have been published on congenital anomalies after exposure to naltrexone during embryogenesis. Three case series comprising reportedly nonoverlapping patients contained 31 infants whose mothers used naltrexone during the first trimester, and there were no congenital anomalies present (Hulse and O'Neil, 2002; Hulse *et al.*, 2001, 2004). Notably, these gravidas were given naltrexone as part of a treatment regimen for heroin addiction. According to its manufacturer, this agent was shown to be embryocidal in animal studies. Independent investigators have reported no increased frequency of congenital anomalies among rats or rabbits exposed during embryogenesis.

OTHER ANALGESICS

Butalbital

Butalbital is a short-acting barbiturate that is contained in a variety (over 40) of available prescription analgesic compounds. Butalbital is usually combined with aspirin or acetaminophen (with or without caffeine). The most common indication for butalbital-containing analgesic compounds is tension headaches. All barbiturates cross the placenta, as do acetaminophen and aspirin. Barbiturate use in the first trimester was not associated with an increase in the frequency of congenital anomalies in exposed offspring. However, barbiturates have been associated with fetal dependence and newborn withdrawal symptoms when used chronically by the mother in the third trimester.

Medical compounds comprised of isometheptene, dichloralphenazine and acetaminophen (Midrin, Amidrin, Migratine) are used to treat vascular headaches or migraines. Isometheptene, a sympathomimetic drug, causes vasoconstriction. Dichloralphenazone is a mild sedative. This combination is commonly used during pregnancy, but no studies of the risk of congenital anomalies are available for two of the components (isometheptene, dichloralphenazine).

Sumatriptan and other triptans

Sumatriptan (Imitrex) is a selective 5-hydroxytryptamine receptor agonist. It is used primarily as acute therapy for migraine headaches. Among 658 infants born to women who used sumatriptan during the first trimester, the frequency of congenital anomalies was no greater than expected (Kallen and Lynger, 2001). According to its manufacturer, it has been shown to cause malformations in rabbits but was not teratogenic in rats. Using the *ex vivo* isolated perfused cotyledon technique, sumatriptan crossed the placenta by passive transport in the *ex vivo* isolated perfused cotyledon technique (Schenker *et al.*, 1995). This drug is listed as an FDA category C agent, but seems to be safe for use during pregnancy (Table 8.2). Other triptans include nartriptan, almotriptan, rizatriptan, zolmitriptan. None have been adequately studied during pregnancy.

SPECIAL CONSIDERATIONS

Labor analgesics

MEPERIDINE

Meperidine provides effective pain relief for 2–4 h in most patients who need systemic labor analgesics. The usual dose is 25–50 mg IV or 50–75 mg IM. Promethazine, in a dose of 25 mg, is also usually given as an adjunct to prevent nausea (Table 8.3).

BUTORPHENOL

Butorphenol is also a very effective narcotic for systemic analgesia and is usually given in a dose of 1–2 mg either IV or IM. This agent provides pain relief for up to 4 h.

Table 8.2 Comparison of Teratogen Information System (TERIS) risk and Food and Drug Administration (FDA) pregnancy risk ratings

Drug	Risk	Risk rating
Acetaminophen	None	B
Butalbital	Unlikely	C*
Butorphanol	Undetermined	C_m^*
Fenoprofen	Undetermined	B*
Fentanyl	Undetermined	C_m^*
Hydrocodone	Unlikely	C*
Hydromorphone	Unlikely	B*
Ibuprofen	Minimal	B_m^*
Indomethacin	None to minimal	B*
Isometheptene	Undetermined	C
Meclofenamate	Undetermined	B*
Meperidine	Unlikely	B*
Methadone	Unlikely	B*
Morphine	Congenital anomalies: unlikely neonatal neurobehavioral Effects: moderate	C_m^*
Nalbuphine	Undetermined	B_m^*
Naloxone	Undetermined	B_m
Naltrexone	Undetermined	C_m
Naproxen	Undetermined	B_m^*
Oxycodone	Undetermined	B_m^*
Oxymorphone	Undetermined	B*
Pentazocine	Unlikely	C*
Phenacetin	None	B
Phenylbutazone	Undetermined	C_m^*
Promethazine	None	C
Propoxyphene	None	C*
Propranolol	Undetermined	C_m^*
Sulindac	Undetermined	B*
Sumatriptan	Unlikely	C_m

Compiled from: Friedman *et al.*, 1990; Briggs *et al.*, 2005; Friedman and Polifka, 2006.

Analgesia following minor procedures

Several oral narcotic agents (hydrocodone, oxycodone) provide satisfactory relief for moderate pain associated with minor surgical procedures, such as dental procedures. Narcotic agents should not be used over a protracted period of time (more than 7 days) late in pregnancy because of the potential for neonatal dependence or withdrawal symptoms.

Headache

Headaches are common during pregnancy and may increase in frequency during gestation. In all headache syndromes, potential identifiable causes of headaches should be ruled out before a long-term treatment plan is implemented. Headache etiology in most patients is unknown. Headaches are divided into two major categories: (1) tension and (2) vascular (migraine). For mild to moderate headaches, aspirin, acetaminophen, ibuprofen, or naproxen usually provide satisfactory relief. Acetaminophen is the preferred analgesic for use during pregnancy. Aspirin should be avoided during pregnancy for hematologic reasons, and especially when headaches occur close to term. Aspirin increases the potential for increased bleeding from salicylcate use. More generally, NSAIDS should not be used after 34 weeks gestational age because of the theoretical potential for premature closure of the ductus arteriosus and other potential adverse effects. If other agents have failed, ibuprofen appears to pose the least risk for increased bleeding and premature ductus closure.

Migraine (vascular) headaches are difficult to treat during pregnancy, and they seem to increase in frequency during gestation. The vasoconstrictive agent, ergotamine, is one of the agents used to treat migraine headaches in the nonpregnant patient; however, it is not recommended for use during pregnancy because it has (1) vasoconstrictive and (2) oxytocin-like actions. Propranolol at a dose of 40 mg or higher per day (several divided doses) has been effective for the treatment of some migraines in the pregnant patient, and poses a negligible risk to the unborn child.

Amitriptyline, a tricyclic antidepressant, has been used to treat migraine headaches in pregnant women. However, this agent should be used as a third line of medical treatment for migraine headaches among pregnant women with vascular headaches who have not responded to analgesics or propranolol.

The combination of isomethertene, dichloralphenazone, and acetaminophen is also used for treatment of migraine headaches during pregnancy. However, the effects of isomethertene and dichloralphenazone are unknown. Importantly, this combination of drugs should be avoided in women with hypertension. The usual dose is two capsules orally at the beginning of an attack and then one capsule every hour; up to five capsules in any one 12-h period (see manufacturer's prescribing recommendations).

Sumatriptan (Imitrex) has been studied sufficiently to state that the risk of congenital anomalies following first trimester exposure is not greater than that in the general population (Kallen and Lygner, 2001).

As emphasized earlier, narcotic analgesics should not be utilized on a chronic basis for headaches because of the potential for addiction in the mother and withdrawal symptoms in the fetus. However, narcotic analgesics may be efficacious for the treatment of an acute migraine episode with little to no risk to the fetus.

Table 8.3 Suggested dosage regimens for some commonly used parenteral narcotic analgesic agents for postoperative pain[a]

Agent	Dosage
Butorphanol	2–4 mg IM q 3–4 h, or 0.5–1 mg IV q 3–4 h
Hydromorphone	1–2 mg IM q 3–4 h, or 0.5–1 mg IV q 3 h
Meperidine	50–100 mg IM q 3–4 h
Morphine	10 mg (5–20 mg) IM q 4 h
Nalbuphine	10 mg IM or IV q 3–6 h
Pentazocine	30 mg IM or IV q 3–4 h

[a]Refer to manufacturer's recommendations.

Analgesia following operative procedures

The most common indication for acute narcotic analgesic therapy is for postoperative pain relief. Women who require surgery during pregnancy can be safely treated with a variety of analgesic agents for postoperative pain with relative safety for the fetus. Two commonly used regimens are meperidine (Demerol), 50–100 mg IM every 3–4 h, or hydromorphone (Dilaudid), 1–2 mg every 3–4 h. Dosage regimens for various parenteral preparations are summarized in Table 8.3.

SUMMARY

Analgesics are not a high-risk drug class for use during pregnancy (Table 8.2). The high-level summary is that none are associated with an increased risk of congenital anomalies, if the risk is known (Table 8.2). The appropriate caveats are that dosage and frequency of dosage must be managed carefully during pregnancy, especially in the third trimester. For example, meperidine probably requires no adjustment in dose or frequency because its pharmacokinetics do not change appreciably from the nonpregnant to pregnant states. In contrast, morphine has a decreased half-life and increased clearance, perhaps indicating a need for upward dose adjustment and or greater frequency (Table 8.3). Important neonatal complications to monitor for are: (1) bleeding disorders (salicylates); (2) neonatal dependence (narcotics and barbiturates); and (3) withdrawal (narcotics and barbiturates). In large doses, maternal respiratory depression may occur with narcotic analgesia. Large analgesic doses are sometimes an attempt to compensate for more rapid metabolism of opiates during pregnancy (Table 8.2).

Key references

Al-Alaiyan S, Seshia M, Casiro O. Neurodevelopmental outcome of infants exposed to indometracin antenatally. *J Perinat Med* 1996; **24**: 405.
CLASP (Collaborative Low-Dose Aspirin Study in Pregnancy) Collaborative Group. Low-dose aspirin in pregnancy and early childhood development. Follow-up of the collaborative low-dose aspirin study in pregnancy. *Br J Obstet Gynaecol* 1995; **102**: 861.
Hulse G, O'Neil G. Using naltrexone implants in the management of the pregnant heroin user. *Aust NZ J Obstet Gynaecol* 2002; **42**: 569.
Hulse GK, O'Neil G, Arnold-Reed DE. Methadone maintenance vs. implantable naltrexone treatment in the pregnant heroin user. *Int J Gynaecol Obstet* 2004; **85**: 170.
Kallen B. Drug treatment of rheumatic disease during pregnancy. *Scand J Rheumatol* 1998; **27** (Suppl. 107): 119.
Kallen B, Lygner PE. Delivery outcome in women who used drugs for migraine during pregnancy with special reference to sumatriptan. *Headache* 2001; **41**: 351.
Little BB. Pharmacokinetics during pregnancy. Evidence-based maternal dose formulation. *Obstet Gynecol* 1999; **93**: 858.
Rasenen J, Jouppila P. Fetal cardiac function and ductus arteriosus during indomethacin and sulindac therapy for threatened preterm labor. A randomized study. *Am J Obstet Gynecol* 1995; **173**: 20.

Regan J, Chambers F, Gorman W, MacSullivan R. Neonatal abstinence syndrome due to prolonged administration of fentanyl in pregnancy. *Br J Obstet Gynaecol* 2000; **107**: 570.

Schenker S, Yang Y, Perez A, Henderson GI, Lee MP. Sumatriptan (Imitrex) transport by the human placenta. *Proc Soc Exper Biol Med* 1995; **210**: 213.

Further references are available on the book's website at http://www.drugsandpregnancy.com

9

Anticonvulsant drugs during pregnancy

Seizure disorders are among the most common serious medical conditions encountered during pregnancy (Cantrell *et al.*, 1994) and are estimated to occur among 0.5–1 percent of all pregnancies (Janz, 1975). It is thought that one million women of childbearing age have a seizure disorder (Yerby, 1991), and an estimated three or four of 1000 gravidas are epileptic (Morrow *et al.*, 2006).

PREGNANCY COMPLICATIONS

Epilepsy has been reported to be associated with an increase in pregnancy complications in both the mother and the fetus (Cantrell *et al.*, 1994). Some of the maternal complications include an increased risk of pregnancy-induced hypertension, preterm delivery, and low birth weight (Bjerkedal and Bahna, 1973; Wilhelm *et al.*, 1990). The major risk to the fetus is an increase in congenital malformations, about two- to three-fold higher than the general population (Yerby, 1994). Specifically, clusters of anomalies seem present with some drugs. For example, neural tubes defects (i.e., spina bifida) are associated with valproic acid and carbemazepine (Yerby, 2000, 2003). Several maternal and fetal complications are associated with epilepsy during pregnancy (Table 9.1).

Antiseizure medications during pregnancy and the occurrence of syndromes (fetal hydantoin syndrome, fetal valproate syndrome) is an area where the emerging field of pharmacogenetics has made progress. The genetic enzyme complement of the gravida and her fetus mediate the effects of these antiseizure medications. Pharmacokinetics are important in the management of pregnancy complicated by epilepsy. Piecemeal information is

Table 9.1 Reported complications of epilepsy and pregnancy

Maternal	Fetal or neonatal
Abruptio placentae	Congenital anomalies
Caesarean delivery	Drug withdrawal
Eclampsia	Feeding difficulties
Hyperemesis gravidarum	Hypoxemia
Hypotonic labor	Low birth weight
Increased seizure activity	Malnutrition
Preeclampsia	Neonatal hemorrhage
Pregnancy-induced hypertension	Perinatal deaths
Preterm delivery	Prematurity
Vaginal bleeding	Stillbirths
	Seizures

Cantrell *et al.*, 1994.

available regarding pharmacokinetics of antiseizure medications during pregnancy (Table 9.2).

EFFECT OF PREGNANCY ON ANTICONVULSANT LEVELS

Physiologic changes associated with pregnancy may affect the metabolism, plasma protein binding, maternal serum level, and clearance of anticonvulsants and other drugs. In one review, pharmacokinetics of several anticonvulsants during pregnancy showed that the levels of phenytoin and phenobarbital decreased during pregnancy and that the clearance of phenytoin, phenobarbital, carbamazepine, and valproate increased during pregnancy (Levy and Yerby, 1985). The level of anticonvulsants during pregnancy for a given dose varies among women and cannot be predicted given the limited data available. Therefore, it is recommended that anticonvulsant levels be monitored throughout pregnancy because seizure activity may increase in some pregnant women (Levy and Yerby, 1985). A survey of the published literature on anticonvulsant pharmacokinetics indicates that dose and frequency of anticonvulsants given during pregnancy to control seizures probably require adjustment (Table 9.2).

Dose and frequency management of anticonvulsant therapy during pregnancy can optimize therapy given the limited information available. Generalizing the findings from studies published on pharmacokinetics of anticonvulsant during pregnancy, it is observed that (1) clearance is increased; (2) steady state concentration is decreased; and (3) plasma protein binding is decreased. These changes indicate that dose adjustment and monitoring levels should be considered because of the expanded volume of distribution associated with pregnancy, the decreased steady state concentrations, and the increased clearance of the drug.

CONGENITAL ANOMALIES AND MATERNAL ANTICONVULSANT THERAPY

Women with epilepsy requiring anticonvulsant therapy are known to have a two- to three-fold increased risk of having an infant with a congenital anomaly (Hill, 1973;

Table 9.2 Pharmacokinetics of antiseizure medications during pregnancy

Agent	n	EGA (weeks)	Route	AUC	V_d	C_{max}	CS_s	$t_{1/2}$	Cl	PPB	Control group[a]	Authors
Carbamazepine	14	16–40	PO						↑			Dam et al. (1979)
Carbamazepine	46	12–40	PO						=		Yes (2)	Bardy et al. (1982)
Carbamazepine	8	30–37	PO				↓		↑		Yes (2)	Bologa et al. (1991)
Carbamazepine	12	12–40	PO				↓		↑		Yes (2)	Froescher et al. (1981)
Carbamazepine	6	8–40	PO				↓		↑		Yes (2)	Battino et al. (1982)
Carbamazepine	9	8–32	PO, IV			=	↓		↓		Yes (2)	Battino et al. (1985)
Carbamazepine	100	6–20	PO								No	Omtzigt et al. (1993)
Carbamazepine	5	8–40	PO				↓		=	↓	Yes (2)	Yerby et al. (1985)
Phenobarbital	5	12–40	PO				↓		=		Yes (2)	Lander et al. (1984)
Phenobarbital	12	8–40	PO				↓		↑		Yes (2)	Battino et al. (1985)
Phenobarbitone	23	12–40	PO						↑		Yes (2)	Bardy et al. (1982)
Phenobarbitone	8	16–40	PO						=		Yes (2)	Dam et al. (1979)
Phenytoin	111	8–40	PO						↑		Yes (2)	Bardy et al. (1982)
Phenytoin	7	16–40	PO						=		Yes (2)	Dam et al. (1979)
Phenytoin	48	1–42	PO				↓				Yes (2)	Dansky et al. (1982)
Phenytoin	3	8–40	PO				↓		=		Yes (2)	Battino et al. (1985)
Phenytoin	15	8–40	PO				↓			↓	Yes (2)	Chen et al. (1982)
Phenytoin	5	16–36	PO, IV						↑		Yes (2)	Lander et al. (1984)
Phenytoin	16	8–40	PO							↓	Yes (1)	Ruprah et al. (1982)
Phenytoin and phenobarbitone	75	8–40	PO							↓	Yes (2)	Chen et al. (1982)
Primidone	10	12–40	PO				=		=		Yes (2)	Bardy et al. (1982)
Primidone	5	8–40	PO								Yes (2)	Battino et al. (1985)
Primidone and phenobarbitone	9	8–40	PO		↑						Yes (2)	Battino et al. (1984)
Primidone	5	33–38	PO		↓	↓			↑		Yes (2)	Bologa et al. (1991)
Primidone	14	10–40	PO				↓	↓	↑		No	Nau et al. (1982a)
Primidone	7	16–40	PO						=		Yes (2)	Dam et al. (1979)
Valproic acid	1	28	PO								No	Nau et al. (1982b)

*Source: Little BB. Obstet Gynecol 1999; **93**: 858.*

EGA, estimated gestational age; AUC, area under the curve; V_d, volume of distribution; C_{max}, peak plasma concentration; C_{ss}, steady-state concentration; $t_{1/2}$, half-life; Cl, clearance; PPB, plasma protein binding; PO, by mouth; ↓ denotes a decrease during pregnancy compared with nonpregnant values; ↑ denotes an increase during pregnancy compared with nonpregnant values; = denotes no difference between pregnant and nonpregnant values; IV, intravenous; IM, intramuscular.
[a]Control groups: 1, nonpregnant women; 2, same individuals studied postpartum; 3, historic adult controls (sex not given); 4, adult male controls; 5, adult male and female controls combined.

Janz, 1975, 1982; Kelly, 1984). A review of approximately 750 000 pregnancies (13 separate cohort studies) indicated that the birth defect rate for newborns of epileptic mothers was 7 percent compared to 3 percent for controls (Kelly, 1984).

ETIOLOGY OF MALFORMATIONS

The pathophysiology of congenital malformations associated with epilepsy is unknown. Evidence suggests that it is a combination of exposure to anticonvulsant medication in an individual with epilepsy who may be 'genetically' susceptible to poor metabolism of the drugs. It is thought that teratogenic effects of certain anticonvulsant drugs may be secondary to a genetic 'defect' (lowered or no activity) in the epoxide hydrolase enzyme system, resulting in an inability to completely metabolize 'toxic' intermediary oxidative metabolites (Bielec et al., 1995; Buehler et al., 1990; Finnell et al., 1992; Jones et al., 1989; Stickler et al., 1985; Van Dyke et al., 2000).

Some anticonvulsants, especially of the phenytoin type, may be associated with folic acid anemia and may also depress vitamin D (Lane and Hathaway, 1985). Therefore, vitamin (D and K) and folic acid supplements have been recommended for the pregnant woman with epilepsy who is taking anticonvulsant medications (Yerby, 2003). Phenytoin and other anticonvulsants may be associated with hemorrhagic disease in the neonate, which may progress to be severe or fatal if it occurs in the first 24 h following delivery (Allen et al., 1980; Lane and Hathaway, 1985). Other than avoiding salicylates during pregnancy, vitamin K supplementation during the last 2 months of pregnancy (10 mg PO) or in the last 2 weeks (20 mg PO) was recommended (Lane and Hathaway, 1985).

SYNDROMES AND ISOLATED CONGENITAL ANOMALIES ASSOCIATED WITH ANTICONVULSANTS

The range of dysmorphic features that have been associated with exposure to anticonvulsants during embryogenesis is wide (Table 9.3). Syndromologists who are 'splitters' assign a new syndrome name to each drug's collection of defects. Those who are 'lumpers' use the 'fetal anticonvulsant syndrome' as an umbrella for all the defects that occur with all anticonvulsants. On balance, each drug seems to have a signature constellation of anomalies, ranging from minor craniofacial dysmorphia to spina bifida (Table 9.3). Dysmorphic features associated with older anticonvulsants have been studied extensively, but newer ones have not been studied as thoroughly.

The overall frequency of congenital anomalies was 4.2 percent among 3607 cases of anticonvulsant exposure during pregnancy in the UK Epilepsy and Pregnancy Register, a prospective, observational, registration, and follow-up study. Decomposing the rates among the congenital anomalies, 6.0 percent of infants exposed to polytherapy had congenital anomalies compared to 3.7 percent among those exposed only to monotherapy during gestation. Valproic acid was associated with a higher frequency of congenital anomalies (6.3 percent) than other anticonvulsants in the study. Notably, high doses (>200 mg) of lamotrigene were associated with an increased frequency of congenital anomalies (5.4 percent). Similarly, high doses of valproic acid (>800 mg) were associated with a 9.1 percent congenital anomaly rate. When valproic acid was a component of

Table 9.3 Syndromic features associated with exposure to antiepileptic drugs (AEDs) during embryogenesis

Drug	Distinctive facies	Facial clefting	Cleft lip/palate	Growth delay	Microcephaly	NTDs	Hypoplastic distal phalanges	CHD	UGD
Carbemazepine	+	–	–	–	+	+	–	–	–
Clorazepam	+	–	–	–	–	–	+	–	–
Diones[a]	+	–	+	+	+	–	–	+	+
Phenobarbital	+	+	+	+	+	–	+	+	–
Phenytoin	+	–	+	+	+	–	+	+	–
Primidone	+	–	–	+	–	–	+	+	–
Valproic acid	+	–	–	+	–	+	+	–	+
New generation AEDs									
Felbamate	?	?	?	?	?	?	?	?	?
Gabapentin	+	–	–	–	–	+	–	–	–
Lamotrigene	–	–	–	–	–	+	–	–	–
Oxcarbazepine	–	–	–	–	–	+	–	–	+
Topiramate	+	–	–	–	–	–	–	–	–
Vigabatrin	?	?	?	?	?	?	?	?	?
Zonisamide	+	–	–	–	–	+	–	+	–

NTDs, Neural tube defects (especially spina bifida); CHD, congenital heart defect; UGD, urogenital defect.

[a]Trimethadione, paramethadione

Compiled from published reports (Dansky and Finnell, 1991; Dieterich et al., 1980; Eller et al., 1997; Hanson 1986; Iqbal et al., 2001; Jager-Roman et al., 1986; Koch et al., 1996; Lajeunie et al., 2001; McMahon and Braddock, 2001; Nulman et al., 1997; Ornoy et al., 1998; Rodriguez-Pinilla, 2000; Samren et al., 1997, 1999; Waters et al., 1994; Williams et al., 2001; Yerby and Devinsky, 1994).

polytherapy, the frequency of congenital anomalies was significantly increased (Morrow et al., 2006).

ANTICONVULSANT POLYTHERAPY

Use of multiple anticonvulsant drugs during pregnancy increases the frequency of fetal malformations. For example, four (7 percent) of 55 newborns with *in utero* exposure to two epileptic drugs had congenital anomalies, compared to six (17 percent) of 36 exposed to three agents and four (25 percent) of 16 exposed to four anticonvulsant agents (Lindhout et al., 1984). Some combinations carry a greater risk than others. Carbamazepine, phenobarbital, and valproic acid (with or without phenytoin) polytherapy was reported to be associated with congenital anomalies in seven (58 percent) of 12 infants compared to only three (7.5 percent) of 40 infants with birth defects who were exposed to other combinations of three or four anticonvulsants (Lindhout et al., 1984). The authors argue that combinations of certain anticonvulsants may result in accumulation of toxic epoxide intermediates. The frequency of congenital anomalies was reported to be 1.6 to 4.2 times higher among fetuses of women taking four anticonvulsants compared to those taking only two (Hauser and Hesdorffer, 1990). Polytherapy for epilepsy during the first trimester is uniformly associated with an increased risk for congenital anomalies (Perucca, 2005).

BIRTH DEFECTS, EPILEPSY, AND ANTICONVULSANTS

Cleft lip and/or palate appear to be the most common malformation encountered in these pregnancies. Among 28 reports there were 73 newborns with cleft lip/palate, an estimated rate of 13.8 percent per 1000 compared to the expected background rate of 1.5 per 1000 (Kelly, 1984). Among infants born to mothers, treated with an anticonvulsant who had epilepsy, compared to infants of untreated mothers with the disease, the rate of cleft lip/palate was 15.9 per 1000 and 1.6 per 1000, respectively. Congenital heart defects appeared to be the second most common malformation encountered, with rates reported to be one in 200 (0.5 percent) compared to an expected rate of one in 300 (0.33 percent) (Kelly, 1984). Several other craniofacial and limb defects may also occur and as the list becomes more exhaustive, almost all types of congenital anomalies have been reported in association with epilepsy (Janz, 1982) or its treatment.

One case of fetal myeloschisis was reported in the offspring of a woman who took 4.8 g of carbamazepine during embryogenesis in a suicide attempt (Little et al., 1993).

ANTICONVULSANT AGENTS

Numerous anticonvulsant agents are Food and Drug Administration (FDA) approved for use in the USA. All anticonvulsant drugs cross the placenta. It is not usually possible for women with epilepsy to discontinue medication preconceptually or during pregnancy. A twofold increase in congenital anomalies was reported in infants exposed to anticonvulsant drugs *in utero*, but there was no drug specificity to the malformations (Speidel and Meadow, 1972). A constellation of anomalies were observed among infants exposed *in utero* to phenytoin; this is referred to as 'the fetal hydantoin syndrome'

(Hanson and Smith, 1975). In the ensuing 30 years, various syndromes were reported in association with (1) phenytoin (Hanson and Smith, 1975), (2) phenobarbitone (Seip, 1976), (3) carbamazepine (Jones *et al.*, 1989), (4) primidone (Rudd and Freedom, 1979), (5) trimethadione (Zackai *et al.*, 1975), and (6) valproic acid (DiLiberti *et al.*, 1984). Some have advocated 'lumping' these into a spectrum of major and minor anomalies to be referred to as 'the fetal anticonvulsant drug syndrome' (Zackai *et al.*, 1975).

Phenytoin

Phenytoin or hydantoin (Dilantin, Diphenylan, Mesantoin, Peganone) is an anticonvulsant, chemically related to the barbiturates, and has been available for over 50 years. Other than epilepsy, it is used to treat arrhythmias, trigeminal neuralgia, and myotonic muscular dystrophy. The 'fetal hydantoin syndrome' was first described in 1975 (Hanson and Smith, 1975), but the association of birth defects with phenytoin was suspected before the syndrome was described. The fetal hydantoin syndrome is characterized by a pattern of multiple minor and major craniofacial and limb anomalies (Box 9.1). Phenytoin is the most commonly prescribed anticonvulsant drug. Hemorrhagic complications in the neonate have also been reported in the offspring of mothers receiving phenytoin (Gimovsky and Petrie, 1986; Solomon *et al.*, 1972). IQ was decreased by approximately 10 points among preschool and school-aged children exposed *in utero* to phenytoin in three prospective studies compared to controls (Gladstone *et al.*, 1992; Scolnick *et al.*, 1994; Vanoverloop *et al.*, 1992). Importantly, none of the children was considered mentally retarded.

Cleft palate, cardiac anomalies, and skeletal defects were increased in the offspring of experimental animals which received phenytoin (Finnell, 1981; Finnell and Chernof, 1984; McClain and Langhoff, 1980).

Box 9.1 Characteristics of the fetal hydantoin syndrome

Craniofacial anomalies	Growth deficiency
Cleft lip/palate	Limb defects
Broad nasal bridge	Hypoplasia of distal phalanges, nails
Hypertelorism	Mental deficiency
Epicanthal folds	

Hanson and Smith, 1975.

Carbamazepine

Carbamazepine (Tegretol) is another widely prescribed anticonvulsant that is also used as an analgesic for trigeminal neuralgia. This agent was thought to be ideal for use during pregnancy, and in one review of 94 exposed infants, the rate of congenital anomalies was not increased over the expected rate (Niebyl *et al.*, 1979). However, recent data indicate that carbamazepine (Jones *et al.*, 1989) is associated with a pattern of congenital anomalies similar to that of phenytoin (Box 9.2). The reason for similarities in malformations is probably

Box 9.2 Characteristics of the fetal carbamazepine syndrome

Craniofacial abnormalities	Growth deficiency
Upslanting palpebral fissures	Limb defects
Short nose	Hypoplasia of distal phalanges, nails
Epicanthal folds	Mental deficiency
	Neural tube defects

Jones *et al.*, 1989; Rosa, 1991.

related to the similarity in toxic intermediates when epoxide hydrolase activity is lowered. However, as with phenytoin, it is uncertain as to whether these anomalies are caused by the disease process itself, the medication, a metabolite, an enzyme deficiency, or a combination thereof (Scialli and Lione, 1989). In 1991, it was reported that neural tube defects may occur in up to 1 percent of offspring of pregnant mothers taking carbamazepine, similar to valproic acid (Rosa, 1991). No decrease in IQ was found in carbemazepine-exposed compared to controls among preschool and school-aged children (Scolnick *et al.*, 1994). A case report of a large lumbar meningomyelocele in a patient given megadose carbamazepine during the period of neural tube closure has been published (Little *et al.*, 1993). In a small case series of carbamazepine-exposed infants (*n* = 23), one infant had an identical neural tube defect (myeloschisis) and multiple other congenital anomalies (Gladstone *et al.*, 1992). An excess risk of spina bifida was demonstrated among 3625 infants from Sweden whose mothers had used carbamazepine during pregnancy (Kallen, 1994).

Anomalies have been reported in the offspring of pregnant animals receiving carbamazepine, including central nervous system anomalies (Finnell *et al.*, 1986; Paulson *et al.*, 1979).

Paramethadione and trimethadione

The dione anticonvulsants, paramethadione (Paradione) and trimethadione (Tridione) were used primarily for the treatment of petit mal seizures. The association between trimethadione and malformed newborns was published in 1970 (German *et al.*, 1970). Following this 1970 report, numerous reports of fetal malformations associated with maternal dione use were published. A review of 65 *in utero* exposures to either trimethadione or paramethadione was summarized in the statement: 'a normal child resulting from such a preg-

Box 9.3 Characteristics of the fetal trimethadione syndrome

Craniofacial abnormalities	Cardiac anomalies
Cleft palate	Growth deficiency
V-shaped eyebrows	Hearing loss
Irregular teeth	Mental deficiency
Epicanthal folds	Microcephaly
Backwards-sloped ears	Simian Creases
	Speech difficulty

Kelly, 1984; Zackai *et al.*, 1975.

nancy is the exception' (Kelly, 1984). No controlled studies have been published of birth defects following exposure during embryogenesis with either of these agents. However, a distinct syndrome has been described for trimethadione (Zackai *et al.*, 1975), termed the 'trimethadione syndrome' (Box 9.3). Note that this syndrome differs from the hydantoin and carbamazepine syndromes only in the absence of distal digital hypoplasia (Kelly, 1984). Dione anticonvulsants are contraindicated for use during pregnancy.

Valproic acid

Valproic acid (Depakane, Myproic Acid, Depakote) is used to treat petit mal seizures. It is also used to treat myoclonic and tonic–clonic (grand mal) seizures. Use of valproic acid and an increased risk of neural tube defects and microcephaly was reported in 1980 (Dalens *et al.*, 1980; Gomez, 1981). Valproic acid during the first trimester increases the risk for neural tube defects to approximately 2 percent, compared to about 0.1 percent (one per 1000) in the general population (CDC, 1983; Jager-Roman *et al.*, 1986; Jeavons, 1982; Koch *et al.*, 1983; Lindhout and Schmidt, 1986; Lindhout *et al.*, 1992; Omtzigt *et al.*, 1992; Padmanabhan and Hameed, 1994; Yerby *et al.*, 1992). Major and minor anomalies comprise the constellation malformations called the 'fetal valproate syndrome' (Box 9.4).

Increased frequency of congenital anomalies was reported in offspring of pregnant animals who received valproic acid (Mast *et al.*, 1986; Moffa *et al.*, 1984).

Box 9.4 Malformations reported to be associated with valproic acid: fetal valproate syndrome

Brachycephaly	Hypospadias
Cleft palate	Low-set ears
Congenital heart defects	Neural tube defects
Hypertelorism	Small nose and mouth

Dalens *et al.*, 1980; DLiberti *et al.*, 1984; Jager-Roman *et al.*, 1986; Jeavons, 1982; Koch *et al.*, 1983; Lindhout and Meinardi, 1984; Lindhout and Schmidt, 1986
Mastroiacovo *et al.*, 1983; Tein and MacGregor, 1985; Thomas and Buchanan, 1981.

Succinimides

Ethosuximide (Zarontin), methsuximide (Celontin), and phensuximide (Milontin) are succinimide anticonvulsants utilized primarily for petit mal seizures. Among more than 90 (42 and 57) infants exposed to ethosuximide during the first trimester, the frequency of congenital anomalies was not increased among the population background risk for epileptics (9–11 percent) (Samren *et al.*, 1997, 1999). Importantly, these drugs are anticonvulsant medications and are probably associated with a higher risk of congenital anomalies than these two small series indicate.

Skeletal and central nervous system and other congenital anomalies have been observed in the offspring of pregnant animals that received ethosuximide (el-Sayed *et al.*, 1983; Sullivan and McElhatton, 1977) or methsuximide (Kao *et al.*, 1979).

Ethosuximide use in late pregnancy has been reported to be associated with neonatal hemorrhage (Bleyer and Skinner, 1976) similar to phenytoin.

Phenobarbital

Phenobarbital is often used in combination with other anticonvulsants. It has also been used for many years in pregnant women for a variety of other indications. There is no firm scientific evidence that phenobarbital is teratogenic, although it is often implicated because of its frequent use with other anticonvulsants. Specifically, facial clefts and heart defects seem to be increased in frequency among infants whose mothers took phenobarbital during the first trimester. Detailed dysmorphic examinations indicated that phenobarbital monotherapy during pregnancy was associated with minor congenital anomalies previously associated with the fetal anticonvulsant syndrome (Holmes *et al.*, 2001). A mild reduction in the IQs of adult males exposed to phenobarbital prenatally was found in one study (Reinisch *et al.*, 1995) and in other investigations (Dessens *et al.*, 2000).

Felbamate

No studies of human neonates born after exposure to felbamate during the first trimester have been published. Two experimental animal studies were published that found no increased frequency of congenital anomalies in rats or rabbits that were exposed during embryogenesis.

Lamotrigine

The FDA warning label for use of lamotrigine during pregnancy indicates a 20- to 30-fold increase in the incidence of nonsyndromic (i.e. isolated) cleft palate with the use of this drug during the first trimester. Congenital anomalies were increased in frequency ($n = 6$, 12 percent) among 51 infants whose mothers took lamotrigine during the first trimester (Lamotrigine Pregnancy Registry, 2004; Mackay *et al.*, 1997; Wilton *et al.*, 1998). Among 414 infants exposed to lamotrigine monotherapy in a registry-based study only 12 (2.9 percent) had congenital anomalies (Lamotrigine Pregnancy Registry, 2004; Tennis and Eldridge, 2002). The frequency of congenital anomalies appeared to be increased among 270 infants whose mothers took lamotrigine polytherapy (combined with one or more other anticonvulsants) during embryogenesis, 16 (5.9 percent). Frequency of major congenital anomalies was greatest among infants whose mothers took lamotrigine with valproic acid during the first trimester (11 of 88, 12.5 percent).

The frequency of congenital anomalies (2.1 percent) was not increased among 390 infants born to women who took lamotrigine monotherapy during the first trimester of pregnancy in another registry-based study (Morrow *et al.*, 2003). No birth defects were reported in 61 infants whose mothers were treated with lamotrigine monotherapy during pregnancy. Four major congenital anomalies (5.9 percent) were found in 68 infants born to women treated with an anticonvulsant polytherapy that contained lamotrigine (Vajda *et al.*, 2003). The frequency of birth defects ($n = 1$, or 2 percent) was not increased among 51 infants born following lamotrigine monotherapy during the first trimester (Sabers *et al.*, 2004). Importantly, at least 16 fetuses or infants with neural tube defects have been reported when the mother took lamotrigine, often in polytherapy with valproic acid or carbamazepine, during the first trimester (Lamotrigine Pregnancy Registry, 2004).

Experimental animal studies of lamotrigene during embryogenesis are equivocal, with a report of no increased frequency of congenital anomalies, and another reporting an increased frequency of birth defects.

Levetiracetam

No epidemiological studies of infants born after exposure to levetiracetam during the first or subsequent trimester of gestation have been published. Nonetheless, the nature of the disease being treated (seizure disorder) and the drug (anticonvulsive agent) raise concerns that infants exposed to levetirecetam during gestation may be at an increased risk of birth defects.

Gabapentin

Congenital anomalies have been reported among 44 women who used gabapentin during pregnancy (Montouris, 2003), but (1) the anomalies (hypospadias, renal agenesis) are not consistent with the fetal anticonvulsant syndrome and (2) it is not clear from the published report precisely when during pregnancy the women were exposed. A case report of an infant with holoprosencephaly and cyclopia whose mother took carbamazepine and gabapentin during pregnancy has been published (Rosa, 1995), but it is unclear what, if any, association this has with prenatal drug exposure. Other isolated case reports have also been published (Bruni, 1998; Morrell, 1996), but their relationship to risks associated with gabapentin use during pregnancy is unknown. A case report described a child whose features resembled the 'fetal anticonvulsant syndrome' and whose mother took gabapentin and valproic acid during pregnancy (Moore et al., 2000).

Experimental animal studies with mice, rats, and rabbits have not found an increased frequency of congenital anomalies among offspring exposed to gabapentin during embryogenesis.

Oxcarbazepine

Important note: oxcarbazepine is an anticonvulsant drug closely related to a known human teratogen, carbamazepine. This drug has been part of a polytherapy regimen in most published reports of its use during pregnancy, confounding its possible causal role.

Among 248 pregnancies exposed to oxcarbazepine monotherapy during pregnancy, there were six congenital anomalies (2.4 percent), which is similar to that expected in the general population. Among 61 infants whose mothers were given polytherapy that included oxcarbazepine, four birth defects (6.6 percent) occurred (Montouris, 2005), which is greater than that in the general population.

Among 35 infants born to epileptic women treated with oxcarbazepine monotherapy in one series, no congenital anomalies were found (Meischenguiser et al., 2004). Among 20 infants born to women who took polytherapy anticonvulsant regimen that included oxcarbazepine, one baby was born with a major cardiac congenital anomaly. One of nine infants born to epileptic women treated in the first trimester with oxcarbazepine monotherapy had multiple major birth defects involving the genitourinary tract (Kaaja et al., 2003). Isolated case reports involving polytherapy (including oxcarbazepine) of single infants with spina bifida, short spine, hypospadias, or limb reduction defects have been published (Lindhout et al., 1992; Lindhout and Omtzigt, 1994). The causal meaning of case reports is not possible to ascertain. Animal teratology studies (one published, Bennett et al., 1996, one unpublished) of oxcarbazepine were negative.

Tiagabine

Among nine infants whose mothers took tiagabine during pregnancy, one infant had a congenital anomaly, but this was not similar to any of the anomalies in the 'fetal anticonvulsant syndrome' (Morrell, 1996).

In unpublished experimental animal studies (rats, rabbits) employing doses much higher than the human dose, and at doses toxic to the mother, there were increased frequencies of congenital anomalies in rats but not rabbits. None of this information is relevant to the assessment of human risk of birth defects following exposure to tiagabine during embryogenesis.

Topiramate

In a case series three normal infants were reported whose mothers were treated with topiramate sometime during gestation (Morrell, 1996). In another case report, a pattern of minor anomalies similar to the 'fetal anticonvulsant syndrome' were observed in an infant whose mother took topiramate monotherapy throughout pregnancy (Hoyme et al., 1998). The relevance of these anecdotal reports, if any, to human risks following exposure to topiramate during embryogenesis is unknown.

The results of studies of rats, mice, and rabbits exposed to topiramate during embryogenesis are conflicting. Rats had limb defects at the highest doses, mice had craniofacial defects, and rabbits had vertebral anomalies. The inconsistent findings and the lack of peer review of these unpublished studies confound any possible interpretation of these data.

Vigabatrin

Among 47 infants born to women who took vigabatrin during the first trimester two (4.3 percent) had congenital anomalies (Wilton et al., 1998).

In several studies, major anomalies were increased among mice exposed to vigabatrin during embryogenesis, and cleft palate occurred among rabbits exposed to maternally and fetotoxic doses. No increased frequency of congenital anomalies was found among rats exposed to vigabatrin during embryogenesis.

Zonisamide

Zonisamide is an anticonvulsant used either in monotherapy or polytherapy to treat a broad spectrum of epileptic conditions (Oguni et al., 1988; Schmidt et al., 1993). In one small prospective case series of 26 infants born to women treated throughout pregnancy with zonisamide as part of a polytherapy anticonvulsant regimen, two infants (7.7 percent) were reported with major congenital anomalies (anencephaly, atrial septal defect) (Kondo *et al.*, 1996). A child whose mother took zonisamide, carbamazepine, phenytoin, sodium valproate, and a barbiturate during pregnancy was reported with features of anticonvulsant embryopathy (Noda *et al.*, 1996).

Increased frequencies of congenital anomalies were found in animal studies of teratogenicity of zonisamide in rats (cardiac), mice (visceral, skeletal), dogs (cardiac), and monkeys (pregnancy wastage) (Terada *et al.*, 1987a,b,c).

SPECIAL CONSIDERATIONS

In general, women with epilepsy should be given preconceptual counseling, and a management plan developed (Box 9.5). If a pregnant woman presents on anticonvulsant therapy, she should be given counseling regarding the two- to three-fold increased risk of malformations. She should also be offered high-resolution ultrasound and alpha-fetoprotein screening at appropriate gestational intervals. It should be emphasized that these techniques, although helpful, may not rule out anticonvulsant embryopathy. Anticonvulsant therapy should be continued if necessary. It may be possible to discontinue medications in certain patients who have been seizure-free for protracted periods of time, especially in patients who have had petit mal seizures. Trimethadione and paramethadione are generally contraindicated during pregnancy, and valproic acid should be avoided if possible. One of the succinimides, ethosuximide, would appear to be a better choice for petit mal seizures in the rare pregnant patient where it is indicated. Monitoring of serum levels of anticonvulsants may be indicated in some pregnant women, especially those with increased seizure activity. A suggested management protocol for pregnant patients with epilepsy is summarized in Box 9.5.

Patients should be counseled that anticonvulsant therapy during pregnancy is associated with risks of serious birth defects. For example, with valproic acid and carbamazepine, the risk for neural tube defects, spina bifida in particular, is increased with exposure during the first trimester (Table 9.4). Risks for other congenital anomalies are increased when associated with exposure to other anticonvulsants during embryogenesis (Table 9.3). Risk for valproic acid-associated neural tube defects is increased at (1) high doses (> 800 mg/day) and (2) polytherapy. Interestingly, recent analyses indicate that the risk for neural tube defects with exposure to oxcarbazepine or to lamotrigene is not different from the risk with carbamazepine (Perucca, 2005).

Table 9.4 Frequency of spina bifida in association with anticonvulsants

	Valproic acid *n/N*	Carbamazepine *n/N*	Other *n/N*
Total	10/740	10/1132	6/4489
Unconfounded total	9/612	9/984	6/4489
Proportion	1/68	1/109	1/748

Number expected (background risk) 1/1500.

n, number affected; *N*, number exposed.

Adapted from Rosa, 1991.

Box 9.5 Suggested protocol for counseling management of pregnant women with epilepsy

Counsel regarding a possible epilepsy-associated two- to three-fold increased risk of malformations above background (3.5–5%)

Indicate that risk for neural tube defects (NTDs) is increased (see Table 9.4), as indicated

Continue anticonvulsants if necessary to control seizures

Seizures may cause congenital anomalies and threaten maternal health; therefore, controlling seizures is a high priority

During embryogenesis [2–10 weeks estimated gestation age (EGA) by menstrual dates, or first 8 weeks of gestation by conception dates] avoid certain anticonvulsants if possible:

- Avoid trimethadione and paramethadione if possible
- Avoid valproic acid if possible
- Avoid carbamazepine if possible
- Avoid polytherapy if possible
- Avoid large anticonvulsant doses, use minimal necessary to control seizures

Discontinue anticonvulsants in only select patients and with neurological medical consultation

Serial high-resolution ultrasound examinations at appropriate intervals

Maternal alpha-fetoprotein screening at appropriate intervals

Serum anticonvulsant level monitoring

Dose titration to achieve therapeutic levels

Bear in mind that pregnancy changes the pharmacokinetics of anticonvulsants, which may indicate the need to adjust dose and/or frequency to prevent maternal seizures

- Clearance is uniformly increased during pregnancy
- C_{ss} (steady state concentration) is lowered
- Plasma protein binding (PPB) is decreased during pregnancy for anticonvulsants that have been studied

Ratings by the FDA Pregnancy Risk Categories and Teratogen Information System (TERIS) Risk for Congenital Anomalies (Table 9.5) provide informative support for clinical decisions.

Pharmacogenetics

The metabolism of folic acid is inhibited by many anticonvulsant drugs. This alteration in folate metabolism is presumed to be provoked by hepatic enzyme induction and folate malabsorption (Janz, 1982; Maxwell *et al.*, 1972). Phenobarbitone, phenytoin, carbamazepine, valproic acid, and primidone have been implicated in these metabolic alterations (Donaldson, 1991). Human and animal studies support the finding that folic acid supplementation decreases the rate of congenital malformations in infants of epileptic mothers who are receiving anticonvulsants during pregnancy (Biale and Lewenthal, 1984; Dansky *et al.*, 1987; Zhu and Zhou, 1989). Therefore, it is recommended that all

Table 9.5 Comparison of Teratogen Information System (TERIS) risk for congenital anomalies and the Food and Drug Administration (FDA) pregnancy risk categories

Drug	TERIS risk	FDA pregnancy risk rating
Phenytoin/Fosphenytoin	Small to moderate	D
Carbamazepine	Small to moderate	D_m
Valproic acid	Fetal valproate syndrome: moderate	D_m
	Neural tube defects: small to moderate	
	Other malformations: small	
	Neurobehavioral abnormalities: small	
Primidone	Small to moderate	D
Trimethadione/		
Paramethadione	High	D
Ethosuximide	Undetermined	C
Methsuximide	Undetermined	C
Phensuximide	Undetermined	D
Phenobarbital	Chronic anticonvulsive treatment: small	D
	occasional, short-term therapy for other	
	reasons: minimal to small	
Zonisamide	Undetermined	NA

Compiled from: Friedman *et al., Obstet Gynecol* 1990; **75**: 594; Briggs *et al.*, 2005; Friedman and Polifka, 2006.

women of childbearing age receive 0.4–0.5 mg per day of folic acid preconceptually and at least through the first trimester of pregnancy. Epileptic mothers with a positive history of neural tube defects or orofacial clefts in previous children, or paternal or maternal family history should be supplemented preconceptually and through the first trimester with 4–5 mg per day of folic acid, especially women taking valproic acid or carbamazepine (Perucca, 2005).

In addition, mothers receiving the above anticonvulsants should be given 20 mg of vitamin K_1 in the final month of pregnancy (Delblay *et al.*, 1982). The newborn should receive 1 mg of vitamin K_1 at birth and again in 12 h. Umbilical cord prothrombin, partial thromboplastin values, and vitamin-K-dependent clotting factors should be evaluated shortly after delivery (Bleyer and Skinner, 1976, Srinivasan *et al.*, 1982). Folic acid and vitamin D supplements should be considered for pregnant women on phenytoin and other similar anticonvulsants, in addition to vitamin K supplementation in the third trimester (Yerby, 2003).

Unfortunately, no anticonvulsant is known to be free from risk. Further, it is not possible to unravel the relationship of the disease being treated, the treatment for the disease, and the genetic complement of the mother and fetus in assessing the risk for birth defects in epileptic pregnancies.

The management of pregnancy in women with epilepsy requires the coordinated efforts of the patient's primary treating physician and her neurologist. With proper management, 90 percent of women with epilepsy can anticipate uneventful pregnancies and normal children.

Key references

Dessens AB, Cohen-Kettenis PT, Mellenbergh GJ, Koppe JG, van de Poll NE, Boer K. Association of prenatal phenobarbital and phenytoin exposure with small head size at birth and with learning problems. *Acta Paediatr* 2000; **89**: 533.

Holmes LB, Harvey EA, Coull BA *et al*. The teratogenicity of anticonvulsant drugs. *N Engl J Med* 2001; **344**: 1132.

Kaaja E, Kaaja R, Hiilesmaa V. Major malformations in offspring of women with epilepsy. *Neurology* 2003; **60**: 575.

Little BB. Pharmacokinetics during pregnancy. Evidence-based maternal dose formulation. *Obstet Gynecol* 1999; **93**: 858.

Montouris G. Gabapentin exposure in human pregnancy. results from the Gabapentin Pregnancy Registry. *Epilepsy Behav* 2003; **4**: 310.

Montouris G. Safety of the newer antiepileptic drug oxcarbazepine during pregnancy. *Curr Med Res Opin* 2005; **21**: 693.

Morrow J, Russell A, Guthrie E *et al*. Malformation risks of antiepileptic drugs in pregnancy: A prospective study from the UK Epilepsy and Pregnancy Register. *J Neurol Neurosurg Psychiatry* 2006; **77**: 193–8.

Perucca E. Birth defects after prenatal exposure to antiepileptic drugs. *Lancet Neurol* 2005; **4**: 781.

Sabers A, Dam M, a-Rogvi-Hansen B *et al*. Epilepsy and pregnancy. Lamotrigine as main drug used. *Acta Neurol Scand* 2004; **109**: 9.

Van Dyke DC, Ellingrod VL, Berg MJ, Niebyl JR, Sherbondy AL, Trembath DG. Pharmacogenetic screening for susceptibility to fetal malformations in women. *Ann Pharmacother* 2000; **34**: 639–45.

Further references are available on the book's website at http://www.drugsandpregnancy.com

10

Psychotropic use during pregnancy

Major psychiatric disorders such as bipolar disorders (0.5–1.5 percent) or schizophrenia (1–1.5 percent) are relatively uncommon during pregnancy (Yonkers *et al.*, 2004). Many women consume some type of psychoactive agent during pregnancy, ranging from 5 to 10 percent. More than one-quarter of women reported symptoms of depression in one large survey (Little and Yonkers, 2001). Thus, physicians treating pregnant women are likely to regularly encounter psychotropic use during pregnancy. Management of psychiatric illness during pregnancy is similar to the nonpregnant state, with notable exceptions. Exceptions are that pharmacokinetics of drugs, including psychotropics, change with the physiological alterations of pregnancy. Additionally, psychotropics include mood stabilizers (valproic acid, carbamazepine, lithium) that are generally agreed to cause major birth defects (i.e., teratogenic), and should be avoided during embryogenesis. Newer antidepressants, serotonin selective reuptake inhibitors (SSRIs) are not associated with significant birth defect risks (Einarson and Einarson, 2005), but may be associated with complications in neonatal adaptation (Kallen, 2004; Oberlander *et al.*, 2004). Mental illness usually does not worsen during pregnancy, and has a prognosis similar to the nongravid state. Importantly, newer antidepressants (e.g., SSRIs) seem to be more effective in women than the older agents (e.g., tricyclics) (Yonkers, 2003).

Depression is an affective disorder that can be unipolar or bipolar. Anhedonia (lack of pleasure) and a depressed mood are major diagnostic criteria. Patients with depression also have physical symptoms (too much or too little sleep, altered appetite, altered activity – decreased motion or agitated pacing, low energy) and cognitive symptoms (ruminative guilty thoughts, suicidal ideation, poor concentration, indecision). Patients with bipolar disorders have periods of mania and depression (American Psychiatric Association, 1993; Yonkers and Cunningham, 1993). The hypothesis at the root of medical treatment of depression is that at least some cases of depression may be caused by an insufficient amount of serotonin and/or norepinephrine in certain areas of the brain. Psychosis is thought to be secondary to elevated amounts of dopamine in certain regions of the brain.

A number of psychotropic agents are available to which pregnant women and their fetuses may be exposed, including antidepressants, antipsychotics, sedatives, hypnotics, and tranquilizers. Pregnancy-associated physiological changes affect pharmacokinetics of most drugs, and psychotropics are not an exception.

PHARMACOKINETICS

The limited data on pharmacokinetics of psychotropics during pregnancy are not consistent. While diazepam has no change in the clearance and increased half-life in gravidas compared to nonpregnant women, oxazepam has a decreased half-life and increased clearance (Table 10.1). Notably, nortriptyline levels are lower in the pregnant state compared to nonpregnant, suggesting that an increase in dose or frequency may be needed to maintain therapeutic levels.

ANTIDEPRESSANTS

Antidepressants can generally be classified into three major groups: (1) tricyclics, (2) selective serotonin re-uptake inhibitors (SSRIs), and (3) monoamine oxidase inhibitors (MOAs) (Box 10.1).

Box 10.1 Commonly used antidepressant agents

Tricyclics
Imipramine (Janimine, Tofranil, Tipramine)
Amitriptyline (Amitril, Elavil, Endep, Emitrip, Enovil)
Desipramine (Norpramin, Pertofrane)
Nortriptyline (Aventyl, Pamelor)
Doxepin (Adapin, Sinequan)
Protriptyline (Vivactil)
Amoxapine (Asendin)
Clomipramine (Anafranil)

Tetracyclics
Maprotiline (Ludiomil)

Monoamine oxidase inhibitors (MAOs)
Isocarboxazid (Marplan)
Phenelzine (Nardil)
Selegeline (MAO A and MAO B activity)
Tranylcypromine (Parnate)

Selective serotonin re-uptake inhibitors (SSRIs)
Citalopram (Celexa)
Escitalopram (Lexapro)
Fluoxetine (Prozac)
Fluvoxamine (Luvox)
Paroxetine (Paxil)
Setraline (Zoloft)

Serotonin norepinephrine reuptake inhibitors (SNRIs)
Duloxetine (Cymbalta)
Venlafaxine (Effexor)

Other
Bupropion (Wellbutrin)
Mirtazepine (Avanza, Norset, Remergil, Remeron, Zispin)
Nefazdone
Trazodone (Desyrel)

Tricyclics

Women of reproductive age are frequently prescribed tricyclic antidepressants, and there has been no apparent decline in prescriptions in recent years (Wen and Walker, 2004).

Table 10.1 Pharmacokinetics during pregnancy of some psychotropic drugs

Agent	n	EGA (weeks)	Route	AUC	V_d	C_{max}	C_{ss}	$t_{1/2}$	CI	PPB	Control group[a]	Authors
Clorazepate	7	37–42	IM		=	↓		↓	↑		Yes (1)	Rey et al. (1979)
Diazepam	14	37–39	IV		↑			↑	=		Yes (1)	Moore and McBride (1978)
Nortriptyline	6	12–40	PO		↑		↓	↑			Yes (2)	Wisner et al. (1993)
Oxazepam	8	40	PO	↑				↓	↑		Yes (3)	Tomson et al. (1979)

Source: Little BB. *Obstet Gynecol* 1999; **93**: 858.

EGA, estimated gestational age; AUC, area under the curve; V_d, volume of distribution; C_{max}, pleak plasma concentration; C_{ss}, steady-state concentration; $t_{1/2}$, half-life; CI, clearance; PPB, plasma protein binding; PO, by mouth; ↓ denotes a decrease during pregnancy compared with nonpregnant values; ↑ denotes an increase during pregnancy compared with nonpregnant values; = denotes no difference between pregnant and nonpregnant values; IV, intravenous; IM, intramuscular.

[a]Control groups: 1, nonpregnant women; 2, same individuals studied postpartum; 3, historic adult controls (sex not given); 4, adult male controls; 5, adult male and female controls combined.

Table 10.2 Summary of psychotropic exposure during the first trimester

	Total	Elective abortions	Miscarriages	Live births	Anomalies n (%)	Source
European network[a]						
Tricyclics						
Amitriptyline	118	18	10	85	1	1.2	
Clomipramine	134	20	22	87	2[c]	2.3	
Imipramine	30	1	3	27	2	7.4	
Nontricyclics						
Amineptine	40	7	7	25	1	4.0	
Fluoxetine	96	15	13	65	2	3.1	
Fluvoxamine	66	9	6	50	1	2.0	
Maprotiline	107	17	11	77	2	2.6	
Mianserin	48	5	7	37	1	2.7	
Viloxazine	23	4	2	17	0	0	
Meta-analysis[b]						
Combined	–	–	–	830	22	2.0	Chan et al., 2005
Bupropion	–	–	–	72	0	0	Chambers et al., 1996; Goldstein, 1995; Patsuzak et al., 1993
Fluoxitine	–	–	–	300	9	3.0	
Paroxetine	–	–	–	222	9	4.1	Kulin et al., 1998
Trazodone/Nefazodone	–	–	–	121	2	1.7	Einarson et al., 2003
Venlafaxine	–	–	–	125	2	1.6	Einarson et al., 2001

[a]European Network of Teratology Services Surveillance of Psychotropics in Pregnancy, Adapted from McElhatton et al., 1996.

[b]Einarson and Einarson, 2005.

–, not analyzed.

Note: Background risk is 3.5–5%.

[c]Excludes one case of Down syndrome.

In a review of the use of psychotropics during pregnancy, Miller (1994a) found no increased risk of teratogenic effects from the use of tricyclics during pregnancy. However, tricyclics may have both fetal and neonatal effects, such as tachycardia, cyanosis, and other withdrawal symptoms (Miller, 1996; Prentice and Brown, 1989). Tricyclics may also cause adverse maternal effects, such as hypotension, constipation, sedation, tachycardia, and light-headedness (Miller, 1996).

IMIPRAMINE

Imipramine is the prototype of tricyclic compounds and is quite effective in the treatment of endogenous depression. It has potent anticholinergic activity. There is little information regarding its safety during pregnancy, and those studies that are available contain only a few cases of first-trimester imipramine exposure during pregnancy. However, there is no indication that imipramine causes significant teratogenic effects (Banister et al., 1972; Crombie et al., 1972; Heinonen et al., 1977; Idanpaan-Heikkila and Saxen, 1973; Kuenssberg and Knox, 1972; Miller, 1994a; Rachelefsky et al., 1972; Scanlon, 1969). There were 30 cases of first-trimester imipramine exposure recently reported, and the frequency of anomalies was not increased (McElhatton et al., 1996) (see Table 10.2).

Although limb reduction defects were reported by Morrow (1972) to be associated with imipramine use during gestation, these observations were, most authorities believe, coincidence, and not causal. Surveillance groups in the USA and Canada examined the histories of hundreds of women who delivered children with limb reduction defects, and concluded that there was insufficient evidence to suggest a cause-and-effect relationship with imipramine (Banister et al., 1972; Rachelefsky et al., 1972). Withdrawal symptoms (transient respiratory, circulatory, and neurological adaptation abnormalities) were reported in three neonates whose mothers were exposed to imipramine during late pregnancy (Eggermont et al., 1972).

Animal studies indicate an increased frequency of congenital anomalies among the offspring of mice, rabbits, and hamsters who received imipramine in doses several times greater than those used in humans (Guram et al., 1980; Harper et al., 1965; Jurand, 1980), but not at lower doses (Harper et al., 1965; Hendrickx, 1975; Larsen, 1963; Wilson, 1974). Changes in development and behavior were observed among the offspring of pregnant rats given one to five times the human dose of imipramine (Ali et al., 1986; Coyle, 1975; Jason et al., 1981). The relevance of these findings to clinical use in humans is unclear.

AMITRIPTYLINE

Amitriptyline is as efficacious as imipramine for depression, but has marked anticholinergic and sedative activity. Among 427 infants born to mothers who took amitriptyline the frequency of birth defects (25, or 5.9 percent) was not increased (Rosa, personal communication, cited in Briggs et al., 2004), but this study is not peer reviewed. One of 89 infants in another study was malformed, and is within the rate for the general population (McElhatton et al., 1996).

The Collaborative Perinatal Project included 21 pregnant women treated with amitriptyline during the first trimester, and there was no increase in congenital malformations noted among the offspring (Heinonen et al., 1977). The European Network of

Teratology Services reported 118 first-trimester exposures to amitriptyline with no increased frequency of malformations (McElhatton *et al.*, 1996; see Table 10.2). Depression of the central nervous system, although transient, has also been reported in a newborn whose mother was exposed to amitriptyline throughout gestation (Vree and Zwart, 1985). Note that the mother had serum levels in the moderately toxic range, whereas the infant's levels were severely toxic.

Animal teratology studies are not consistent. Thus, the relevance of these findings in animals to therapeutic use in humans is unknown.

DESIPRAMINE

Desipramine is an active metabolite of imipramine used to treat depression. The anticholinergic and sedative effects of desipramine are less than those of imipramine. Among 31 infants whose mothers filled prescriptions for desipramine during the first trimester, there was one malformed infant (Rosa, personal communication, cited in Briggs *et al.*, 2004). Neonatal withdrawal symptoms have been observed with desipramine when taken throughout gestation (Webster, 1973).

NORTRIPTYLINE

Nortriptyline is chemically similar to amitriptyline. Two (3.3 percent) of 61 infants whose mothers had prescriptions for nortriptyline had birth defects (Rosa, personal communication, cited in Briggs *et al.*, 2004). However, this study was not peer reviewed. The active precursor of nortriptyline, amitriptyline, is discussed above. There is a single case report of a newborn with limb reduction anomalies and a dermoid cyst born to a mother who was treated with 30 mg nortriptyline daily in the early first trimester (Bourke, 1974). This is probably not a causal relationship. Maternal use of nortriptyline has been associated with transient urinary retention in the newborn (Shearer *et al.*, 1972).

DOXEPIN

Doxepin has the same characteristics as the other tricyclics. Doxepin is as effective as imipramine and amitriptyline in treating depression, although it has a stronger sedative effect than the other two drugs. No reports have been published on studies of congenital anomalies among the infants born to women treated with doxepin during the first trimester. The frequency of congenital anomalies was not increased among rats and rabbits exposed to doxepin during embryogenesis (Owaki *et al.*, 1971a,b). However, at doses 40 to 100 times those used in humans, an increase in fetal loss and neonatal death was found.

PROTRIPTYLINE, AMOXAPINE, AND CLOMIPRAMINE

There are no available teratologic studies in animals or epidemiological studies of malformations among the newborns of pregnant women treated with these tricyclic agents. No data on protriptyline use in pregnancy are published. Amoxapine is a metabolite of loxapine, an antipsychotic and antidepressant. Among 19 infants, there were three (15.8 percent) with congenital anomalies (Rosa, personal communication, cited in Briggs *et al.*, 2004), which seems high compared to the expected rate of 5.3 percent. However, this study was not peer reviewed and this is a very small number of exposed infants.

The frequency of congenital anomalies was not increased among 134 pregnancies exposed to clomipramine during the first trimester (McElhattan et al., 1996; see Table 10.2). Seizures and abnormalities of perinatal adaptation have been reported in clomipramine-exposed newborns (Cowe et al., 1982; Ostergaard and Pedersen, 1982). Withdrawal symptoms (increased irritability, alternating hypertonia and hypotonia, hyperreflexia, cyanosis, and hypothermia) were described in a newborn 1 day after delivery; these resulted from clomipramine use by the mother during late pregnancy (Boringa et al., 1992). An increased frequency of central nervous system and other anomalies was found among the offspring of pregnant mice exposed to clomipramine in doses 36 times those used in humans (Jurand, 1980). Persistent changes of behavior were found in the offspring of pregnant rats treated with this agent in doses greater than those used clinically (de Ceballos et al., 1985; Drago et al., 1985; File and Tucker, 1983).

MAPROTILINE

Maprotiline is a tetracyclic antidepressant. The frequency of congenital anomalies was not increased among 107 pregnancies exposed to maprotiline during the first trimester (McElhatton et al., 1996; see Table 10.2). Teratology studies in animals have failed to demonstrate any adverse fetal effects (Esaki et al., 1976; Hirooka et al., 1978).

Newer antidepressants or selective serotonin re-uptake inhibitors

This relatively new class of antidepressants includes fluoxetine, paroxetine, and sertraline. Fluoxetine (Prozac) is probably the most commonly used and best-known agent in this group.

Meta-analysis of seven published studies revealed no increased risk for congenital anomalies among infants whose mothers took newer antidepressants (Table 10.2) in the first trimester (Einarson and Einarson, 2005). Recently, problems in neonatal adaptation (Chambers et al., 1996; Costei et al., 2002; Kallen, 2004; Oberlander et al., 2004) and symptoms of a neonatal withdrawal syndrome (Nordeng et al., 2001) were described in infants born to women who used SSRIs in late pregnancy. No adequate studies have been published of infants born following exposure to escitalopram, venlafaxine, or duloxetine during pregnancy. Of 125 infants born to women who took venlafaxine during pregnancy, the frequency of congenital anomalies was not increased. However, the neonatal behavioral alterations noted above may comprise a withdrawal syndrome. Some authorities have anecdotally noted similar symptoms of abstinence among adults who abruptly discontinue SSRI use. Furthermore, it is suggested by some psychiatrists that infants antenatally exposed to SSRIs, and perhaps other antidepressants, remain at risk for depression as teenagers and adults.

FLUOXETINE

Fluoxetine (Prozac) acts primarily by inhibiting serotonin reuptake by neurons (Goldstein et al., 1991). Although there are no large epidemiological studies of fluoxetine in pregnant women, the manufacturer's registry has collected outcome information on 184 pregnancies exposed to this agent (Goldstein et al., 1991). Of these, 35 resulted in spontaneous abortions and 41 pregnancies were electively terminated. Of the 114 live-born infants, 93 were normal, nine were premature, nine had perinatal complications, and three had malformations of a nonspecific type. One of these infants had major cardiac malformations and was born to a mother who took fluoxetine in the second trimester, after the period of embryonic cardiac development. The spontaneous abortion rate of 19 percent and malformation rate of 2–3 percent is similar to the rate of these complications in the general population.

A review of pregnancy outcomes following first-trimester exposure to fluoxetine, found no increase in congenital malformations (Pastuszak et al., 1993). Similarly, there was no increased frequency of anomalies among 96 first-trimester-exposed pregnancies in a European study (McElhatton et al., 1996; see Table 10.2). Meta-analysis indicated no increased risk of congenital anomalies among 300 infants exposed to fluoxetine during the first trimester (Einarson and Einarson, 2005). The frequency of congenital anomalies was not increased among 174 infants whose mothers used fluoxetine throughout pregnancy (including first trimester) (Chambers et al., 1996). The rate of preterm delivery was significantly increased in the fluoxetine-exposed group. No differences in IQ or neurodevelopment were found compared to matched controls at 1.5–3 years of age among 43 children whose mothers took fluoxetine during pregnancy (Nulman and Koren, 1996).

Problems in neonatal adaptation have been reported with SSRI use in late pregnancy.

PAROXETINE AND SERTRALINE

Paroxetine and sertraline are listed as FDA category B drugs. The frequency of congenital anomalies was not increased above background among 394 infants exposed to paroxetine during the first trimester (Diav-Citrin et al., 2002; Ericson et al., 1999; Inman et al., 1996; Kulin et al., 2002; McElhatton et al., 1996; Wilton et al., 1998). However, as recently as July 2006, the manufacturer of Paxil (paroxetine) reported that first trimester use increased the risk of birth defects by between two and three times, with the risk of congenital heart defects being doubled. This contradicts prior studies of the drug's use during the first trimester.

Similarly, the frequency of birth defects was not increased among infants born to 326 women who took sertraline during the first trimester (Chambers et al., 1999; Hendrick et al., 2003; Kulin et al., 2002; Wilton et al., 1998).

Problems in neonatal adaptation termed the 'neonatal adaptation syndrome' was described in infants exposed to paroxetine in late pregnancy (Costei et al., 2002).

CITALOPRAM

Citalopram is an SSRI used to treat depression. Among 125 pregnancies with 114 live born infants whose mothers took citalopram during the first trimester, there was one (0.9 percent) congenital anomaly (Sivojelezova et al., 2005). The authors concluded that the drug was not associated with congenital anomalies with exposure during early pregnancy, but that use of citalopram in late pregnancy was associated with increased frequency of poor neonatal adaptation, recently reported with other SSRIs (Chambers et al., 1996; Costei et al., 2002; Kallen, 2004; Nordeng et al., 2001; Oberlander et al., 2004).

Other nontricyclic antidepressants

Data have been published for other nontricyclic antidepressants that are not discussed above. No increased frequency of congenital anomalies was found among 40, 66, 48, and 23 pregnancies exposed during the first trimester to amineptine, fluvoxamine, mianserin, and viloxazine, respectively (McElhatton *et al.*, 1996; see Table 10.2).

BUPROPION AND TRAZODONE

Burpropion is an antidepressant that is also used in tobacco smoking cessation treatment. It was not associated with an increased risk of congenital anomalies among 354 infants born to women who used bupropion during the first trimester and reported to a registry, 12 (3.4 percent) of whom were malformed (Bupropoin Registry, 2004). Bupropion is a category B drug.

Trazodone is an antidepressant that is also given for its sedative activity. First-trimester exposure to trazodone in 112 infants was not associated with an increased frequency of congenital anomalies (Rosa, personal communication, cited in Briggs *et al.*, 2004), although this study is not peer reviewed. In another investigation that was peer reviewed, 121 women took trazodone or nefazodone during the first trimester. The frequency of congenital anomalies was not increased above that expected in the general population (3.5 percent) (Einarson *et al.*, 2003). Trazodone is a category C drug.

Monoamine oxidase inhibitors

The monoamine oxidase inhibitors are also used for treating depression. There are no large epidemiological studies available regarding the safety of these agents during pregnancy. Only 21 pregnancies with early exposure to the monoamine oxidase inhibitors have been published, and there was an apparent increase in malformations associated with the use of these agents (Heinonen *et al.*, 1977). However, it is impossible to draw clinically useful information from such data because the sample size is too small.

Animal teratology studies undertaken with with monoamine oxidase inhibitors are not consistent, with some reporting no increase in the frequency of birth defects with tranylcypromine (Poulson and Robson, 1963), while others reported an increase in both the mortality rate and stillbirth rate in the isocarboxazid group (Werboff *et al.*, 1961). An increase in placental infarcts occurred in pregnant rats who received iproniazid during gestation (Poulson *et al.*, 1960). Decreased fertility was reported in the offspring of rats treated with nialamide (Tuchmann-Duplessis and Mercier-Parot, 1963). No animal teratology studies have been published on the monoamine oxidase inhibitor, phenelzine.

These agents are generally not used during pregnancy because of potential adverse maternal side effects, and are category C drugs. Women on drugs in this class must follow a diet low in tyramine. Failure to do so may result in hypertensive crisis (Yonkers and Cunningham, 1993). Importantly, monoamine oxidase inhibitors given with meperidine, or other similar agents, may cause hyperthermia (Yonkers and Cunningham, 1993).

ANTIPSYCHOTICS

Antipsychotics are used to treat psychosis of any cause, including psychotic depression, bipolar disorder, substance-induced hallucinations, or delirium-induced psychosis. 'Off-label' these medications are used to augment antidepressants and antianxiolytics. These drugs are continued only as long as the underlying cause of psychosis is present because of the tardive dyskinesia associated with these medications. Antipsychotics were formerly called neuroleptics or major tranquilizers.

Commonly used antipsychotics or neuroleptic agents, with the exception of clozapine (Box 10.2), are dopamine antagonists (Yonkers and Cunningham, 1993). These agents have numerous side effects including anticholinergic effects such as constipation, dryness, and orthostatic hypotension, and extrapyramidal side effects such as akathisia (Miller, 1996; Yonkers and Cunningham, 1993). These agents may also cause marked sedation.

Antipsychotics may cause transient neonatal side effects including withdrawal symptoms and extrapyramidal dysfunction (hand posturing, tremors, and irritability) (Auerbach *et al.*, 1992; Miller, 1994a, 1996; Sexson and Barak, 1989).

Two major confounders make it problematic to evaluate possible associations of antipsychotics and congenital malformations. First, many of these agents are used for indications other than psychosis (hyperemesis, anxiety) where lower doses may be used (Yonkers and Cunningham, 1993). Second, the psychiatric disease itself may be associated with an increased frequency of malformations (Elia *et al.*, 1987).

Butyrophenones

HALOPERIDOL

Haloperidol is a butyrophenone derivative. It has pharmacological properties similar to the piperazine phenothiazines, although it is not chemically related to them. Haloperidol is used as a major tranquilizer to treat psychosis, Tourette's syndrome, mania, and severe hyperactivity. In lower doses than for psychosis, it is also used to treat nausea or anxiety. In a cohort study of 98 pregnant women who received haloperidol for hyperemesis gravidarum (90 during early pregnancy), there were no obvious congenital anomalies or adverse fetal effects noted (van Waes and van de Velde, 1969). These patients received 0.6 mg haloperidol twice a day for differing durations, which is less than the dose typically used in the treatment of psychiatric illnesses. Among 56 infants whose mothers took haloperidol during the first trimester, the frequency of congenital anomalies was not increased (3, or 5.4 percent) (Rosa, personal communication, cited in Briggs *et al.*, 2004).

Two cases of newborns with limb reduction malformations after haloperidol exposure during the first trimester have been published (Dieulangard *et al.*, 1966; Kopelman *et al.*, 1975), but a cause–effect relation cannot be made from such anecdotal observations.

Box 10.2 Commonly used antipsychotic agents

Chlorpromazine (Thorazine)	Trifluoperazine (Stelazine)
Clozapine (Clozaril)	
Fluphenazine (Prolixin, Permitil)	*Newer antipsychotics*
Haloperidol (Haldol, Decanoate)	Amisulpride (Solian)
Loxapine (Loxitane, Daxolin)	Aripiperazole (Abilify)
Mesoridazine (Serentil)	Clozapin (Clozaril)
Molindone (Moban, Lidone)	Olanzapine (Zyprexa)
Perphenazine (Etrafon, Trilafon)	Risperidone (Risperdal)
Thioridazine (Mellaril)	Sertindol (Serdolect)
Thiothixene (Navane)	Ziprasidone (Geodon)

Several researchers have noted an association between large doses of haloperidol in pregnant animals and adverse fetal effects and pregnancy losses (Druga *et al.*, 1980; Gill *et al.*, 1982; Szabo and Brent, 1974), but not at lower doses (Bertelli *et al.*, 1968; Hamada and Hashiguchi, 1978). The pertinence of animal studies to the clinical use of haloperidol in human pregnancy is unclear.

LOXAPINE

Loxapine is a dibenzoxazepine derivative used to treat schizophrenia. No information on the use of this tricyclic antipsychotic during pregnancy in humans has been published. In mice and rats whose mothers were treated with loxapine during embryogenesis, a low incidence of exencephaly and an increase in fetal loss was observed in only one mouse litter out of 20 studied (Mineshita *et al.*, 1970).

Phenothiazines

Phenothiazines are related drugs with potent adrenergic-blocking action. Pharmacologic effects include central nervous system depression, prolonged effects of narcotic or hypnotic drugs, and hypotensive, antiemetic and antispasmodic activity.

CHLORPROMAZINE

Chlorpromazine is a phenothiazine derivative used to treat psychoses and has tranquilizing and sedative effects. It is also used as an antiemetic during pregnancy. Two well-described side effects – hypotension and extrapyramidal tract symptoms – of this drug need special attention. The frequency of congenital anomalies was not increased among 140 infants born to women exposed to this agent during the first trimester of pregnancy (Heinonen *et al.*, 1977). In a cohort study of 264 pregnant women who took chlorpromazine for hyperemesis gravidarum in the first trimester, the frequency of congenital anomalies was not increased (Farkas and Farkas, 1971). One study reported an increase in the frequency of congenital anomalies in offspring exposed to chlorpromazine compared to controls (Rumeau-Rouquette *et al.*, 1977). However, the 3.5 percent incidence of malformations in the chlorpromazine group is no higher than is expected in the general population (3.5–5 percent). The frequency of congenital anomalies or pregnancy loss in 52 pregnancies was not increased among those exposed to chlorpromazine. However, three infants were reported with respiratory distress delivered from mothers treated with 500–600 mg per day (Sobel, 1960). A case of congenital defects involving the heart in association of phenothiazine use during gestation was reported (Vince, 1969), but this is anecdotal and its meaning unknown.

Transient newborn neurological dysfunction was reported by several investigators in association with chlorpromazine use during pregnancy (Hammond and Toseland, 1970; Hill *et al.*, 1966; Levy and Wisniewski, 1974; Tamer *et al.*, 1969). Extrapyramidal signs in exposed infants include muscle rigidity, hypertonia, and tremor.

Some investigators reported an increase in congenital anomalies in animals exposed to this antipsychotic during embryogenesis (Brock and von Kreybig, 1964; Jones-Price *et al.*, 1983b; Singh and Padmanabhan, 1978; Yu *et al.*, 1988), but others have not found such an increase (Beall, 1972; Jelinek *et al.*, 1967; Jones-Price *et al.*, 1983a; Robertson *et al.*, 1980).

FLUPHENAZINE

Fluphenazine is a piperazine phenothiazine that appears to be relatively safe to use during gestation. Among 226 infants whose mothers who took fluphenazine (as an antiemetic) during the first trimester, the frequency of congenital anomalies was not increased (King *et al.*, 1963). Extrapyramidal signs in the newborn were observed several weeks after delivery of a newborn exposed to fluphenazine *in utero* (Cleary, 1977). Malformations were not increased in the offspring of pregnant rats exposed to this phenothiazine during organogenesis compared to controls (Jahn and Adrian, 1969) or in those exposed throughout pregnancy (Adrian, 1973).

MESORIDAZINE

Mesoridazine, a piperidyl phenothiazine, is the major active metabolite of thioridazine and is an effective antipsychotic agent. No reports are published regarding the safety of its use during the first trimester. Phenothiazines that have been studied appear to be safe to use during gestation. Mesoridazine was given to pregnant rats and rabbits in doses 12 times those used in humans and no increased frequency of congenital anomalies among the offspring was found (Van Ryzin *et al.*, 1971).

PERPHENAZINE

Perphenazine is a piperazine phenothiazine tranquilizer used to treat psychoses, and in lower doses helps control nausea and vomiting. Among the infants of 63 pregnant women who received perphenazine during the first trimester, the frequency of congenital anomalies was not increased (Heinonen *et al.*, 1977). In an unpublished study of 140 infants exposed to this drug during the first trimester, the frequency of congenital anomalies was not increased above the expected rate in the general population (Rosa, personal communication, cited in Briggs *et al.*, 2004).

An increased frequency of chromosomal abnormalities (breaks and rearrangements) in peripheral blood lymphocytes in patients taking perphenazine was found in one study (Nielen *et al.*, 1969), but the relevance of this to gametic chromosomes is unknown. No reports examining the effects of somatic chromosomal breaks on the gametes or children of these patients have been published. Typically, somatic chromosomes are not conserved because they have no genetic progeny. Only breaks in gametic chromosomes are directly relevant to reproduction or genetic toxicity. Offspring of pregnant rats treated with perphenazine had an increased frequency of cleft palate and micromelia (Beall, 1972; Druga, 1976). Suppression of the mother's appetite was thought to play a causative role in the cleft palate teratogenic effect (Szabo and Brent, 1974, 1975).

THIORIDAZINE

Thioridazine is one of the most frequently used phenothiazine tranquilizers and is the prototype piperidine compound. Thioridazine is used to treat psychoses, emotional disorders, and severe behavioral problems. A small series of 23 newborns exposed to this medication during the first trimester was reported and no congenital defects were found (Scanlon, 1972). Offspring of mice and rats were given this phenothiazine in doses greater than those used in humans during embryogenesis; an increased frequency of cleft palate was observed (Szabo and Brent, 1974). Frequency of cleft palate was not increased in frequency when pregnant mice and rats were given forced feedings (Szabo and Brent, 1975).

THIOTHIXENE

Thiothixene is a thioxanthine tranquilizer used to treat psychosis. Chemical structure and pharmacological activity of thiothixene are similar to the piperazine phenothiazine compounds. First-trimester exposure to thiothixene was not associated with an increased frequency of congenital anomalies among 38 infants in one study (Rosa, personal communication, cited in Briggs et al., 2004). The frequency of congenital anomalies was not increased among offspring of pregnant mice or rabbits given 20–180 times the typical human dose of thiothixene during embryogenesis (Owaki et al., 1969a, 1969b).

MOLINDONE

Molindone is an indole derivative that is not related chemically to the phenothiazines, butyrophenones, or thioxanthenes, but is an effective antipsychotic drug. No studies have been published of birth defects in newborns that were exposed to molindone *in utero*, and no studies in animals evaluating its teratogenic effects are available.

LITHIUM SALTS AND BIPOLAR TREATMENT

Bipolar disorder is treated with mood stabilizers (lithium, anticonvulsants, antipsychotics) with an adjuvant antidepressant if necessary. Lithium is effective in the prophylaxis and treatment of affective psychiatric disorders.

Of all the psychotropic agents currently available, lithium has received the greatest attention as a possible teratogen. Cardiovascular system anomalies, particularly Ebstein's anomaly, have been reported to be increased among the infants of mothers that received lithium carbonate during the first trimester (Nora et al., 1974), but the question of the magnitude of these risks has been questioned (Cohen et al., 1994). Ebstein's anomaly is induced between weeks 2 and 6 postconception.

Three congenital anomalies were reported among 60 infants exposed to lithium *in utero*. This is no different from the incidence in the general population (Schou and Amidsen, 1971). Among 50 women who reportedly received lithium during gestation, one infant had myelomeningocele, one had unilateral hernia, and none had congenital heart defects (Cunniff et al., 1989). No maternal history of lithium ingestion was found among 40 infants with Ebstein's anomaly and in 44 with tricuspid atresia (Kallen, 1971).

The risk of Ebstein's anomaly and other birth defects was reevaluated, and the risk of cardiac anomalies appears to be much less than estimated in previous studies (Cohen et al., 1994; Miller, 1994a, 1996). The early recommendation that women who take lithium salts during early gestation should undergo prenatal diagnosis with fetal echocardiography (Allan et al., 1982) is still valid (Yonkers et al., 2004). The risk of birth defects associated with lithium was probably overestimated in the past (Yonkers et al., 2004). The risk is 'likely to be weak if it exists' and the 'data certainly do not support the 30-fold increased risk of Ebstein's anomaly suggested by the Register of Lithium Babies' (Moore, 1995). Nonetheless, first-trimester exposure to lithium is an indication for a fetal echocardiogram, targeting the competence and function of the tricuspid valve.

Table 10.3 Lithium exposure during first trimester and congenital anomalies

	Exposed N	Non-heart anomalies n/N	%	Heart anomalies n/N	%	Ebstein's anomaly n/N	%
Cohort studies							
Background		35/1000	3.5	8/1000	0.8	1/20 000	0.005
Weinstein (1980)	225	7/225	3.1	18/225	8.0	6/225	2.7
Jacobsen *et al.* (1992)	138	3/138	2.2	0/138	0	1/138[a]	0.8
Kallen and Tandberg (1983)	59	11/59	18.6	4/59	6.8	0/59	0

	Ebstein's anomaly Lithium exposure		Unaffected control Lithium exposure	
	Yes	No	Yes	No
Case–control studies				
Kallen (1988)	69	0	128	0
Edmonds and Oakley (1990)	34	0	34	0
Zalzstein *et al.* (1990)	59	0	168	0
Correa-Villasenor *et al.* (1994)	44	0	3572	0

[a]The case of Ebstein's anomaly was a therapeutic abortion.

Adapted from Yonkers *et al.*, 1998.

No increase in physical or mental anomalies was found in a follow-up study of 60 school-aged children that were exposed to lithium *in utero* (Schou, 1976). Lithium toxicity, including cardiac, hepatic, and neurological abnormalities, has been reported in newborns of mothers who took lithium salts at term (Morrell *et al.*, 1983; Woody *et al.*, 1971). Diabetes insipidus and polyhydramnios are also complications attendant to lithium-exposed pregnancies.

An increased frequency of cleft palate, eye and ear defects, and fetal loss among the offspring exposed to lithium carbonate *in utero* has been observed in animal teratology studies (Smithberg and Dixit, 1982; Szabo, 1970; Wright *et al.*, 1971). Inconsistencies in animal teratology studies of lithium make it impossible to interpret these data for use in evaluation of human exposures.

SEDATIVES, HYPNOTICS, AND TRANQUILIZERS

Barbiturates

Barbiturates are a family of drugs that are all salts of barbituric acid. To varying degrees, these drugs have analgesic, sedative, and hypnotic actions (Box 10.3). In addition, they have anticonvulsant action.

PHENOBARBITAL

Phenobarbital is a barbiturate used to treat seizure disorders. In the past this drug was used for mild anxiety or sedation, but it is now rarely used for that purpose today.

Administration of phenobarbital is usually via the oral route, but it may be given parenterally if necessary.

Possible teratogenic effects of phenobarbital and phenytoin were suspected early (Janz and Fuchs, 1964). The risk for the pregnant woman treated with phenobarbital and other seizure medications of having an infant with congenital malformations is two to three times greater than that of the general population. It is not clear whether the increased risk is secondary to the anticonvulsants, genetic factors, the seizure disorder itself, or possibly a combination of these factors (Kelly, 1984).

Evidence implicates anticonvulsants as the etiology (Hanson and Buehler, 1982). An increased frequency of minor and major congenital anomalies was found among offspring of pregnant women who received phenobarbital during gestation for seizure disorders compared to women who received the drug for other reasons (Hanson and Buehler, 1982). The frequency of congenital anomalies was not increased in several studies of children born to women who were treated with phenobarbital for epilepsy when compared to the offspring of women with epilepsy who were not treated (Greenberg et al., 1977; Nakane et al., 1980; Robert et al., 1986; Rothman et al., 1979). In an analysis of phenobarbital monotherapy exposure separately (i.e., no other concomitant anticonvulsants), the frequency of congenital anomalies was not always increased (Nakane et al., 1980). In a multinational European collaborative study of 250 infants born to women with epilepsy, the frequency of congenital malformations was the same among those who received phenobarbital monotherapy and those who received monotherapy with other anticonvulsants (Bertollini et al., 1987). A slight, but significant, reduction in birth weight and head circumference was found among 55 newborns born to epileptic women who used phenobarbital during gestation, compared to newborns of women without epilepsy (Mastroiacovo et al., 1988). Notably, a similar effect on head circumference was observed among the newborns of women with epilepsy who received no treatment, implicating the disease. No increased frequency of congenital malformations was found among the offspring of over 1400 pregnant women who received phenobarbital during the first trimester (Heinonen et al., 1977).

Box 10.3 Commonly used sedatives, hypnotics, and tranquilizers

Barbiturates
Amobarbital (Amytal)
Aprobarbital (Alurate)
Butalbital
Mephobarbital (Mebaral)
Pentobarbital (Nembutal)
Phenobarbital
Secobarbital (Seconal)

Benzodiazepines
Alprazolam (Xanax)
Chlordiazepoxide (Librium)
Clonazepam (Klonopin)
Diazepam (Valium)
Lorazepam (Ativan)

Oxazepam (Serex)

Miscellaneous sedatives and hypnotics
Chloral hydrate
Eszopiclone (Lunesta)
Ethchlorvynol (Placidyl)
GHB – gammahydroxy butyrate
Hydroxyzine (Vistaril, Atarax)
Meprobamate (Equanil, Equagesic, Miltown, Deprol)
Methaqualone (Quaalude, Sapor, Parest)
Ramelteon (Rozerem)
Zaleplon (Sonata)
Zolipidem (Ambien)

Characteristic dysmorphic features of the fetal hydantoin syndrome are commonly seen in newborns of women with epilepsy treated with both phenytoin and phenobarbital during gestation, and are discussed in Chapter 9 in the section on antiseizure medications during pregnancy. Sporadic reports of similar dysmorphic features among the infants of women with epilepsy who received phenobarbital monotherapy have been published (Robert *et al.*, 1986; Seip, 1976).

The frequency of cleft palate, cardiovascular defects, and other congenital malformations were increased among the offspring of pregnant mice or rats given phenobarbital in doses greater than those used in humans (Finnell *et al.*, 1987; Fritz *et al.*, 1976; Nishimura *et al.*, 1979; Sullivan and McElhatton, 1977; Vorhees, 1983). Malformations observed included facial anomalies similar to those observed in human newborns delivered to women with epilepsy who received anticonvulsants during gestation. A decrease in the number of specific brain cells and changes in neonatal behavior have been observed in animal studies of gestational exposure to the drug (Bergman *et al.*, 1980; Takagi *et al.*, 1986; Vorhees, 1983, 1985). The relevance of these observations to the clinical use of phenobarbital in humans is unknown.

Transient neonatal sedation or withdrawal symptoms that include hyperactivity, irritability, and tremors have been observed among newborns exposed to phenobarbital during pregnancy (Desmond *et al.*, 1972; Koch *et al.*, 1985). Hemorrhagic disease of the newborn has been associated with phenobarbital use during pregnancy and typically begins within the first 24 h of life (Gimovsky and Petrie, 1986; Mountain *et al.*, 1970). The exact cause of this hemorrhagic defect is unknown, but is probably related to phenobarbital induction of fetal liver microsomal enzymes that deplete fetal vitamin K and suppress the synthesis of vitamin-K-dependent clotting factors II, VII, IX, and X. In contrast, maternal phenobarbital therapy immediately before delivery has been used to prevent intraventricular hemorrhage in premature newborns (Morales and Koerten, 1986; Shankaran *et al.*, 1986).

A follow-up study of 114 adult males whose mothers used phenobarbital while pregnant showed lowered IQ scores by approximately 7–10 points, and it was concluded that phenobarbital exposure during early development can have long-term deleterious cognitive effects. However, detrimental environmental conditions (i.e., maternal epilepsy) may intensify such negative outcomes (Reinisch *et al.*, 1995).

AMOBARBITAL

Amobarbital, a barbiturate, is an effective sedative usually administered orally. The frequency of major and minor congenital anomalies was not increased among 298 infants born to women treated with amobarbital exposure during the first trimester (Heinonen *et al.*, 1977). Amobarbital use during the first trimester was possibly associated with cardiovascular defects (seven cases), inguinal hernia (nine cases), clubfoot (four cases), genitourinary anomalies (three cases), and polydactyly in Black infants (two cases). In a survey including over 1300 women exposed to multiple agents, of whom 175 infants were exposed to amobarbital during the first trimester, the frequency of congenital anomalies was increased (Nelson and Forfar, 1971). Authorities in the field generally believe that this drug is not likely to be a teratogen and that the significant associations may be due to chance and conducting multiple statistical comparisons (Friedman and Polifka, 2006).

APROBARBITAL

Aprobarbital is a barbiturate used as a sedative and hypnotic agent. No information has been published regarding its safety for use during pregnancy. Furthermore, no studies in animals evaluating the teratogenic effects of aprobarbital have been published.

BUTALBITAL

A number of analgesic compounds contain butalbital, a short-acting barbiturate with hypnotic and sedative properties. Among 112 infants whose mothers took butalbital during the first trimester, no increased frequency of congenital anomalies was found among the offspring (Heinonen *et al.*, 1977). Transient neonatal withdrawal was reported in association with butalbital use late in gestation (Ostrea, 1982). No animal studies of possible teratogenic effects of butalbital have been published.

PENTOBARBITAL

Pentobarbital is an effective, short-acting barbiturate that is used as a hypnotic and seda-tive agent, and is typically given orally. Among 250 infants whose mothers took pento-barbital during the first trimester, the frequency of congenital malformations was not increased (Heinonen *et al.*, 1977). Similarly, among more than 50 newborns born to women exposed to pentobarbital during the first trimester of gestation, the frequency of birth defects was no greater than expected (Jick *et al.*, 1981).

Skeletal and craniofacial defects, as well as fetal loss, were increased among the off-spring of pregnant mice, golden hamsters, and rabbits given pentobarbital many times the doses that are used in humans (Hilbelink, 1982; Johnson, 1971; Setala and Nyyssonen, 1964). Changes in behavior and decreased brain–body weight ratios were reported among the offspring of pregnant rats administered 20–40 times the human dose of pentobarbital during embryogenesis (Martin *et al.*, 1985). The relevance of these findings in animals to the clinical use of this barbiturate in humans is unknown.

MEPHOBARBITAL

Mephobarbital, which is used as an anticonvulsant and sedative, is metabolized by the liver to phenobarbital and thus has similar properties. Results in a Japanese multi-institutional study that included the frequency of congenital anomalies in a cohort of 111 infants born to pregnant epileptics who used mephobarbital during the first trimester, were similar to those for the infants of pregnant epileptics treated with other medications (Nakane *et al.*, 1980). In a small case series, the frequency of congenital malformations was no greater among the newborns of 17 epileptic mothers exposed to mephobarbital during the first trimester of pregnancy than among the newborns of epileptic mothers who received no treatment (Annegers *et al.*, 1974). No animal teratol-ogy studies of mephobarbital have been published.

SECOBARBITAL

Secobarbital is as effective as pentobarbital and is generally administered orally. Among 378 infants born to women who took secobarbital during the first trimester, the fre-quency of congenital anomalies was not increased (Heinonen *et al.*, 1977). One report of an infant with neonatal withdrawal symptoms of hyperirritability and seizures associated with maternal use of large doses of secobarbital throughout gestation has been published (Bleyer and Marshall, 1972).

Benzodiazepines

Benzodiazepines are minor tranquilizers with mild anticonvulsant and sedation properties (Box 10.3). These agents differ in potency and duration of effect, and indications for their use are based upon these features. They are commonly used anxiolytic agents. Of these, diazepam is probably the most frequently used drug.

DIAZEPAM

Diazepam is a benzodiazepine used as a tranquilizer, skeletal muscle relaxant, and preanesthetic medication. Diazepam is also used to treat alcohol withdrawal and as an adjunct to anticonvulsants in the treatment of seizure disorders. It is the most extensively used drug in the benzodiazepine family.

Inconsistencies in the currently available epidemiological data on the risk of congenital anomalies among newborns of women who were exposed to diazepam during gestation, confound the issue. Diazepam use during the first trimester was not associated with an increased frequency of malformations among the newborns of more than 150 women in two cohorts, or among 60 newborns of women who used the drug in the first trimester (Aselton et al., 1985; Crombie et al., 1975; Jick et al., 1981).

In contrast, first-trimester diazepam use was increased almost threefold among 1427 infants with congenital malformations compared to controls in one study (Bracken and Holford, 1981), but not in another case–control study that included 417 newborns with multiple congenital malformations (Czeizel, 1988). A hypothesized 'benzodiazepine embryofetopathy' (typical facial features, neurological dysfunction, and other anomalies) (Laegreid et al., 1987, 1989) is not widely accepted in the human teratology community.

Some early evidence suggested that maternal use of diazepam or other benzodiazepines during the first trimester of gestation was associated with facial clefts in the infants (Aarskog, 1975; Safra and Oakley, 1975; Saxén, 1975; Saxén and Saxén, 1975); more extensive studies have not confirmed this association. Among the infants of women who had first-trimester exposure to antineurotics (mainly diazepam) the frequency of congenital anomalies was not increased (Crombie et al., 1975; Rosenberg et al., 1983; Shiono and Mills, 1984). On balance, the possible risk of cleft lip or palate in the infant of a women exposed to diazepam during the first trimester, if increased at all, is less than 1 percent. Notably, family history of congenital anomalies is a confounder in at least two of these studies.

Maternal use of diazepam or related compounds during the first trimester of pregnancy and an increased risk for cardiovascular anomalies was observed in two case–control studies involving 773 infants (Bracken and Holford, 1981; Rothman et al., 1979). However, in a reanalysis, no significant association was found (Bracken, 1986). In a follow-up study of 298 infants with congenital heart defects, no association with first-trimester diazepam was found (Zierler and Rothman, 1985). The risk for congenital heart disease among the infants of women who have first-trimester exposure to diazepam, is probably not increased, but if it is increased the magnitude is small (< 1–2 percent).

Diazepam is readily transferred across the placenta to the human fetus and becomes concentrated in the fetal compartment with a 2:1 ratio (Erkkola *et al.*, 1974). Apnea, hypotonia, and hypothermia were observed in newborns of women who took diazepam during the third trimester of pregnancy or peripartum (Cree *et al.*, 1973; Gillberg, 1977; Owen *et al.*, 1972; Speight, 1977). Tremors, irritability, and hypertonia similar to neonatal narcotic withdrawal was observed in some infants chronically exposed *in utero* during the third trimester to diazepam (Rementeria and Bhatt, 1977). Loss of beat-to-beat fetal heart rate variability was associated with diazepam exposure during late pregnancy (Scher *et al.*, 1972) and decrease in fetal movement (Birger *et al.*, 1980). The effect of prenatal exposure to this drug and any untoward central nervous system function in later life is unknown. A few reports of normal infants born to women who took toxic doses of diazepam during gestation, with the majority of cases occurring after the first trimester have been published (Cerqueira *et al.*, 1988; Czeizel, 1988).

Animal studies indicate that diazepam is a teratogen in mice and hamsters, but only when doses hundreds of times greater than those used in humans are administered (Kellogg, 1988; Weber, 1985).

CHLORDIAZEPOXIDE

Chlordiazepoxide is a benzodiazepine tranquilizer that has less potency than diazepam on a milligram basis. It also has less anticonvulsant, muscle relaxant and sedative properties, but is effective in treating alcohol withdrawal. In several cohort studies, the frequency of congenital defects was not increased among more than 480 newborns whose mothers had first-trimester exposure to chlordiazepoxide (Crombie *et al.*, 1975; Hartz *et al.*, 1975; Heinonen *et al.*, 1977; Kullander and Kallen, 1976a, 1976b). Two case–control studies reported no association between maternal use of this benzodiazepine in the first trimester and congenital defects (Bracken and Holford, 1981; Rothman *et al.*, 1979). In contrast, in a small cohort study an association was reported between congenital malformations in 35 infants and maternal use of chlordiazepoxide in the first 42 days of gestation (Milkovich and van den Berg, 1974). However, there was no pattern to the anomalies observed.

Maternal chlordiazepoxide was associated with neonatal withdrawal beginning on day 26 of life (Athinarayanan *et al.*, 1976), which is an unusually long lag time for such an effect. Withdrawal symptoms included extreme tremulousness and irritability. Chlordiazepoxide given to pregnant hamsters in doses greater than those used in humans during embryogenesis resulted in an increased frequency (dose-dependent) of central nervous system anomalies and maternal toxicity (Guram *et al.*, 1982). The frequency of congenital anomalies was not increased among the offspring of pregnant rats given benzodiazepine, but fetal loss, growth retardation, and skeletal variants were increased in frequency with higher doses (Buttar, 1980; Saito *et al.*, 1984).

LORAZEPAM

Lorazepam is a benzodiazepine class minor tranquilizer. The drug is used as an anti-anxiolytic and hypnotic drug. It is also used as a preanesthetic medication because of its amnesic action. In a case–control study, a significant association between first-trimester exposure to lorazepam and anal atresia was published (Bonnot *et al.*, 1999), but the meaning of the association is unclear. Placental transfer of lorazepam was reported by several investigators (de Groot *et al.*, 1975; Kanto *et al.*, 1980; McBride *et al.*, 1979).

Transient neonatal hypotonia was observed in newborns of women who took lorazepam late in gestation, either chronically or intrapartum (McAuley et al., 1982; Whitelaw et al., 1981). Intravenously administered maternal lorazepam in hypertensive gravidas was associated with low Apgar scores, hypothermia, poor feeding, and a requirement for assisted ventilation in the infant. No congenital anomalies were reported among the offspring of pregnant rats and mice given up to 4 mg/kg.day lorazepam during organogenesis (Esaki et al., 1975).

ALPRAZOLAM

Alprazolam is a benzodiazepine tranquilizer. The rate of malformations was approximately 5 percent in over 400 births reported to the manufacturer (St Clair and Schirmer, 1992). In a case–control study from Hungary, the association between alprazolam exposure and congenital anomalies was slightly elevated, but not significantly so (Eros et al., 2002). Several series containing more than 300 pregnancies followed through teratogen information services found no apparent increase in congenital anomalies (Friedman and Polifka, 2006) This agent, as other benzodiazepines, may cause hypotonia and hypothermia in the newborn (Yonkers and Cunningham, 1993).

OTHER BENZODIAZEPINES

Oxazepam and clonazepam are benzodiazepine tranquilizers. Among 89 infants born to women who used oxazepam during the first trimester, there were no congenital anomalies (Ornoy et al., 1998). Small numbers of first-trimester exposure to clonazepam are published in clinical case series, but they are confounded by concomitant use of other known teratogens (anticonvulsants), as well as small sample sizes and sample selection bias (Friedman and Polifka, 2006).

Congenital anomalies were not increased in frequency among the offspring of pregnant rabbits or rats administered oxazepam in doses greater than those used in humans (Owen et al., 1970; Saito et al., 1984). Changes in behavior were observed among the offspring of pregnant mice given oxazepam in doses four to 42 times those used clinically (Alleva and Bignami, 1986).

MISCELLANEOUS

Hydroxyzine

Hydroxyzine is a piperazine antihistaminic compound that is used to treat anxiety, pruritus, nausea, and vomiting. The frequency of congenital anomalies in a double-blind controlled study was not increased among 74 newborns exposed *in utero* to hydroxyzine (50 mg/day) during the first trimester (Erez et al., 1971). Birth defects were not increased in frequency among 50 infants born to women who used hydroxyzine during the first trimester (Heinonen et al., 1977). Hydroxyzine has been shown to be a teratogen in rats (Giurgea and Puigdevall, 1968; King and Howell, 1966).

Chloral hydrate

Chloral hydrate is an effective hypnotic and sedative agent. There is a paucity of information regarding the safety of chloral hydrate use during pregnancy. However, among

71 infants born to women who used chloral hydrate during the first trimester, the frequency of congenital anomalies was not increased (Heinonen *et al.*, 1977). No gross external defects were observed in pregnant mice with chloral hydrate in doses less than one to five times the human dose (Kallman *et al.*, 1984).

Ethchlorvynol

Ethchlorvynol is a tertiary acetylenic alcohol and is used as an oral hypnotic and sedative agent. No studies have been published regarding the frequency of congenital malformations among newborns of women exposed to ethchlorvynol during gestation. Symptoms of neonatal withdrawal were observed in the newborn of a woman who was treated with ethchlorvynol as a hypnotic during the last 3 months of gestation. Neonatal withdrawal symptoms observed were jitteriness, irritability, and hypotonia (Rumak and Walravens, 1973). No animal studies evaluating the teratogenic effects of ethchlorvynol are published, but behavioral changes were observed among the offspring of pregnant rats treated with ethchlorvynol in doses greater than those used in humans (Peters and Hudson, 1981).

Meprobamate

Meprobamate is a carbamate tranquilizer that is useful in the treatment of anxiety but seems to be less effective than the benzodiazepines. The most common side effect is drowsiness. Inconsistencies in studies of the possible teratogenic effects of meprobamate in humans make it difficult to assess the risk of congenital anomalies with exposure to the drug in therapeutic doses during embryogenesis. Reports of an association between maternal use of this drug during the first trimester of pregnancy and a variety of congenital defects in newborns have been published, but the association is weak, and in no two studies was the same defect present. Among 66 infants born to women exposed to meprobamate in the first 42 days after their last menstrual period, congenital anomalies were increased fourfold (Milkovich and van den Berg, 1974). No apparent pattern of congenital anomalies was identified, but there were five infants with congenital heart disease. The frequency of hypospadias was increased among the 186 male infants born to women treated with meprobamate during the first trimester of pregnancy (Heinonen *et al.*, 1977), but the finding was disregarded because of the small sample size. Accordingly, the relationship is probably a random finding, not representing a causal link. A third study had an increased frequency of major congenital anomalies among the newborns of more than 50 pregnant women given meprobamate during the first trimester (Jick *et al.*, 1981), but no other details are available. Other studies have failed to find an association between the first-trimester use of meprobamate and congenital malformations. Among 356 pregnant women given meprobamate during the first trimester, the frequency of congenital anomalies was not increased (Heinonen *et al.*, 1977). Another cohort study of congenital anomalies among 207 infants whose mothers used meprobamate during the first trimester failed to find an association (Belafsky *et al.*, 1969). However, it should be noted that these studies analyzed only therapeutic dose exposures for infants examined for birth defects.

Table 10.4 Teratogen Information System (TERIS) and Food and Drug Administration (FDA) pregnancy risk ratings

Drugs	TERIS risk	FDA Pregnancy risk rating
Alprazolam	Unlikely	D_m
Amitriptyline	Unlikely	C_m
Amobarbital	None to minimal	D*
Amoxapine	Undetermined	C_m
Aprobarbital	Undetermined	C
Bupropion	Undetermined	B_m
Butalbital	Unlikely	C*
Chloral hydrate	Unlikely	C_m
Chlordiazepoxide	Unlikely	D
Chlorpromazine	Unlikely	C
Clomipramine	Unlikely	C_m
Clonazepam	Undetermined	D_m
Clozapine	Undetermined	B_m
Desipramine	Undetermined	C
Diazepam	Minimal	D
Doxepin	Undetermined	C
Ethchlorvynol	Undetermined	C_m
Fluoxetine	Unlikely	C_m
Fluphenazine	Unlikely	C
Haloperidol	Unlikely	C_m
Hydroxyzine	Unlikely	C
Imipramine	Unlikely	D
Isocarboxazid	Undetermined	C
Lithium	Small	D
Lorazepam	Undetermined	D_m
Loxapine	Unlikely	C
Maprotiline	Undetermined	B_m
Mephobarbital	Unlikely	D_m
Meprobamate	Minimal	D
Mesoridazine	Undetermined	C
Molindone	Undetermined	C
Nortriptyline	Undetermined	D
Oxazepam	Unlikely	D
Pentobarbital	Unlikely	D_m
Perphenazine	Unlikely	C
Phenelzine	Undetermined	C
Phenobarbital	Chronic anticonvulsive	D
Phenytoin/fosphenytoin	Small to moderate	D
Protriptyline	Undetermined	C
Secobarbital	None	D_m
Sertraline	Unlikely	B_m
Thioridazine	Unlikely	C
Thiothixene	Undetermined	C
Tranylcypromine	Undetermined	C
Trazodone	Unlikely	C_m
Trifluoperazine	Unlikely	C

Compiled from: Friedman *et al.*, *Obstet Gynecol* 1990; **75**: 594; Briggs *et al.*, 2005; Friedman and Polifka, 2006.

The frequency of birth defects was not increased among the offspring of pregnant mice, rats, or rabbits given meprobamate in doses greater than those used in humans (range 2.5–16 times) (Brar, 1969; Clavert, 1963; Werboff and Dembicki, 1962). In other studies when doses 16 times greater than those used in humans were administered to rabbits, and doses 2.5 or 20 times the typical dose in humans were given to pregnant rats, fetal and neonatal loss was increased (Bertrand, 1960; Clavert, 1963; Werboff and Kesner, 1963).

Methaqualone

Methaqualone (Quaalude, Sopor, Parest) is an effective hypnotic and sedative agent and is not presently commercially available. No clear medicinal advantage of methaqualone over the other available hypnotics can be shown and the drug is commonly abused by drug-dependent people. Tolerance to the drug develops in abusers. No published reports are available that analyze the possible association of the use of methaqualone during pregnancy with congenital malformations. However, its use during gestation is not recommended because of its abuse potential. The frequency of congenital anomalies was not increased among rats or rabbits whose mothers were administered 200 mg/kg methaqualone orally (rabbits) from days 1 to 29 or 100 mg/kg (rats) from days 1 to 20 (Bough et al., 1963) (Table 10.4).

Electroconvulsive therapy

High-voltage electrical shock is used to treat some psychiatric disorders, although it may also occur in accidental electrocution. The mechanism of action of electroconvulsive therapy is unknown. However, it is clearly understood that the seizure produced by electroconvulsive therapy is necessary for therapeutic efficacy (Ottosson, 1962a, 1962b). Electroconvulsive therapy was used safely in the treatment of depression in a pregnant woman following expanded clinical guidelines that included the presence of an obstetrician during treatment, endotracheal intubation, low-voltage, nondominant therapy with electrocardiographic and electroencephalogram monitoring, Doppler ultrasonography of fetal heart rate, tocodynamometer recording of uterine tone, arterial blood gases during and after treatment, glycopyrrolate (anticholinergic of choice) use during anesthesia, and weekly nonstress tests (Wise et al., 1984). The frequency of birth defects among the newborns of 318 women who received electroconvulsive therapy during gestation has not increased (Impastato et al., 1964).

Reports of uterine contractions, vaginal bleeding, and transient benign fetal cardiac arrhythmias have been published (Miller, 1994b; Rabheru, 2001). Miscarriage was reported following a third electroconvulsive therapy session in the first trimester of pregnancy (Moreno et al., 1998). One infant was described with hydrops fetalis and meconium peritonitis after the mother received electroconvulsive therapy during the third trimester of pregnancy (Gilot et al., 1999). As is usually the case with isolated reports, it is not possible to evaluate any causal links with anecdotal data.

No animal studies evaluating the teratogenic effects of high-voltage electrical shock have been published.

SPECIFIC CONDITIONS

Depression

Management of depression during pregnancy should be undertaken in consultation with a psychiatrist and/or psychologist (Yonkers, 2003). Although psychotherapy or hospitalization in a supportive environment is the first consideration in treatment (Spinelli, 2001; Yolles, 2001), antidepressant therapy may be necessary if these regimens are unsuccessful (Yolles, 2001; Robinson *et al.*, 1986). Indeed, antidepressant medications are indicated in the pregnant woman whose depression is so severe that it threatens her life and the life of her unborn child (Yolles, 2001; Yonkers 2003). Since the medications used in the treatment of depression have potential fetal risks and may result in obstetric complications and long-lasting sequelae, the minimal effective antidepressant dose should be initiated and maintained. Most antidepressants have established therapeutic serum levels that can be monitored.

No antidepressant has proven safety for use during gestation, although some are better studied than others. Thus the selection of an antidepressant is dependent upon a patient's past response, side effects, and potential teratogenic effects of the particular agent. However, it is recommended that one uses an agent that has been relatively well studied during pregnancy and that has relatively few side effects (Miller, 1994a, 1996). These include desipramine, nortriptyline, and fluoxetine. The older antidepressants may have lower efficacy in women than the newer SSRI drugs. Women seem to respond better to fluoxetine, sertraline, and other SSRIs (Yonkers, 2003).

The usual starting dosages for imipramine, amitriptyline, and desipramine are 25–50 mg daily at bedtime. The dose can be increased to 25–50 mg daily every week, if warranted, to a maximum dose of 300 mg daily. The initial dosage for nortriptyline is 10–25 mg PO q d and can be increased by 10 mg each week if necessary to a maximum dose of 150 mg daily (Bryant and Brown, 1986). However, if the pregnant patient's depression is not improved on these older drugs, it is recommended to use one of the SSRIs. In fact, it may be beneficial to begin therapy with a well-studied SSRI such as fluoxetine (Yonkers, 2003).

Therapeutic response usually occurs within 10–14 days and includes improved sleep and appetite, as well as return of normal routine activities and mood elevation (Bryant and Brown, 1986). If there is absolutely no response to therapy after 2–3 weeks, one should consider an alternative antidepressant. It is recommended that tapering of the antidepressant dose begin approximately 2–3 weeks prior to delivery, to minimize neonatal effects. To prevent anticholinergic withdrawal symptoms (chills, malaise, muscle aches, diarrhea, and nightmares) in the mother, the dose should be reduced by 50 mg every 3–4 days (Blackwell, 1981). The starting dose of fluoxetine is 10–20 mg/day (Yonkers and Cunningham, 1993).

Psychosis

Management of psychosis during pregnancy frequently requires hospitalization because of the patient's confusion, hostility, disorientation, anxiety, and possible suicidal tendencies. Psychiatric consultation and psychological evaluation are mandatory for patients with psychosis. Antipsychotic agents are frequently necessary in the treatment of psychosis. The agent of choice for acute psychotic reactions is haloperidol 1–5 mg PO (or IM) every 6–8 h. Chlorpromazine is another agent that is used in the acutely psychotic patient with a starting dose of 100 mg PO every 8–12 h. Upon achievement of a stable dose, chlorpromazine can be administered once daily at bedtime. Some authorities recommend high-potency agents, haloperidol or trifluoperazine, over the low-potency neuroleptics (Miller, 1994a, 1996). The daily dose of haloperidol (Haldol) is 5–10 mg/day and of trifluoperazine (Stelazine), 10–40 mg/day (Yonkers and Cunningham, 1993).

Lithium may be necessary for manic-depressive disorders or manic disorders. For acute mania, the initial dosage is 0.6–2.1 g/day in three divided doses. Monitoring of the serum levels is mandatory, with adjustments in the dosage as indicated to maintain serum levels of 0.8–1.5 mEq/L. Recently, reevaluation of lithium use during early pregnancy led to marked lower estimated risk for birth defects, specifically for Ebstein's anomaly. The drug is currently recommended for use during pregnancy, avoiding weeks 2–6 of embryonic development if possible (Yonkers *et al.*, 1998, 2004).

Electroconvulsive therapy is warranted when all else fails. Although carbamazepine and valproic acid are used effectively to treat mania, these drugs are not recommended for use during pregnancy.

Key references

Bupropion Pregnancy Registry. *Interim Report. 1 September 1997 through 29 February 2004*. Wilmington: Inveresk, June 2004.

Diav-Citrin O, Shechtman S, Weinbaum D, Arnon J, Wajnberg R, Ornoy A. Pregnancy outcome after gestational exposure to paroxetine. a prospective controlled cohort study. *Teratology* 2002; **65**: 298.

Einarson T, Einarson A. Newer antidepressants in pregnancy and rates of major malformations. A meta-analysis of prospective comparative studies. *Pharmacoepidemiol Drug Saf* 2005; **14**: 823.

Hendrick V, Smith LM, Suri R, Hwang S, Haynes D, Altshuler L. Birth outcomes after prenatal exposure to antidepressant medication. *Am J Obstet Gynecol* 2003; **188**: 812.

Little BB. Pharmacokinetics during pregnancy. Evidence-based maternal dose formulation. *Obstet Gynecol* 1999; **93**: 858.

Little BB, Yonkers KA. Epidemiology of psychiatric disorders and the importance of gender. In: Yonkers KA, Little BB (eds). *Treatment of Psychiatric Disorders in Pregnancy*. London: Arnold Publishers, 2001.

Rabheru K. The use of electroconvulsive therapy in special patient populations. *Can J Psychiatry* 2001; **46**: 710.

Yolles JC. Psychotropics versus psychotherapy. an individualized plan for the pregnant patient. In: Yonkers KA, Little BB (eds). *Treatment of Psychiatric Disorders in Pregnancy*. London: Arnold Publishers, 2001:1.

Yonkers KA. Special issues related to the treatment of depression in women. *J Clin Psych* 2003; **64** (Suppl. 18): 8.

Yonkers KA, Little BB, March D. Lithium during pregnancy. Drug effects and their therapeutic implications. *CNS Drugs* 1998; **9**: 261.

Yonkers KA, Wisner KL, Stowe Z et al. Management of bipolar disorder during pregnancy and the postpartum period. *Am J Psychiatry* 2004; **161**: 608.

Further references are available on the book's website at http://www.drugsandpregnancy.com

11

Antihistamines, decongestants, and expectorants during pregnancy

Upper respiratory infections, sinusitis, rhinitis, hay fever, nasal congestion, and a variety of 'allergic maladies' are frequent during pregnancy. The 'common cold' is the most frequent respiratory ailment encountered in pregnant women, and the most frequent indication for an antihistamine decongestant and/or expectorant regimen (Hornby and Abraham, 1996). There is no curative therapy against rhinoviruses, but the symptoms can be relieved until the illness runs its course.

A variety of antihistamines are available and most are used in combination with a sympathomimetic amine, such as pseudoephedrine with its decongestant activity. These agents are given for symptomatic relief in pregnant women. Dose and systemic effects are important considerations. Intranasal routes of administration are equally, if not more, effective than oral administration. Importantly, the nasal route reduces dose delivered to the fetus while adequately treating the patient's symptoms (Hornby and Abrahams, 1996).

DECONGESTANTS

All the commonly used decongestants have been assigned Food and Drug Administration (FDA) pregnancy risk rating (Table 11.1).

Pseudoephedrine

Pseudoephedrine hydrochloride is the preferred agent for pregnant women who require a decongestant (Hornby and Abrahams, 1996). It is the most frequently used sympathomimetic and is usually taken as a decongestant. It is also frequently combined with different antihistamines in 'common cold' or 'sinus' medications. Epidemiological studies of more than 1000 first-trimester human pregnancies exposed to pseudoephedrine indicate no association with congenital anomalies (Aselton et al., 1985; Heinonen et al., 1977; Jick et al., 1981).

Table 11.1 Some commonly used decongestants

Drug	FDA class
Decongestants	
Ephedrinea	C
Naphazoline	C
Oxymetazoline	C
Phenylephrine	C
Phenylpropanolamine	C
Pseudoephedrine	C
Tetrahydrozoline	C
Xylometazoline	C
Expectorants	
Guaifenesin	None
Iodinated glycerol	X
Potassium iodide	D
Terpin hydrate	None
Antitussives	
Benzonatate	C[a]
Codeine	C
Dextromethorphan	C

FDA, Food and Drug Administration

[a]See Chapter 7.

Ephedrine (Ephedra, Ma Huang, over-the-counter weight loss/energy pill) used in large doses is associated with sudden cardiac death in adults, and based upon anecdotal information should be avoided during pregnancy because of potential adverse maternal and fetal effects, including tachycardia and serious adverse cardiovascular events, such as heart attack, stroke, and fetal vascular disruption.

Phenylephrine and phenylpropranolamine

Phenylephrine and phenylpropranolamine are decongestants in common use and are frequently combined with antihistamines in cold and flu remedies. Phenylephrine (Neo Synephrine) may also be used in nasal sprays. According to their manufacturer, these agents may interfere with uterine blood flow and thus should be used with caution in women with conditions already associated with decreased uterine blood flow, such as hypertension. A weak, possible association of phenylephrine and phenylpropranolamine with congenital anomalies was found in the Collaborative Perinatal Project among 1249 and 726 pregnancies, respectively (Heinonen *et al.*, 1977). It is unlikely that either agent is causally related to congenital malformations in first-trimester-exposed fetuses.

In another study of more than 225 infants exposed during the first trimester, no such association was found (Aselton *et al.*, 1985; Jick *et al.*, 1981). No adverse effects were found among offspring in animal studies regarding the teratogenicity of these two agents. Phenylephrine may also be used for the treatment of acute hypotension.

Oxymetazoline, xylometazoline, and naphazoline

Oxymetazoline, xylometazoline, and naphazoline are sympathomimetic agents used as decongestants in long-acting nasal sprays (Afrin, Allerest, Dristan, 4-Way). The frequency of congenital anomalies was not increased among more than 250 infants whose mothers took oxymetazoline during the first trimester (Aselton *et al.*, 1985; Jick *et al.*, 1981). Similarly, among 432 infants whose mothers took xylometazoline in the first trimester, the frequency of congenital anomalies was not increased (Aselton *et al.*, 1985; Jick *et al.*, 1981). No studies have been published regarding naphazoline use during pregnancy.

Table 11.2 Antihistamines

Generation	FDA class
First generation	
Azatadine (Optimine)	C
Bromodiphenhydramine (Ambenyl)	C
Brompheniramine	C
Buclizine (Bucladin)	C
Carbinoxamine (Clistin)	C
Chlorpheniramine	B
Clemastine (Tavist)	B
Cyclizine (Marezine)	C
Cyproheptadine (Periactin)	B
Dexchlorpheniramine (Polaramine)	B
Dimenhydrinate	C
Diphenhydramine	B
Diphenylpyraline (Hispril)	C
Doxylamine (Unisom)	B
Meclizine (Antivert, Bonine)	C
Methdilazine	B
Phenindamine (Nolahist)	C
Promethazine	C
Pyrilamine (Dormarex, Sommicaps, Sominex)	C
Terfenadine (Seldane)	C
Trimeprazine	C
Tripelennamine (PBZ)	B
Triprolidine (Actidil, Bayidy)	C
Second generation	
Astemizole	C
Cetirizine	B
Cromolyn sodium	B
Desloratadine	–
Ebastine	–
Fexofenadine	C
Ipratropium	B
Loratadine	B

Table 11.3 Congenital anomalies and first-trimester antihistamine exposure

Antihistamine	Percent congenital anomalies (%)	*n/N*
First generation		
Azatadine	4.7	6/127
Brompheniramine	5.9	16/271
Chlorphenamine (chlorpheniramine)	6.9	96/1388
Clemastine	3.7	110/2847
Cyproheptadine	4.2	12/285
Dexchlorpheniramine	4.6	50/1080
Diphenhydramine	4.7	154/3286
Hydroxyzine	6.0	60/995
Tripelennamine	6.0	6/100
Triprolidine	1.4	9/628
Second generation		
Astemizole	1.8	2/114
Cetirizine	4.0	38/950
Loratadine	3.8	81/2147
Terfenadine	4.0	88/2195

n, number of infants with a congenital anomaly who were exposed to antihistamine during the first trimester; *N*, number of mother–infant pairs exposed to antihistamine during the first trimester.

Compiled from Gilbert *et al.*, 2005. Most of these studies were controlled and only the numbers of exposed are shown here for illustrative purposes without odds ratios and comparative data.

ANTIHISTAMINES

Antihistamines and some popular proprietary preparations are listed in Table 11.2. These medications act primarily by competing with histamine for H_1-receptor binding. Chemically they are related to local anesthetics and may be used as such. Other effects of some members of this group include sedation, antiemesis, antimotion sickness, and antidyskinesia.

The primary difference between the first-generation and second-generation antihistamines is the sedative effect. Second-generation antihistamines are also referred to as the nonsedating antihistamines.

The FDA pregnancy risk categories for antihistamines are given in Table 11.3. Adapted from a recent review, the percentage of congenital anomalies shows the generally accepted nonteratogenic nature of antihistamines in human exposure (Gilbert *et al.*, 2005). Most authorities consider antihistamines to be safe for use during pregnancy, but it is prudent to rely on research for specific agents rather than blanket statements about drug classes. One report suggested that antihistamines as a group may be associated with an increased frequency of retrolental fibroplasia in premature infants (Zierler and Purohit, 1986).

Propylamine derivatives

Propylamine derivatives include brompheniramine, chlorpheniramine, dexchlorpheniramine, and triprolidine. Of all antihistamines analyzed in the Collaborative Perinatal

Project, only brompheniramine was found to be weakly associated with congenital defects in 65 offspring, and it is unlikely that it was causative (Heinonen *et al.*, 1977). In a larger study of 270 infants born following first-trimester exposure to brompheniramine, there was no increased frequency of congenital anomalies (Aselton *et al.*, 1985; Jick *et al.*, 1981). Meta-analysis of all available data on brompheniramine indicate it is not a human teratogen (Seto *et al.*, 1993) and this finding is supported by a recent review (Gilbert *et al.*, 2005) that included more information than the meta-analysis (Table 11.3).

Chlorpheniramine was not associated with an increased frequency of congenital anomalies; neither was the closely related agent dexchlorpheniramine (Gilbert *et al.*, 2005; Heinonen *et al.*, 1977). In one survey of 275 infants exposed to this drug in the first trimester, chlorpheniramine was not associated with an increased frequency of malformations (Gilbert *et al.*, 2005; Jick *et al.*, 1981). According to its manufacturer, this antihistamine was not teratogenic in animal studies, although the study has not been published.

Triprolidine was not associated with an increased frequency of malformations in the offspring of 628 women who took this drug in the first trimester (Aselton *et al.*, 1985; Gilbert *et al.*, 2005; Jick *et al.*, 1981). No animal teratology studies have been published regarding this agent.

Ethanolamine/ethylamine derivatives

Of 2847 infants exposed to clemastine during the first trimester, there was no increased frequency of congenital anomalies (Table 11.3). No human studies have been published regarding the use of bromodiphenhydramine and carbinoxamine, and neither have animal teratology studies with either drug been published. The frequency of malformations was not increased in one animal study of carbinoxamine (Maruyama and Yoshida, 1968).

In a large case–control study (23 757 cases; 39 877 controls), the risk of congenital anomalies was not increased among 2640 infants born to women who used dimenhydrate during the first trimester (Czeizel and Vargha, 2005). Dimenhydrinate exposure during embryogenesis was not associated with an increased frequency of congenital anomalies in one animal study (McColl *et al.*, 1965).

Diphenhydramine was not associated with an increased frequency of congenital anomalies among 865 pregnancies exposed during the first trimester (Aselton *et al.*, 1985; Heinonen *et al.*, 1977). No studies regarding the use of bromodiphenhydramine during pregnancy have been published. Ten normal infants whose mothers were exposed to bromodiphenhydramine during gestation were included in the Collaborative Perinatal Project (Heinonen *et al.*, 1977), but this number is too small to interpret. Importantly, ethanolaminide derivatives have been reported to have oxytocic-like effects when used parenterally (Hara *et al.*, 1980; Klieger and Massart, 1965; Rotter *et al.*, 1958).

Doxylamine was one of the main components of the popular antinausea drug, Bendectin (along with pyridoxine and dicyclomine). Some investigators reported an association of Bendectin use in pregnancy and diaphragmatic hernias (Bracken and Berg, 1983), congenital heart disease, and pyloric stenosis (Aselton *et al.*, 1985; Eskenazi *et al.*, 1982). Other researchers found no such association with congenital anomalies following exposure during embryogenesis (Mitchell *et al.*, 1981, 1983; Zierler and Rothman, 1985). The frequency of congenital anomalies was not increased among more than 1100 infants exposed to doxylamine (an antihistamine component of Bendectin) during the first trimester of pregnancy (Heinonen *et al.*, 1977). No association was found between doxylamine and congenital heart disease in a case-controlled study (Zierler and Rothman, 1985), nor were malformations found to be increased in frequency in one animal teratology study of doxylamine (Gibson *et al.*, 1968). Considering the millions of women who have used Bendectin during the first trimester of pregnancy without scientific evidence of adverse fetal effects, it is extremely unlikely that doxylamine or the components of Bendectin are human teratogens. Drugs such as Bendectin that do not cause birth defects, but are associated with lawsuits are called 'litogens,' i.e., lawsuit-inducing (Brent, 1983).

In summary, doxylamine is a safe drug for use during pregnancy.

Piperadine derivatives

The frequency of congenital anomalies was not increased among 127 infants whose mothers took azatadine during the first trimester. Similarly, among 285 infants whose mothers took cyproheptadine during the first trimester, the frequency of congenital anomalies was not increased (see Table 11.3). There are no epidemiological studies of adverse fetal effects, including congenital malformations, in the offspring of mothers who took diphenylpyraline during pregnancy. Animal teratology studies of cyproheptadine are not consistent (de la Fuente and Alia, 1982; Rodriguez-Gonzalez *et al.*, 1983; Weinstein *et al.*, 1975). No animal teratology studies of azatadine have been published.

Ethylenediamine derivatives

In a survey of 100 and 112 offspring exposed to tripelennamine and pyrilamine, respectively, during the first trimester, the frequency of congenital anomalies was not increased (Heinonen *et al.*, 1977). Pyrilamine was associated with an increased rate of fetal loss in animal studies (Bovet-Nitti *et al.*, 1963; Naranjo and de Naranjo, 1968). No animal teratology studies on tripelennamine have been published.

SECOND-GENERATION ANTIHISTAMINES

Butyrophenone derivatives

The only member in this group is terfenadine (Seldane). Among 134 infants born to women who used terfenadine during the first trimester, there was no increased frequency of congenital anomalies (Schick *et al.*, 1994). In a recent review, the frequency of congenital anomalies among 2194 infants whose mothers took terfenadine during the first trimester was not increased (see Table 11.3). Terfenadine is not recommended for nursing mothers as it has been associated with decreased pup weight in rat studies (data from the manufacturer).

Other second-generation antihistamines

Among 950 infants whose mothers took cetirizine during the first trimester the frequency of congenital anomalies was not increased. Similarly, astemizole exposure during the first trimester was not associated with an increased frequency of congenital anomalies among 114 infants. Loratidine, an FDA category B drug, exposure during the first trimester was not associated with a higher than expected frequency of congenital anomalies (see Table 11.3). These drugs seem safe for use during pregnancy, with greater confidence assigned to those drugs whose studies have the larger denominators (e.g., loratidine) (Gilbert *et al.*, 2005).

Piperazine derivatives

Cyclizine, buclizine, and meclizine are used primarily as antiemetics, although they also have antihistamine action. Among over 1000 infants who were exposed to meclizine in the first trimester, the frequency of congenital anomalies was not increased (Heinonen *et al.*, 1977). In addition, the risk of congenital anomalies was not increased by first-trimester exposure to meclizine in one cohort and three case–control studies (Greenberg *et al.*, 1977; Mellin, 1964; Milkovich and van den Berg, 1976; Nelson and Forfar, 1971). First-trimester exposure to cyclizine among 111 infants was not associated with an increased frequency of congenital anomalies (Milkovich and van den Berg, 1976). No studies have been published on the use of buclizine during pregnancy.

In a rat study, the frequency of craniofacial and skeletal malformations was increased among fetuses exposed to meclizine during embryogenesis (King, 1963). No birth defects were found in the offspring of monkeys who received 10 times the usual human dose of meclizine during embryogenesis (Courtney and Valerio, 1968; Wilson and Gavan, 1967).

Phenindamine

No animal or human studies regarding congenital anomalies and the use of phenindamine in pregnant women have been published. However, it is closely related to chlorpheniramine which has been studied during pregnancy and found not to increase the risk for birth defects (Table 11.4).

EXPECTORANTS AND ANTITUSSIVES

Expectorants

Guaifenesin is the major expectorant used currently, and is a major component of most cough mixtures. There are no animal teratology studies available. Guaifenesin use during the first trimester in more than 1000 human pregnancies was not associated with an increased risk of congenital anomalies (Aselton, 1985; Heinonen *et al.*, 1977; Jick *et al.*, 1981). Other mucolytic agents or drugs that act as an expectorant include potassium iodide or iodinated glycerol. It is well known that iodine-containing agents cross the placenta freely and may result in fetal goiter. Therefore, iodide-containing agents are contraindicated for use during pregnancy.

Antitussives

Dextromethorphan is commonly used as an antitussive. It was used by 300 pregnant women during the first trimester and the frequency of congenital anomalies was not

Table 11.4 Teratogen Information System (TERIS) risk for congenital anomaly and Food and Drug Administration (FDA) pregnancy risk category

Drugs	TERIS risk	FDA risk rating
Astemizole	Unlikely	C_m
Azatadine	Undetermined	B_m
Bendectin	None	NA
Benzonatate	Undetermined	NA
Bromodiphenhydramine	Undetermined	C
Brompheniramine	None	C_m
Buclizine	Undetermined	C
Carbinoxamine	Undetermined	C
Chlorpheniramine	Unlikely	B
Chlorphenirmine	Unlikely	B
Clemastine	Undetermined	B_m
Cyclizine	Unlikely	B
Cyproheptadine	Undetermined	B_m
Dextromethorphan	None	C
Dicyclomine	None	B_m
Dimenhydrinate	Unlikely	B_m
Diphenhydramine	Unlikely	B_m
Diphenylpyraline	Undetermined	NA
Doxylamine	None	A
Guaifenesin	None	C
Hydroxyzine	Unlikely	C
Iodinated glycerol	Undetermined	X_m
Meclizine	Unlikely	B_m
Naphazoline	Undetermined	NA
Oxymetazoline	Unlikely	C
Phenindamine	Undetermined	C
Phenylephrine	None to minimal	C
Pseudoephedrine	None to minimal	C
Pyridoxine	None	NA
Pyrilamine	None	C
Terfenadine	Unlikely	C_m
Triprolidine	Unlikely	C_m
Xylometazoline	Unlikely	NA

NA, not available.

Compiled from: Friedman *et al., Obstet Gynecol* 1990; **75**: 594; Briggs *et al.*, 2005; Friedman and Polifka, 2006.

increased (Heinonen *et al.*, 1977). Numerous narcotics are used in cough preparations, including codeine, hydrocodone, and hydromorphone. Chronic use of narcotic agents may result in neonatal addiction, withdrawal, and respiratory depression. However, narcotics are not associated with an increased frequency of congenital anomalies. Also, acute use of narcotic antitussives is not associated with neonatal addiction or congenital anomalies.

Benzonatate (Tessalon) is a local anesthetic-like compound and acts as an antitussive by anesthetizing the stretch receptors in the respiratory passage. No human studies are available on which to base an evaluation of adverse fetal effects.

Note: Many cough preparations contain ethyl alcohol and may cause adverse fetal effects if used chronically. Case reports of fetal alcohol syndrome have been published in which the mother abused cough preparations during pregnancy. However, it is unlikely that short-term use carries significant risk. Alcohol is discussed in further detail in Chapter 16.

SPECIAL CONSIDERATIONS

Viral upper respiratory infections (the common cold)

Pregnant women with colds usually do not require specific therapy, especially in the first trimester. If symptomatic therapy is indicated, pregnant women with the common cold can be treated with acetaminophen, in combination with a decongestant and an antihistamine, and a combination of an antitussive and expectorant. Pseudoephedrine and chlorpheniramine are the preferred treatments (Hornby and Abrahams, 1996). If a nasal spray is deemed necessary, agents containing oxymetazoline, xylometazoline, or naphazoline are reasonable, since minimal systemic absorption occurs. Antitussive/expectorant compounds containing iodide are contraindicated. Other, noniodinated preparations offer equally effective alternative medication (Tables 11.1 and 11.2).

Allergic rhinitis/sinusitis

Chlorpheniramine compounds are preferable for first-line use in pregnant women because they are better studied. The histamine H_1-receptor antagonist astemizole (Hismanal) and terfenadine (Seldane) have been studied in the first trimester in pregnant women (Table 11.3), and are probably safe.

Pruritis/urticaria

Diphenhydramine is well studied during pregnancy and is a safe agent to use (Table 11.3). Its oxytocic effects do not appear to be as pronounced as dimenhydrinate (Hara *et al.*, 1980). Other medications found to be safe and effective in the treatment of pruritus are hydroxyzine or dexchlorpheniramine (Drugs and Pregnancy Study Group, 1994) (Table 11.3).

Motion sickness/vertigo

Dimenhydrinate is a commonly used agent, although it may have some oxytocic properties. It has been studied during the first trimester of human pregnancy and was not associated with an increased frequency of congenital anomalies (Czeizel and Vargha, 2005).

Drug-induced dyskinesia

The antimuscarinic and sedative effects of diphenhydramine make it the ideal agent for the treatment of drug-induced dyskinesia in the pregnant patient. Its use during pregnancy has been studied extensively, and there were no apparent untoward effects (Table 11.3).

Key references

Czeizel AE, Vargha AEP. A case–control study of congenital abnormality and dimenhydrinate usage during pregnancy. *Arch Gynecol Obstet* 2005; **271**: 113.

Gilbert C, Mazzotta P, Loebstein R, Koren G. Fetal safety of drugs used in the treatment of allergic rhinitis. A critical review. *Drug Safety* 2005; **28**: 707.

Hornby PJ, Abrahams TP. Pulmonary pharmacology. *Clin Obstet Gynecol* 1996; **39**: 17.

Further references are available on the book's website at http://www.drugsandpregnancy.com

12

Nutritional and dietary supplementation during pregnancy

A balanced 'nonfad' diet should provide pregnant women with an adequate complement of nutrients during pregnancy. Prenatal vitamin supplements are usually given, but there is no clear consensus that they are needed. Under the Hippocratic dictum of 'do no harm,' prenatal vitamin supplements are not harmful in recommended daily allowance (RDA) doses. Vitamin supplements for pregnant women should, along with dietary intake, approximate the RDA set by the Food and Drug Administration (FDA) (Table 12.1). Iron is the only nutrient for which supplementation during pregnancy is invariably required.

PROTEIN-CALORIE REQUIREMENTS AND SUPPLEMENTS

During a normal pregnancy, women should gain between 22 and 27 lbs. Calories required during pregnancy increase (approximately 300–500 calories per day) only marginally above the needs of nonpregnant women (2100 calories daily). Composition of the 2400 to 2600 calories should be comprised of 74 g of protein. A reasonably balanced diet provides adequate protein and calories during pregnancy (ACOG, 1993). Under special circumstances, protein-calorie supplementation is warranted. Gravidas who follow a vegetarian diet or are otherwise nutritionally restricted (e.g., gluten intolerant), may require supplementation. When considering the gravid vegetarian, it is extremely important to distinguish between the strictly vegetarian (e.g., Buddhist) and the lacto-ovo vegetarian (e.g., Seventh Day Adventists). Lacto-ovo vegetarians do not consume animal flesh-derived foods (i.e., meat and fish) from their diets, but do consume animal products (i.e., eggs and dairy products). Nonlacto-ovo vegetarians eat only plant-derived foods and are

Table 12.1 National Research Council recommended daily dietary allowances for women before and during pregnancy and lactation

Nutrient	Nonpregnant[a]	Pregnant	Lactating
Kilocalories	2200	2500	2600
Protein (g)	55	60	65
Fat-soluble vitamins			
A (µg RE)[b]	800	800	1300
D (µg)	10	10	12
E (mg TE)[c]	8	10	12
K (µg)	55	65	65
Water-soluble vitamins			
C (mg)	60	70	95
Cobalamin, B_{12} (µg)	2.0	2.2	2.6
Folate (µg)	180	400	280
Niacin (mg)	15	17	20
Pyridoxine, B_6 (mg)	1.6	2.2	2.1
Riboflavin (mg)	1.1	1.5	1.6
Thiamin (mg)	1.3	1.6	1.8
Minerals			
Calcium (mg)	1200	1200	1200
Iodine (µg)	150	175	200
Iron (mg)	15	30	15
Magnesium (mg)	280	320	355
Phosphorus (mg)	1200	1200	1200
Zinc (mg)	12	15	19

[a]For nonpregnant females age 15–18 years.
[b]1 µg retinol = 1 retinol equivalent (RE).
[c]TE, tocopherol equivalent.
From the National Academy of Science, 1989; current as of January 2006.

at high risk of inadequate protein-calorie nutrition. Special action from the clinician to ensure an adequate intake of the essential amino acids and folate must be taken. A professional nutritionist should be involved to help manage meal plans during pregnancy for the strict vegetarian. Nonlacto-ovo vegetarians may also suffer from various other nutrient deficiencies, specifically of vitamins of the A and B group.

VITAMINS

'Super-vitamin' preparations or megadose regimens, such as Centrum, should not be used during pregnancy for reasons discussed below.

Vitamin A

Vitamin A is an essential nutrient, and the recommended supplement of vitamin A (approximately 8000 IU per day; Table 12.1) is usually consumed. The risk of birth defects and adverse fetal effects is probably nil with maternal intake of 10 000 IU or less of vitamin A daily. However, megadoses of vitamin A, taken by some individuals for undocumented health advantages, are often encountered in practice. No data to support large-dose vitamin A are published in the scientific literature. Investigators analyzed the teratogenicity of high vitamin A intake of pregnant women and found that one in about 57 children had a malformation in cranial neural crest formation associated with high dose vitamin A (> 10 000 IU supplements per day) (Rothman *et al.*, 1995). The prevalence of malformations among infants born to mothers who ingested 5000 IU or less of food and supplements of vitamin A per day was significantly lower than the high-dose group (Rothman *et al.*, 1995). The vitamin A dose associated with an increased risk for congenital anomalies is unknown; however, more than 10 000 IU daily may significantly increase that risk.

Important note: Current RDA of 10 000 IU of vitamin A includes dietary intakes, not just supplementation.

Water-soluble vitamin A supplements are beta-carotene derived from vegetables. Other vitamin A supplements (retinoic acid, discussed above) are fat soluble, and usually fish liver derived. Beta-carotene vitamin A probably has a higher clearance rate than retinoic acid because it is water soluble. Beta-carotene presumably poses much less, if any, teratogenic risk compared to similar amounts of retinoid acid-derived vitamin A (or Retinol). Anecdotal data (case reports) support the hypothesized association of birth defects with high-dose retinoic acid-derived vitamin A. Case reports describe urinary tract and craniofacial complex congenital anomalies among infants whose mothers who took > 40 000 IU or more of vitamin A during pregnancy (Bernhardt and Dorsey, 1974; Mounoud *et al.*, 1975; Pilotti and Scorta, 1965). Findings among infants whose mothers used megadoses of vitamin A analogs (isotretinoin, etretinate) support the existence of a retinoic acid embryopathy (see Chapter 14).

Offspring of rats, mice, hamsters, pigs, and dogs whose mothers were given vitamin A (doses up to 5000 times RDA) during embryogenesis had increased frequencies of congenital anomalies that were dose related (Cohlan, 1951; Kalter and Warkany, 1961; Kochhar, 1964; Marin-Padrilla and Ferm, 1965; Palludan, 1966; Wiersig and Swenson, 1967; Willhite, 1984). As with human case reports, anomalies in animal studies were also heterogeneous (brain, cardiac, eye, and craniofacial anomalies) and not consistent with a syndrome.

Despite the purely anecdotal nature of direct information on large doses of vitamin A during early pregnancy, an increased risk of congenital anomalies seems highly likely. On balance, the negative information regarding the association of birth defects and high-dose vitamin A is the apparent lack of a pattern of congenital anomalies observed (highly heterogeneous collection of defects). The high frequency of congenital anomalies with isotretinoin and etretinate – vitamin A congeners – exposure during embryogenesis offers evidence that vitamin A megadoses during pregnancy increase the risk of congenital anomalies (see Chapter 14).

Vitamin D

Vitamin D is produced by skin exposed to ultraviolet light and is integral to normal calcium metabolism. Notably, vitamin D deficiency is associated with rickets. Skeletal anomalies comparable to rickets in humans were found in rats born to mothers who were vitamin D deficient during gestation (Warkany, 1943). No congenital anomalies were observed in a clinical case series of 15 children born to hypoparathyroid women who took more than 200 times the RDA of vitamin D throughout pregnancy (Goodenday and Gordon, 1971).

Defects with high-dose vitamin D parallel those seen in Williams syndrome – supravalvular aortic stenosis, unusual facies, and infantile hypercalcemia – in the human (Chan et al., 1979; Friedman and Mills, 1969; Friedman and Roberts, 1966). Williams syndrome was speculated to be caused by the use of megadoses of vitamin D during pregnancy (Friedman, 1968), but the available data do not support this (Forbes, 1979; Warkany, 1943). Interestingly, rats and rabbits born to mothers given several thousands of times the human RDA of vitamin D during gestation had cardiovascular and cranio-facial anomalies (Friedman and Mills, 1969).

Vitamin B group

NIACIN

Vitamin B_3, niacin, is naturally present in many foods. Prescriptions for vitamin B_3 are usu-ally for doses 200–400 times the RDA to treat hyperlipidemia. No studies have been pub-lished of congenital anomalies among infants born to mothers who took niacin during the first trimester. No increased frequency of congenital anomalies was found in rats and rab-bits born to mothers given large doses of niacin during organogenesis (Takaori et al., 1973).

PANTOTHENATE

Pantothenate is an essential cofactor in metabolism of carbohydrates, proteins, and fats. It contributes to the composition of coenzyme A. Pantothenate is nearly ubiquitous in a well-balanced diet.

No reports have been published of infants born to women who took more than the RDA of pantothenate during pregnancy, or of the effects of megadoses of pantothenate on ani-mals are not published. However, deficiency of pantothenate during pregnancy in rats, mice, and swine was associated with an excess of intrauterine deaths and brain, eye, limb, and heart defects among offspring exposed during gestation (Kalter and Warkany, 1959; Kimura and Ariyama, 1961; Lefebvres, 1954; Nelson et al., 1957; Ullrey, et al., 1955).

PYRIDOXINE

Pyridoxine (vitamin B_6), another essential nutrient, is an enzyme cofactor. Dietary pyri-doxine requirements are increased among pregnant women (Table 12.1).

No investigations have been published on the frequency of congenital anomalies among infants born to women who took megadoses of pyridoxine during pregnancy. In one animal study, congenital anomalies were not increased in frequency among rats born to mothers given many times the RDA for pyridoxine during pregnancy (Khera, 1975). Pyridoxine deficiency during pregnancy was associated with digital defects and cleft palate in mice and rats (Davis et al., 1970; Miller, 1972).

THIAMINE

Vitamin B_1 (thiamine) is an essential dietary component because it is a coenzyme. No studies of high doses of thiamine during human pregnancy have been published. Congenital anomalies were not increased in frequency among offspring of rats given up to 140 times the RDA of thiamine during pregnancy (Morrison and Sarett, 1959;

Schumacher *et al.*, 1965) or about 50 times the rat daily requirement. Thiamine deficiency was associated with an increased frequency of fetal death and decreased fetal weight gain among pregnant rats (Nelson and Evans, 1955; Roecklein *et al.*, 1985).

CYANOCOBALAMIN

Vitamin B_{12}, also known as cyanocobalamin, is also an essential nutrient. Megadose cyanocobalamin (about 260 times RDA) is used to treat pernicious anemia. The frequency of congenital anomalies among infants whose mothers took megadoses of vitamin B_{12} during pregnancy has not been published. Malformations were not increased in frequency among the offspring of mice treated during pregnancy with 5250–10 500 times the RDA of cyanocobalamin (Mitala *et al.*, 1978). Cyanocobalamin deficiency among offspring of rats treated with megadoses of cyanocobalamin had increased frequencies of hydrocephalus, eye defects, and skeletal anomalies (Grainger *et al.*, 1954; Woodard and Newberne, 1966).

VITAMIN C

Vitamin C (ascorbic acid) is an essential nutrient. Deficiency of vitamin C causes scurvy. No increase in the use of vitamin C was found in a case–control study of the use of vitamin C during the first trimester by mothers of 175 infants with major congenital anomalies and 283 with minor anomalies compared to the control group (Nelson and Forfar, 1971). Embryofetal effects of megadoses of vitamin C during pregnancy have not been published. Two infants born to women who took more than six times the RDA of vitamin C during pregnancy had scurvy (Cochrane, 1965).

The frequency of congenital anomalies was not increased among mice and rats born to mothers treated with hundreds to several thousand times the RDA of vitamin C during embryogenesis (Frohberg *et al.*, 1973). An increased frequency of fetal death was found in offspring of mice fed 4800 times the RDA of ascorbic acid during embryogenesis (Pillans *et al.*, 1990). Increased dietary requirements for vitamin C was found in guinea pigs born to mothers who were given several hundred times the RDA throughout pregnancy; increased clearance apparently caused the need for more vitamin C (Cochrane, 1965; Norkus and Rosso, 1975, 1981).

VITAMIN E

Vitamin E is another essential nutrient. If caloric intake is adequate, vitamin E deficiency is extremely rare. No studies of vitamin E use during human pregnancy have been published. Among rats and mice born to mothers given vitamin E in doses up to thousands of times the RDA, the frequency of congenital anomalies was not increased (Hook *et al.*, 1974; Hurley *et al.*, 1983; Krasavage and Terhaar, 1977; Sato *et al.*, 1973). In contrast, the frequency of cleft palate was increased among mice born to mothers given several-hundred times the human RDA of vitamin E during embryogenesis (Momose *et al.*, 1972).

OTHER ESSENTIAL NUTRIENTS

Folic acid

Folic acid is an essential nutrient and acts as a coenzyme. It has been shown that folic acid is extremely important in normal embryonic development, specifically the neural tube complex. Pregnancy elevates the RDA for folic acid.

'On March 5, 1996, the US Food and Drug Administration (FDA) required that manufacturers fortify enriched cereal-grain products with 140 µg of folic acid per 100 g of cereal-grain product by January 1, 1998' (Grosse et al., 2005). Subsequent analysis has shown a reduction in neural tube defects (NTDs) on a national scale of 20–30 percent, and a resulting associated monetary saving of $312–425 million annually. Direct cost avoidance was $88–145 million per year for an annual investment of $23 million. The return on investment (ROI) for the associated economic impact and direct cost avoidance were minimally 13.6 and 3.8, respectively. What follows is the scientific background to an apparently very effective public health intervention to reduce birth defects (neural tube defects) through improved population level nutrition intervention, providing needed folic acid supplementation.

Folic acid supplementation and deficiency during pregnancy with infant outcome was investigated in a number of published studies, but results were inconsistent. No congenital anomalies were found among 44 treatment infants whose mothers took 15 times the RDA throughout pregnancy to prevent the recurrence of a NTD (Laurence et al., 1981). However, there were two NTDs in the treatment noncompliance group and four in the placebo control group. Other studies have analyzed folic acid supplements at doses similar to the RDA, and the occurrence of neural tube defects was not more frequent than expected.

Folic acid supplements given in prospective studies to prevent NTDs have shown a decreased risk of neural tube defects (Bower and Stanley, 1989; Smithells et al., 1981, 1983, 1989). Daily intake of folic acid was found to reduce the occurrence and recurrence of NTDs in 5502 women in a randomized controlled study (Czeizel and Dudas, 1992; Czeizel et al., 1994). Folic acid antagonists, such as aminopterin, are well-known human and animal teratogens. Numerous teratology studies using rats and mice have consistently shown that folic acid deficiency is associated with an increased frequency of various congenital anomalies (Shepard, 1995). Daily periconceptional intake of 0.4 mg of folic acid by women before and during early pregnancy in a case–control study decreased the risk of NTD occurrence in their infants by 50 percent (Werler et al., 1993).

Conversely, retrospective studies have not found a reduced risk of neural tube defects with folic acid supplementation during pregnancy (Mills et al., 1989; Milunsky et al., 1989). Folic acid deficiency was associated with adverse pregnancy outcome in one study (Dansky et al., 1987), but not in two others (Pritchard et al., 1970, 1971).

In 1992, the US Centres for Disease Control (CDC) issued the recommendation that women of childbearing should consume 0.4 mg of folic acid per day. However, it was cautioned that women should consume less than 1.0 mg per day of the supplement. The untoward effects of hypervitaminosis B_{12} are not well studied, especially during pregnancy. For this reason, folate intake among women who are of childbearing age should regulate their intake to 0.4 mg or less than 1 mg per day (MMWR, 1992). In 1996, the US FDA issued the requirement that manufacturers fortify enriched cereal-grain products with 140 µg of folic acid per 100 g (Grosse et al., 2005).

Iron

Iron is an essential dietary metal and its requirements during pregnancy increase as gestation age advances. Scholl et al. (1992) found that iron-deficiency anemia was related to low energy levels and a lower mean corpuscular volume among 800 pregnant women at their first prenatal care visit. Preterm delivery was doubled and the incidence of delivering a low-birth weight baby was tripled among the iron deficiency anemic women. Need for iron supplementation usually occurs 20–28 weeks gestation. Iron supplementation (60–100 mg daily) is needed because the normal diet cannot supply the required amounts. It is also recommended that the iron supplement be given alone and not as a component of prenatal vitamins because of lower absorption from multivitamin preparations (Cunningham *et al.*, 1989). Anecdotally, iron overdose is a common suicide attempt method during pregnancy. A prudent practice for high-risk patients is to provide only a 1-week supply at a time, which limits access to toxic doses of iron. Toxic doses are between 3 and 6 g of iron supplements. Iron supplement megadoses are among the more commonly used medications in suicide gestures, which is discussed in Chapter 14, Drug overdoses during pregnancy.

Congenital anomalies were not increased in frequency among 66 infants born to women who received parental iron supplementation during the first trimester. No complications or malformations were found among more than 1800 infants whose mothers received iron supplementation at any time during pregnancy (Heinonen *et al.*, 1977). Similarly, the frequency of congenital anomalies or complications was no different than the general population among 1336 infants born to either women who received iron supplements when they were anemic or women who routinely received the supplement during the second and third trimester of pregnancy (Hemminki and Rimpela, 1991). Therefore, it may be prudent to limit prescriptions to a 1-week course per refill in gravidas with a history of suicide gestures, although no abnormalities were observed in a group of 19 children whose mothers had ingested overdoses of iron during the last two trimesters of pregnancy (McElhatton *et al.*, 1991).

Animal data regarding iron use during pregnancy are inconsistent. Rats born to mothers given up to 100 times the usual therapeutic dose of iron during embryogenesis showed frequency of congenital anomalies no different from controls (Flodh *et al.*, 1977; Tadokoro *et al.*, 1979). Central nervous system anomalies were increased in frequency above control levels among mice and rabbits whose mothers were given comparably large doses of iron during embryogenesis (Flodh *et al.*, 1977; Kuchta, 1982).

Calcium

Calcium is an essential nutrient required for normal physiological function and fetal growth. A balanced diet provides the required amount of calcium.

The frequency of congenital anomalies was not increased among more than 1000 infants born to women who received calcium supplements during the first trimester, or among more than 3500 infants whose mothers took supplements after the first trimester (Heinonen *et al.*, 1977). A slight, but significant excess of nonspecific central nervous system abnormalities was reported. The heterogeneity of the defects suggests that the association may be a chance occurrence of multiple comparisons.

Among rats, rabbits, and mice whose mothers were given twice the RDA of calcium during embryogenesis, the frequency of congenital anomalies was no greater than controls (McCormack *et al.*, 1979). Fetal death and growth retardation occurred more frequently in the offspring of pregnant rats given about 1600 mg/kg.day of calcium chloride (Hayasaka *et al.*, 1990).

Special considerations

NEURAL TUBE DEFECTS

There is highly compelling evidence that occurrence and recurrence of NTDs can be decreased by folic acid supplementation, as discussed earlier. Risk of NTD recurrence was decreased in several different studies in England when a combination vitamin regimen that contained folic acid and seven other vitamins was given to women who had given birth to a child with a NTD in a previous pregnancy (Smithells *et al.*, 1981, 1983, 1989; MRC Vitamin Study Research Group, 1991). The group concluded that, 'Folic acid supplementation starting before pregnancy can now be firmly recommended for all women who have had an affected pregnancy and public health measures should be taken to ensure that the diet of all women who may bear children contains an adequate amount of folic acid,' (MRC Vitamin Study Research Group, 1991). This has led to a cost-effective and significant reduction in the occurrence of NTDs in the USA.

Nutritional summary

In conclusion, iron supplements during pregnancy are definitely necessary. Folic acid supplements are also a universal necessity. The gravid vegetarian or one who is following a 'fad' diet is a special concern and a nutritional assessment should be undertaken to assure adequate intake. Prenatal vitamins should probably be given, although there is no consensus on whether they are necessary. At RDA doses, such preparations will not cause harm and may be of benefit. Following Hippocrates to above all do 'no harm,' prenatal vitamins should be given. Megadose regimens are clearly contraindicated.

GASTROINTESTINAL MEDICATIONS DURING PREGNANCY

Gastrointestinal disorders occur frequently during pregnancy, often in response to the pregnancy-related physiological changes. Nausea, with or without vomiting is the most common gastrointestinal disorder of early pregnancy. In the extreme form (i.e., hyperemesis gravidarum), vomiting may result in significant weight loss and dehydration. Pyrosis or 'heartburn' is a very common symptom in pregnancy and is related to increased gastroesophageal reflux secondary to decreased muscular tone in the lower esophagus. Gastrointestinal disorders that may be associated with pregnancy, but occur with about the same frequency in nongravid women, include peptic ulcer disease, inflammatory bowel disease, and gallbladder disease – cholelithiasis and cholecystitis (Cunningham, 1994). Medications to treat gastrointestinal disorders, including antacids, anticholinergics, antiemetics, antiflatulents, and laxatives, are discussed in this section. Corticosteroids, which may be useful in the therapy of inflammatory bowel disease, are discussed in Chapter 4.

Antacids

Antacids are classified based on their content: aluminum, calcium, magnesium, magaldrate, sodium bicarbonate, and combinations of any of these. Antacids are the most common over-the-counter and prescribed gastrointestinal medications used by pregnant women. Combinations of aluminum hydroxide and magnesium hydroxide are used in popular commercial preparations (e.g., Maalox, Mylanta, Riopan, and Gelusil). Calcium carbonate is also a very popular antacid (e.g., Tums, Titralac, Rolaids, and Chooz).

No human or animal teratology studies have been published regarding antacids. Antacids are associated with little, if any, significant risk for congenital anomalies or fetal risk when used in moderation. Chronic use of high-dose antacids has been associated with adverse effects such as hypercalcemia, hypermagnesemia, or hypocalcemia.

Histamine receptor antagonists

Histamine receptor antagonists are systemic agents used to reduce gastric acidity. Currently available preparations include cimetidine, ranitidine, famotidine, and nizatidine (Table 12.2). A primary use of these agents in pregnant women before general anesthesia is as a prophylaxis against aspiration. Histamine receptor antagonists are also used to treat peptic ulcer disease, which is uncommon in pregnant women. H_2-receptor antagonists (i.e., inhibitors of gastric acid production) are also useful in pregnant women with severe forms of reflux esophagitis unresponsive to the usual antacids (Cunningham, 1994). These agents are known to cross the placenta (Howe et al., 1981; Schenker et al., 1987).

Among 237 infants born to women who took cimetidine during the first trimester of pregnancy, the frequency of congenital anomalies was not increased (Ruigomez et al., 1999). In another study the frequency of congenital anomalies was increased among 113 infants exposed to cimetidine during the first trimester (Garbis et al., 2005). First-trimester ranitidine exposure was reported in 335 infants and the frequency of congenital anomalies was not increased above controls (Garbis et al., 2005). Similarly, congenital anomalies in infants born to 300 women who took ranitidine during embryogenesis were not increased over controls (Ruigomez et al., 1999). Among infants born to 58 women who used famotidine in the first trimester, the frequency of congenital anomalies was no higher than that expected in the general population (Kallen, 1998). In one study of 75 infants whose mothers took famotidine during the first trimester, the frequency of congenital anomalies detected at birth was no higher than would be expected in the general population (Garbis et al., 2005). However, two elective terminations occurred in the famotidine group because they had NTDs. The relevance of these data is unknown because of the small sample size; the authors felt that timing of famotidine exposure excluded a causal association with the neural tube defects (Garbis et al., 2005). Data have been published on a small number of first-trimester exposures to nizatidine

Table 12.2 Histamine receptor antagonists

Agent	Brand name
Cimetidine	Tagamet
Famotidine	Pepcid
Nizatidine	Axid
Ranitidine	Zantac
Rozatidine	

(n = 15) and roxatidine (n = 15) and there were no congenital anomalies (Garbis *et al.*, 2005). Nizatidine is closely related to cimetidine.

Histamine receptor antagonists were not associated with an increased frequency of malformations or adverse fetal effects in several animal teratology studies involving rodents (Brimblecombe *et al.*, 1985; Higashida *et al.*, 1983; Hirakawa *et al.*, 1980; Tamura *et al.*, 1983). Several reports regarding the use of these agents as premedications prior to Caesarean section found an increased frequency of complications (Gillett *et al.*, 1984; Hodgkinson *et al.*, 1983; Mathews *et al.*, 1986; Thorburn and Moir, 1987), but these exposures are not relevant to the risk for congenital anomalies.

Therefore, data suggest that histamine receptor antagonists may be used safely in the first trimester of pregnancy in humans and with apparent safety for both mother and fetus in the latter half of pregnancy.

Proton pump inhibitors

OMEPRAZOLE, LANSOPRAZOLE, AND ESOMEPRAZOLE

Omeprazole (Prilosec) is a proton pump inhibitor (PPI) and blocks the production of gastric acid. Among 295 infants whose mothers were exposed to omeprazole during embryogenesis, the frequency of congenital anomalies was no greater than among controls (Kallen, 1998). Ninety-one infants were born to women who took omeprazole during the first trimester and the frequency of congenital anomalies was no greater than expected (Lalkin *et al.*, 1998). Among 233 infants exposed during the first trimester to omeprazole, the frequency of congenital anomalies was not significantly greater than unexposed controls (Diav-Citrin *et al.*, 2005). A case report of an omeprazole overdose during pregnancy that resulted in a normal infant has been published (Ferner and Allison, 1993). Also, there is a small case series (n = 3) in which mothers were treated with omeprazole chronically, and all three infants were healthy in the neonatal period (Harper *et al.*, 1995). No congenital anomalies were found among rat pups born to mothers given many times the usual human dose of omeprazole during embryogenesis, although growth retardation was present (Shimazu *et al.*, 1988).

Among 55 infants exposed to lansoprazole during the first trimester, the frequency of congenital anomalies was not increased. In the same investigation, the frequency of congenital anomalies among infants exposed to pantoprazole during the first trimester was no greater than controls (Diav-Citrin *et al.*, 2005).

No epidemiological studies of esomeprazole during first trimester of pregnancy have been published. Notably, esomeprazole is the sinister racemate of omeprazole. Clinically, the advantage of esomeprazole over omeprazole is that the *S*-racemate isomer is cleared from the body more slowly, decreasing dose frequency (Kendall, 2003). It is tempting to deduce that esomeprazole is safe because a closely related drug (omeprazole) is apparently safe based upon 538 first-trimester exposures. However, it is imperative that we bear in mind that an isomer of thalidomide, the most notorious human teratogen ever discovered, was not associated with birth defects.

Proton pump inhibitors seem to be safe for use during pregnancy. Omeprazole (Prilosec) is the best studied and should be the drug of choice. Esomeprazole (Nexium) has not been adequately studied to assess its safety for use during pregnancy.

Antiemetics

Most pregnant women experience at least some degree of nausea during the first trimester; most can be managed without medication. A variety of medications can be used in women requiring therapy for protracted vomiting or vomiting resulting in dehydration.

Phenothiazides

Phenothiazides are used for several medical indications (nausea, vomiting, psychotic disorders, mild pain). This drug class is also effective as an antidyskinetic and a mild sedative. Prochlorperazine, chlorpromazine, and promethazine are the most commonly used phenothiazine derivatives used to treat nausea and vomiting during pregnancy. Phenothiazine use during pregnancy may be associated with extrapyramidal symptoms in the mother as well as the fetus, but these adverse effects are uncommon (Hill *et al.*, 1966; Levy and Wiseniewski, 1974). The phenothiazide class does not seem to be associated with an increased frequency of congenital anomalies when used during gestation.

Promethazine

Promethazine is sold under several proprietary names, but Phenergan is the known brand. It is also used with meperidine during labor and for post-Caesarean section pain. Among over a hundred infants whose mothers took promethazine in the first trimester, the frequency of malformations was not increased (Heinonen *et al.*, 1977). Neither was the frequency of malformations increased in two other studies that included several-hundred women who used the drug during their first trimester (Aselton *et al.*, 1985; Farkas and Farkas, 1971). The frequency of malformations was also not increased in the offspring of animals exposed to this agent (King *et al.*, 1965).

Chlorpromazine

The frequency of birth defects was not increased among infants of more than 400 women who took chlorpromazine during embryogenesis (Farkas and Farkas, 1971; Heinonen *et al.*, 1977). The frequency of congenital anomalies was not increased among rodents whose mothers were given large doses of the drug during embryogenesis (Beall, 1972; Jones-Price *et al.*, 1983; Robertson *et al.*, 1980).

Prochlorperazine

Published studies include over 3000 women who took prochlorperazine during pregnancy, involving over 1000 exposed during the first trimester (Heinonen *et al.*, 1977; Jick *et al.*, 1981; Kullander and Kallen, 1976; Milkovich and van den Berg, 1976). The frequency of congenital anomalies was not increased in the offspring of women who took the drug in the first trimester.

The frequency of cleft palate was increased in the offspring of pregnant animals given large doses of prochlorperazine during embryogenesis (Roux, 1959; Szabo and Brent, 1974). The significance of this finding in humans is unknown.

Piperazine derivatives

Cyclizine, buclizine, and meclizine are piperazine derivatives used for their antiemetic and anti-histamine properties. The frequency of congenital anomalies was not increased in association with the exposure to cyclizine or meclizine during the first trimester in the Collaborative Perinatal Project in more than 1000 infants (Heinonen *et al.*, 1977). Among 111 infants whose mothers took cyclizine in the first trimester, no increase in congenital anomalies was found (Milkovich and van den Berg, 1976). More detailed discussion of these agents is given in Chapter 11. No studies have been published on buclizine during pregnancy.

Doxylamine-pyridoxine

The combination of doxylamine–pyridoxine (Bendectin) has received considerable attention over the past decade as a possible teratogen. Until it was taken off the market, Bendectin was the most commonly prescribed antiemetic for hyperemesis during pregnancy. There have been reports of an association of Bendectin use with diaphragmatic hernias (Bracken and Berg, 1983) and with congenital heart disease and pyloric stenosis (Aselton *et al.*, 1985; Eskenazi and Bracken, 1982). Reports refuting such an association (Mitchell *et al.*, 1981, 1983; Zierler and Rothman, 1985) have also been published. Among more than 1100 infants exposed to doxylamine (Bendectin) during the first trimester of pregnancy, the frequency of congenital anomalies was not increased (Heinonen *et al.*, 1977). No statistically significant association was found between doxylamine and congenital heart disease in a large case–control study (Zierler and Rothman, 1985). Animal teratology studies are also negative (Gibson *et al.*, 1968).

Millions of women used Bendectin during the first trimester of pregnancy with no apparent epidemic of birth defects or adverse fetal effects. Therefore, it seems very unlikely that either doxylamine or pyridoxine is a significant human teratogen. It is generally accepted that neither Bendectin nor its components caused birth defects in human infants.

Unfortunately, it does appear that Bendectin was a significant 'litogen,' i.e., capable of inducing lawsuits (Brent, 1983, 1985; Holmes, 1983).

Other

Ondansetron (Zofran) is a 5-hydroxytryptamine (5-HT$_3$) receptor agonist and is a very potent antiemetic. It is most often utilized for severe nausea and vomiting associated with cancer chemotherapy. It has also been utilized for severe hyperemesis gravidarum (World, 1993; Guikontes *et al.*, 1992), and the authors have also had experience with the successful use of this agent for severe hyperemesis gravidarum. Among 176 infants born to women who used ondansetron during pregnancy, six (3.6 percent) major malformations occurred, and this is no different from the control group (Einarson *et al.*, 2004). In unpublished studies, this agent was not teratogenic in animal studies (information provided by the manufacturer). It is an FDA pregnancy risk category B drug.

Prokinetic agents

Prokinetic agents stimulate upper gastrointestinal tract motility and are utilized primarily for the treatment of gastrointestinal reflux. Two agents are currently available in this class: cisapride (Propulsid) and metoclopramide (Reglan). Among 88 infants born to women who used cisapride during the first trimester, the frequency of congenital anomalies was not increased (Bailey *et al.*, 1997). Metoclopramide is also used as an antiemetic, especially for postoperative nausea. Among 175 infants born to women who used metoclopramide during the first trimester, the frequency of congenital anomalies was 4.4 percent, which was no different from the control rate, 4.8 percent (Berkovitch *et al.*, 2002). According to the manufacturer, metoclopramide was not teratogenic in rats or rabbits (unpublished data). Interestingly, cisapride is listed as a category C drug and metoclopramide as a category B drug. In view of the data, both prokinetic agents appear safe for use during pregnancy, keeping in mind that metoclopramide has a larger cohort size and more power.

Anticholinergics

Anticholinergics are mainly used as antispasmodics and in the therapy of gastrointestinal diseases (ulcer disease, irritable bowel disease). Some of these medications are utilized for other nongastrointestinal indications, such as cardiac arrhythmias or urologic disorders. This class of preparations (Table 12.3) is known to cross the placenta.

Table 12.3 Anticholinergics

Agents	Brand names
Atropine	
Belladonna	
Clidinium	Quarzan
Dicyclomine	Bentyl, Byclomine, Dibent, Di-Spaz
Glycopyrolate	Robinul
Hexocyclium	Tral Filmtabs
Homatropine	Homapin
Hyoscyamine	Cystospaz, Levsinex, Levsin, Anaspaz, Neoquess, Bellafoline
Isopropamide	Darbid
Mepenzolate	Cantil
Methantheline	Banthine
Methscopolamine	Pamine
Oxyphencyclimine	
Oxyphenonium	
Propantheline	Norpanth, Pro-Banthine
Scopolamine	
Tridihexethyl	Pathilon

ATROPINE

Atropine is an anticholinergic that is utilized for a variety of indications, such as cardiac arrhythmias (especially bradycardia), Parkinsonism, asthma, biliary tract diseases, as an antidote for organophosphate insecticide poisoning, and as a preanesthetic agent. The frequency of congenital anomalies was not increased among more than 450 women who received this agent in early pregnancy (Heinonen *et al.*, 1977; Jick *et al.*, 1981). Skeletal anomalies were reported to be increased in one animal study (Arcuri and Gautieri, 1973). Such anomalies have not been reported to date in humans and the data suggest atropine is a safe drug for use during pregnancy.

SCOPOLAMINE

Scopolamine is an anticholinergic agent similar to atropine, and like atropine, may be utilized as a preoperative medication. It may also be used as an antiemetic and for motion sickness. The frequency of congenital anomalies was no different from control in the offspring of the almost 400 women who received this medication in early pregnancy (Heinonen et al., 1977). The frequency of birth defects was not increased among the offspring of rodents given doses much larger than the human dose during embryogenesis (George et al., 1987).

HOMATROPINE AND METHSCOPOLAMINE

No information has been published regarding the use of the anticholinergics homatropine (an ophthalmic preparation) or methscopolamine (used for cardiac arrhythmias, functional bowel disease, and ulcer disease) during pregnancy for experimental animals or humans.

BELLADONNA

Belladonna is a naturally occurring anticholinergic and is used to treat several conditions: functional bowel disorders, motion sickness, dysmenorrhea. Among more than 500 infants born to women who took belladonna during the first trimester, the frequency of major congenital anomalies was not increased (Heinonen et al., 1977). There was an association with minor malformations, but the meaning of this finding is unknown. No animal teratology studies of this agent have been published.

GLYCOPYROLATE

Glycopyrolate is used for several indications: ulcer disease, functional bowel syndrome, and as a preanesthetic agent. No publications on human or animal exposure to this agent during pregnancy have been published.

DICYCLOMINE

Used primarily for the treatment of spastic or irritable colon, dicyclomine was at one time used in combination with doxylamine and pyridoxine in the popular antiemetic preparation, Bendectin. No increase in the frequency of congenital anomalies was found in the offspring of about 100 women who used this agent in early pregnancy (Aselton et al., 1985). The frequency of malformations was not increased in the offspring of animals given dicyclomine in doses several times that of the human dose during embryogenesis (Gibson et al., 1968).

HYOSCYAMINE

Hyoscyamine is used to treat spasmodic bowel diseases and asthma. Over 300 women were exposed to hyoscyamine in early pregnancy, and their infants did not have an increased frequency of birth defects (Heinonen et al., 1977). No animal teratology studies have been published on hyoscyamine.

ISOPROPAMIDE

This agent is used as an adjunct to treat ulcer disease and is also used for the treatment of spastic bowel disorders. Congenital anomalies were not increased in frequency in the offspring of 180 women who took the drug during early pregnancy (Heinonen *et al.*, 1977). No published animal teratology studies are available regarding isopropamide.

PROPANTHELINE

Very little information is available regarding the use of this agent during early pregnancy. Only 33 women who took this drug during early pregnancy are included in the Collaborative Perinatal Project database, and the frequency of congenital anomalies in their infants was not increased (Heinonen *et al.*, 1977).

OTHER AGENTS

No epidemiological studies of congenital anomalies in infants born to women who took clidinium, hexocyclium, mepenzolate, tridihexethyl, oxyphencyclimine, or methantheline during pregnancy have been published. No animal teratology studies of these agents have been published.

Appetite suppressants

Appetite suppressants are not indicated during pregnancy. It is not unusual to encounter pregnant women who used these medications during early pregnancy before they knew that they were pregnant, because these agents are commonly used by women of reproductive age. Numerous available commercial preparations and some common appetite suppressants are listed (Box 12.1).

Box 12.1 Appetite suppressants

Amphetamine	Fenfluramine	Phendimetrazine
Benzphetamine	Mazindol	Phenmetrazine
Diethylpropion	Methamphetamine	Phentermine

AMPHETAMINES, DEXTROAMPHETAMINES, AND METHAMPHETAMINES

These controlled substances are used in a variety of medications for the treatment of hyperactivity, short attention span syndrome, narcolepsy, and as an appetite suppressant for morbid obesity. They are not recommended for use during pregnancy or in breast-feeding mothers because of potential adverse effects. These stimulants are discussed in further detail in Chapter 16.

BENZPHETAMINE

No information has been published on teratogenicity of the use of benzphetamine (Didrex) in pregnant women.

DIETHYLPROPION

Use of diethylpropion (M-Orexic, Nobesine, Tenuate) in early pregnancy was not associated with an increased frequency of congenital anomalies among infants born to several-hundred women (Bunde and Leyland, 1965; Heinonen *et al.*, 1977). Diethylpropion was not teratogenic in one animal study (Cohen *et al.*, 1964).

Although appetite suppressants are generally not recommended for use during pregnancy, this agent is listed as an FDA category B.

PHENDIMETRAZINE

At least 36 different commercial preparations of this agent are available in the USA, but no epidemiological studies have been published of human infants born following its use during pregnancy. No animal teratology studies of phendimetrazine (Prelu-2) have been published. It should be listed as a category C drug because of lack of information.

PHENTERMINE AND FENFLURAMINE

Among 98 infants born to women who took phentermine/fenfluramine during the first trimester, the frequency of both minor and major congenital anomalies was comparable to the control group frequency (Jones *et al.*, 2002).

MAZINDOL

No human reproduction studies with mazindol (Mazanor) have been published.

DEXFENFLURAMINE

Dexfenfluramine is a dextroisomer of fenfluramine, a serotoninergic agent. Information on dexfenfluramine and exposure during pregnancy have not been published.

ANTIFLATULENTS, LAXATIVES, AND ANTIDIARRHEALS

Gastric motility is decreased during pregnancy (Little, 1999) and constipation is a relatively common complaint in pregnant women. Various iron preparations may also contribute to constipation in the pregnant patient. Laxatives are frequently used during pregnancy. The majority of such agents are absorbed very little, if at all, from the gastrointestinal tract. Overall, they should have no systemic effects or pose any serious threat to the fetus.

Antiflatulents

SIMETHICONE

Simethicone (Phazyme, Myliam, Gas-X, Gas Relief) is the most commonly used antiflatulent. There are no human or animal reproductive studies available. Simethicone is logically not expected to cause systemic effects or have access to the fetal–placental unit, because simethicone is not absorbed from the gastrointestinal tract. It is contained in several antacid preparations.

CHARCOAL

No information has been published regarding the use of charcoal during pregnancy, although activated charcoal capsules and tablets are used for relief of gas. Notably, it is not absorbed systemically.

From a practical standpoint, it has no clear indications for use during pregnancy, neither does this agent offer any advantage over simethicone. However, it should be used without hesitation when it is needed in the treatment of acute poisoning.

CALCIUM CARBONATE

This agent in combination with magnesium hydroxide (Mylanta) is utilized as both an antacid and an antiflatulent. This combination can be used safely in pregnancy, avoiding chronic high doses which pose a risk (hypercalcemia, etc).

Laxatives and purgatives

Laxatives/purgatives can generally be divided into several classes depending on the mode of action: (1) emollients and softeners; (2) bulk-forming agents; (3) stimulants; and (4) saline, hyperusmetic, or lubricant agents (Box 12.2). Fortunately, there are few side effects associated with the use of these agents. Allergic reactions are rare. Chronic use of the agents should be avoided because diarrhea and electrolyte imbalances may occur.

Box 12.2 Laxatives and purgatives

Emollients and softeners
Docusate sodium (Colace plus numerous others) plus combinations
Docusate calcium (Surfak, Pro-Cal-Sof) plus combinations
Docusate potassium (Dialose, Diocto-K, Kasof)
Bulk-forming agents
Psyllium (Metamucil, Konsyl-D, Pro-Lax, Serutan, plus several others)
Methylcellulose (Citrucel, Cologel)
Malt soup extract (Maltsupex)
Polycarbophil (Fibercan, Equalactin, Mitrolan)
Stimulants
Castor oil
Bisacodyl (Dulcolax plus others) plus combinations
Casanthrunol (Black-Draught) plus combinations
Cascara sagrada plus combinations
Phenolphthalen (Ex-Lax plus others) plus combinations
Senna (Senokot plus others) plus combinations
Saline, hyperosmotic, or lubricant agents
Mineral oil (Kondremul plus others) plus combinations
Glycerin
Lactulose (Chronulac plus others)
Magnesium citrate (Citroma; Citro-Nesia)
Magnesium hydroxide (Milk of Magnesia) plus combinations

DOCUSATE

This agent is an emollient-type laxative used either singly as a stool softener or in combination with other laxatives. Congenital anomalies were not increased in frequency among the offspring of over 800 women who utilized this agent in early pregnancy (Aselton *et al.*, 1985; Heinonen *et al.*, 1977; Jick *et al.*, 1981). Docusate is not absorbed systemically.

CASANTHRANOL AND CASCARA SAGRADA

The anthraquinone cathartics belong to the stimulant class of laxatives. They are used as monotherapy or in combination with other laxatives. Congenital anomalies were not increased in frequency among offspring of mothers who utilized either casanthranol (21 patients) or cascara sagrada (53 patients) in early pregnancy (Heinonen *et al.*, 1977).

SENNA

Senna is also an anthraquinone laxative. No human reproduction studies have been published. It is very unlikely that it poses any risk to the fetus because this agent is minimally absorbed from the gastrointestinal tract.

PHENOLPHTHALEIN

Phenolphthalein (Ex-Lax, Feen-A-Mint, Atophen, Medilax, Modone, Espotabs) is a commonly utilized agent in commercial preparations. In one mouse study, decreased litter size and fertility were observed, but no somatic effects (Anonymous, 1997).

LACTULOSE

This agent is utilized as a laxative and for lowering serum ammonia in cases of hepatic encephalopathy. Although there are no human reproduction studies, this agent is not absorbed from the gastrointestinal tract for the most part, and thus is unlikely to be associated with adverse fetal effects.

MINERAL OIL

Mineral oil is a lubricant laxative. There are no published human epidemiological or animal teratology studies with this agent. However, chronic use of mineral oil as a laxative might interfere with the absorption of fat-soluble vitamins such as vitamin K and D, and thus theoretically could have adverse fetal effects.

CASTOR OIL

There are no published human epidemiological or animal teratology studies with this agent. There are also no reports of an association of adverse fetal effects with the use of castor oil during pregnancy. It has been a commonly held belief that this agent would stimulate labor and it is often utilized for this purpose in women close to term. However, little scientific data support the use of this agent as a potent stimulant of labor.

Antidiarrheal agents

Unlike constipation, diarrhea is an uncommon complaint of pregnancy and is usually secondary to medications (especially antibiotics), infections (bacterial, viral, and para-

Box 12.3 Antidiarrheal medications

Bulk agents
  Absorbents
  Kaolin and pectin (Kaopectate)
Opioid agents

site), and abuse of laxatives or lactose intolerance. Fortunately, most cases of acute diarrhea are self-limited and require no specific therapy. Patients should maintain adequate hydration. Antidiarrheals can generally be divided into three major categories – bulk-forming agents, absorbents, and opiates (Box 12.3).

BULK-FORMING AGENTS

These agents are utilized primarily for chronic diarrhea and are listed in Box 12.3. None of these agents are absorbed systemically. Therefore, embryofetal exposure does not occur and there is no associated risk.

ABSORBENTS

The combination of kaolin and pectin (Kaopectate) is probably the antidiarrheal agent most commonly used, including during pregnancy. Its main mode of action is reported to be via absorbent action. There are no epidemiological studies regarding the use of this agent in pregnant women. However, since very little, if any, of it is absorbed from the gastrointestinal tract, it seems very unlikely that this antidiarrheal poses a significant risk to either mother or fetus.

OPIOID AGENTS

Kaolin and pectin have also been combined with opium and belladonna (Amogel-PG, Donnagel-PG, Donnapectolin-PG, Quiagel-PG) and with paregoric (kapectolin with paregoric, parepectolin). The addition of belladonna and opioid agents results in decreased gastrointestinal mobility. There is little available information regarding the use of opium-containing agents in pregnant women. There were only 36 women with early pregnancy exposure included in the Collaborative Perinatal Project database, but there was no evidence of a significant increase in the frequency of congenital anomalies (Heinonen et al., 1977). Almost 100 women were exposed to paregoric in early pregnancy with no significant increase in frequency of congenital anomalies (Aselton et al., 1985). There is, however, the possibility of addiction and withdrawal syndrome in neonates whose mothers use this agent on a chronic basis.

Another commonly used antidiarrheal is the combination of diphenoxylate and atropine (Lomotil and others). Diphenoxylate is a compound similar to meperidine and acts primarily to reduce intestinal motility. Of interest is the fact that atropine is included in this preparation in an effort to prevent abuse. Although there is a case report of an infant born with congenital heart disease whose mother used this agent during pregnancy (Ho et al., 1975), there are no large epidemiologic studies regarding its use during pregnancy. Moreover, there were less than 10 patients who utilized this agent in early pregnancy included in the Collaborative Perinatal Project (Heinonen et al., 1977). None of the offspring of these women had malformations.

LOPERAMIDE

This antidiarrheal agent works by decreasing intestinal motility. No human reproduction studies have been published. According to its manufacturer, loperamide was not teratogenic in rats and rabbits. It is an FDA category B drug.

Teratogen Information System (TERIS) and FDA risk ratings for congenital anomalies

The TERIS and FDA risk ratings for drugs in this chapter provide a reasonable summary of risks that are supported by the medical literature. Most of the supporting literature for Table 12.4 has been discussed above.

SPECIAL CONSIDERATIONS

Most agents utilized for gastrointestinal disease can be safely used in pregnant women, especially after the first trimester.

Nausea and vomiting

All pregnant women probably experience nausea to some degree in early pregnancy. Nausea and vomiting or 'morning sickness' are common symptoms of pregnancy during the first trimester, but most pregnant women do not require antiemetic therapy. Frequent small meals may prove a beneficial way to manage nausea without medical intervention. Fortunately, hyperemesis gravidarum, the most severe form of pregnancy-associated nausea and vomiting occurs in only a small percentage of gravidas. Women with hyperemesis gravidarum may require hospitalization and intravenous hydration, and antiemetic therapy. One of the most effective antiemetic agents for nausea and vomiting associated with pregnancy was doxylamine plus pyridoxine (Bendectin). However, this agent is no longer available because of the fear of litigation. When antiemetics are indicated, promethazine suppositories (or occasionally orally) in doses of 25 mg should be used. Other agents which may prove useful for hyperemesis gravidarum are described in Box 12.4.

Such agents as prochlorperazine, promethazine, chlorpromazine, and thiethylperazine may be associated with extrapyramidal side effects manifested by dystonia, torticollis, and oculogyric crisis. If it occurs, this unusual syndrome of adverse effects can be treated with diphenhydramine (Benadryl). Importantly, chlorpromazine may be associated with significant hypotension when given intravenously. Therefore, suppositories are the preferred route of administration.

In severe cases of hyperemesis gravidarum in which other agents are largely ineffective, ondansetron (Zofran) 32 mg intravenously as a single dose may be effective. It is also available in oral form (8 mg twice a day), but this is much less likely to be effective in cases of hyperemesis gravidarum where almost everything taken orally is vomited.

Reflux esophagitis

Reflux esophagitis resulting in heartburn or pyrosis is very common in pregnancy and is thought to be secondary to decreased gastroesophageal sphincter tone with resultant

Table 12.4 Teratogen Information System (TERIS) risk rating for congenital anomalies and Food and Drug Administration (FDA) pregnancy risk: category rating for nutritional supplements and gastrointestinal drugs

Drugs	TERIS risk	FDA pregnancy risk rating
Aminopterin	Moderate to high	X
Amphetamine	Unlikely	C
Ascorbic acid (vitamin C)	None	A*
Beta-carotene	Low dose: none	C
Calcium salts	Unlikely	NA
Chlorpromazine	Unlikely	C
Cimetidine	Unlikely	B
Cisapride	Undetermined	C
Cyanocobalamin	Undetermined	NA
Dexfenfluramine	Undetermined	C
Diethylpropion	None	NA
Famotidine	Unlikely	B
Fenfluramine	Undetermined	NA
Folic acid	None	A*
Iron	None	NA
Isotretinoin	High	X_m
Mazindol	Undetermined	NA
Methamphetamine	Unlikely (therapeutic dose)	NA
Metoclopromide	Unlikely	B
Niacin	Undetermined	A*
Nizatidine	Undetermined	B
Omeprazole	Unlikely	C
Pantothenate	Undetermined	NA
Phendimetrazine	Unlikely	NA
Phentermine	Undetermined	C
Prochlorperazine	None	NA
Promethazine	None	C
Pyridoxine	None	A
Ranitidine	Unlikely	B
Retinol (vitamin A)	Low dose: none	A*
	High dose: undetermined	
Thiamine	Undetermined	A*
Vitamin D	Unlikely	A*
Vitamin E	Undetermined	A*

NA, not available.

Compiled from: Friedman et al., Obstet Gynecol 1990; **75**: 594; Briggs et al., 2005; Friedman and Polifka, 2006.

gastric acid reflux. Therapy consists primarily of one of the antacid preparations discussed in the previous section. Frequent small feedings and elevation of the head of the bed at night may be beneficial. An H_2-receptor antagonist or omeprazole, as well as metoclopramide, may also prove useful for severe forms of reflux. Esomeperazole and omeprazole are the most popular treatments for reflux esophagitis, and omeprazole is well studied during pregnancy.

Box 12.4 Therapy for nausea and vomiting of pregnancy[a]

Chlorpramazine
- Suppositories, 50–100 mg q 8 h
- Oral, 10–25 mg q 4 h
- Parenteral, 12.5–25 mg IM q 4 h

Ondansetron
- Intravenous, 32 mg as a single dose once a day
- Oral, 8 mg bid

Prochlorperazine
- Suppositories, 5–10 mg two to three times per day
- Oral, 5–10 mg tid or gid
- Parenteral, 5–10 mg IM q 4 h

Promethazine
- Suppositories, 12.5–25 mg q 4 h
- Oral, 5–10 mg tid or gid
- Parenteral, 25 mg IM q 4 h

Thiethylperazine
- Suppositories, 10 mg gd to tid
- Oral, 10 mg qd to tid
- Parenteral, 10 mg IM qd to tid

Trimethobenzamide
- Suppositories, 200 mg tid or gid
- Oral, 250 mg tid or gid
- Parenteral, 200 mg IM tid or gid

[a]See manufacturer's recommendations.

Peptic ulcer disease

Peptic ulcer disease is not common during pregnancy and active ulcer disease may actually improve during pregnancy. The mainstay of therapy in patients with ulcer disease is reduction of gastric acid production. This can be accomplished with either antacids or the H_2-receptor antagonists. The most popular treatment is with PPIs.

Any of the antacids described can be used in pregnant women with peptic ulcer disease, but preference should be given to the best studied during pregnancy (i.e., ranitidine or omeprazole). The usual dosing regimen is given after meals and at bedtime. It is not generally recommended that pregnant women with inactive or asymptomatic disease be treated with 'prophylactic' antacids.

The H_2-receptor antagonists cimetidine and ranitidine inhibit gastric acid secretion and may be used to treat peptic ulcer disease in pregnant women. Cimetidine is usually given in a dose of 300 mg orally four times a day, while ranitidine is usually given in a dose of 150 mg orally twice a day. Omeprazole may also be used with twice daily dosing.

Diarrhea

Most cases of acute diarrhea require no specific therapy other than ensuring adequate hydration. When antidiarrheal therapy is required, the combination of kaolin and pectin

Box 12.5 Therapy for uncomplicated diarrhea of pregnancy[a]

Diphenoxylate and atropine, 2.5–5 mg orally three to four times per day.

Kaolin, pectin, belladonna, opium, 30 mL initial dose, followed by 15 mL q 3 h.

Kaolin, pectin, paregone, 15–30 mL after each diarrheal episode.

Kaolin plus pectin, 60–120 cc of regular strength orally after each diarrheal episode.

Loperamide, 20 mL or two caplets after first diarrheal episode. Then 10 mL or 1 caplet after each diarrheal episode, not exceeding 40 mL or four caplets in 24 h.

[a]From manufacturer's recommendation.

(Kaopectate) can be used safely. If this fails and a stronger medications is indicated, an opioid-like preparation can be utilized (Box 12.5). However, narcotic preparations should not be used chronically, especially in pregnant women.

Traditional antidiarrheal medication should be used cautiously in pregnant women with diarrhea of an infectious etiology (i.e., *Escherichia coli*, shigella, and salmonella). It is generally accepted that infections may be increased in severity or prolonged when treated with these agents.

Diarrhea secondary to bacterial agents may or may not need specific antimicrobial therapy, and, when necessary, therapy should be directed towards the specific organism (see Chapter 2, Antimicrobials during pregnancy: bacterial, viral, fungal, and parasitic indications).

Diarrhea secondary to protozoan disease (i.e., amebiasis and giardiasis) can be treated with metronidazole (500 or 750 mg tid for 5–10 days for the former, and 250 mg tid for 5–10 days for the latter). Therapy need not be delayed until after the first trimester as first-trimester use of metronidazole does not increase the risk for congenital anomalies.

Celiac disease

Celiac disease is a characterized by diarrhea, bloating, anemia, weight loss, and gluten intolerance. Usually, folic acid, iron, and other essential nutrients are not adequately absorbed from the gastrointestinal tract. Patients usually improve when placed on a gluten-free diet. One large series of 94 women with celiac disease during pregnancy showed that with untreated celiac disease there were nine times more miscarriages than among women on a gluten-free diet. Low birth weight was approximately six times more frequent among untreated women compared to those maintained on a gluten-free diet. Severity of celiac disease during pregnancy was apparently not related to pregnancy outcome; maintenance of a gluten-free diet during gestation was the important determinant of pregnancy outcome (Ciacci *et al.*, 1996).

Inflammatory bowel disease

Ulcerative colitis and Crohn's disease commonly occur in pregnant women. Among 30 percent of more than 1000 pregnant women with inactive inflammatory bowel disease, the condition worsened during pregnancy. Of the 320 patients with active disease at the start of pregnancy, 143 (45 percent) became worse, 84 (26 percent) remained the same, and 93 (29 percent) improved (Miller, 1986).

Ulcerative colitis, a chronic disease of unknown etiology, is associated with two life-threatening conditions: fulminant disease and adenocarcinoma of the colon. Ulcerative colitis therapy includes sulfasalazine (Azulfidine), glucocorticoids, azathioprine, and mercaptopurine. Sulfasalazine is comprised of sulfapyridine and aminosalicylic acid, and usually used for mild or moderate disease (Hanauer, 1996). Sulfapyridine, a sulfanamide, crosses the placenta (Azad and Truelove, 1979) and theoretically could cause hyperbilirubinemia or kernicterus, but there are no publications of these complications. According to its manufacturer, the usual initial treatment dose is 0.5–1 g orally four times a day for active disease, and maintenance doses are usually lower.

Glucocorticoids (e.g., prednisone) in large doses may be necessary for active disease. Azathioprine, an immunosuppressant, may be necessary in the small number of patients who do not respond to the usual regimen. Cyclosporine has also been used to treat patients refractory to intravenous steroids (Hanauer, 1996).

Aminosalicylate, metronidazole, corticosteroids, azathioprine, and cyclosporine may also be used to treat pregnant patients with Crohn's disease.

Key references

Berkovitch M, Mazzota P, Greenberg R *et al.* Metoclopramide for nausea and vomiting of pregnancy. A prospective multicenter international study. *Am J Perinatol* 2002; **19**: 311.

Diav-Citrin O, Arnon J, Shechtman S *et al.* The safety of proton pump inhibitors in pregnancy. a multicentre prospective controlled study. *Aliment Pharmacol Ther* 2005; **21**: 269

Einarson A, Maltepe C, Navioz Y, Kennedy D, Tan MP, Koren G. The safety of ondansetron for nausea and vomiting of pregnancy. a prospective comparative study. *BJOG* 2004; **111**: 940.

Grosse SD, Waitzman NJ, Romano PS, Mulinare J. Reevaluating the benefits of folic acid fortification in the United States. Economic analysis, regulation, and public health. *Am J Public Health* 2005; **95**: 1917.

Jones KL, Johnson KA, Dick LM, Felix RJ, Kao KK, Chambers CD. Pregnancy outcomes after first trimester exposure to phentermine/fenfluramine. *Teratology* 2002; **65**: 125.

Kallen B. Delivery outcome after the use of acid-suppressing drugs in early pregnancy with special reference to omeprazole. *Br J Obstet Gynaecol* 1998; **105**: 877.

Lalkin A, Loebstein R, Addis A *et al.* The safety of omeprazole during pregnancy. A multicenter prospective controlled study. *Am J Obstet Gynecol* 1998; **179**: 727.

Little BB. Pharmacokinetics during pregnancy. Evidence-based maternal dose formulation. *Obstet Gynecol* 1999; **93**: 858.

Rothman KUJ, Moore LL, Singer MR, Nguyen US, Mannino S, Milunsky A. Teratogenicity of high vitamin A intake. *N Engl J Med* 1995; **333**: 1369.

Ruigomez A, Garcia Rodriguez LA, Cattaruzzi C *et al.* Use of cimetidine, omeprazole, and ranitidine in pregnant women and pregnancy outcomes. *Am J Epidemiol* 1999; **150**: 476.

Further references are available on the book's website at http://www.drugsandpregnancy.com

13

Use of dermatologics during pregnancy

Dermatologic disorders are frequent among pregnant women, but few conditions are unique to pregnancy. However, pruritic urticarial papules and plaques of pregnancy, herpes gestation, and papular dermatitis of pregnancy do occur and are unique to pregnancy.

A number of dermatologic preparations are available for local and systemic use. Most of these agents can be used with little or no risk to the unborn child. Two of the most potent human teratogens known, etretinate and isotretinoin, are dermatologic drugs.

Six major categories of dermatologic preparations are reviewed: (1) vitamin A derivatives, (2) antibiotics, (3) antifungals, (4) antiseborrheics, (5) adrenocorticosteroids, and (6) keratolytics, astringents, and defatting agents. Dermatologic conditions unique to pregnancy and common dermatologic conditions that may occur during pregnancy are discussed under Special Considerations.

VITAMIN A DERIVATIVES

Three retinoic acid derivatives, vitamin A analogs (two oral agents and one topical agent), are currently available to treat cystic acne, acne vulgaris, or psoriasis. Isotretinoin (Accutane) and etretinate (Tegison) are oral preparations, and tretinoin (Retin-A) is a topical agent.

Isotretinoin

Except for thalidomide, isotretinoin is the drug with greatest teratogenic potential of all the medications to which pregnant woman may be exposed in the first trimester. The 'retinoic acid embryopathy' is a distinct pattern of anomalies that has been described in several reports encompassing over 80 offspring of women exposed to this agent during

Box 13.1 Characteristic anomalies in offspring of mothers exposed to isotretinoin (accutane)

Anotia	Cleft palate	Microtia
Cardiovascular defects	Eye anomalies	Thymic abnormalities
Central nervous system	Limb reduction	
anomalies	Micrognathia	

the first trimester of pregnancy (Coberly *et al.*, 1996; Lammer, 1985, 1987; Medical Letter, 1983; MMWR, 1984; Rizzo *et al.*, 1991; Rosa, 1983, Rosa *et al.*, 1986; Thompson and Cordero, 1989). Among 94 infants who were born to women who used isotretinoin in early pregnancy, 28 percent had major congenital anomalies (Chen *et al.*, 1990; Dai *et al.*, 1992). In this series, 18 percent of the pregnancies resulted in spontaneous abortions. The constellation of anomalies is called retinoic acid embryopathy (Box 13.1). Postnatal intellectual development of infants apparently unaffected (without major or minor congenital anomalies) at birth was subnormal at 5 years of age (IQ less than 85) in 47 percent of 31 (Adams and Lammer, 1993; Adams *et al.*, 1991, 1992).

Clinicians are concerned about the risks associated with pregnancy among patients who recently discontinued taking isotretinoin. This agent has a short half-life of 10–12 h, and the risk of congenital anomalies is not increased in the offspring of women who discontinued this medication within days of conception (Dai *et al.*, 1989). The terminal elimination half-life of isotretinoin is 96 h.

Major and minor anomalies were found in animal teratology studies with isotretinoin, similar to the pattern of malformations seen in human retinoic acid embryopathy (Agnish *et al.*, 1984; Kamm, 1982; Kochhar and Penner, 1987; Kochhar *et al.*, 1984; Webster *et al.*, 1986).

Etretinate

Etretinate is an oral retinoid used to treat psoriasis. A significant complication of use of this medication in women of reproductive age is that it may be detected in serum at therapeutic levels for at least 2 years after cessation of therapy (DiGiovanna *et al.*, 1984). The manufacturer reports that etretinate is detected at near-therapeutic levels for 3–7 years following cessation of therapy (Hoffman-LaRoche, personal communication). No epidemiological studies have been published of etretinate use by pregnant women. Of 43 pregnancies exposed to etretinate, there were 14 pregnancy terminations and five had malformations similar to retinoid embryopathy. Twenty-nine live-born infants were reported, of whom six had major congenital anomalies (Geiger *et al.*, 1994). Case reports are published of neural tube, other central nervous system, and limb reduction defects in the offspring of mothers exposed to this drug during embryogenesis (Happle *et al.*, 1984; Lammer, 1988; Rosa *et al.*, 1986; Verloes *et al.*, 1990). In one published case report, a fetus with a hypoplastic leg was born to a mother who conceived several months after discontinuing etretinate (Grote *et al.*, 1985).

Conceptions after etretinate exposure may pose serious risks of birth defects because the drug has an indeterminate half-life. although the elimination half-life is published as

100 to 120 days for etretinate, therapeutic levels of the drug have been detected as long as 2 years after discontinuation. The manufacturer has offered pro bono testing for etretinate in women of reproductive age who used this drug. In the ideal situation, this should be done preconceptually.

Animal teratology studies have produced teratogenic effects with etretinate similar to those observed in the retinoic acid embryopathy, such as limb, genitourinary, neural tube, and cloacal defects (Mesrobian et al., 1994). The implication of this with regard to human teratogenicity is unknown. Obviously, this drug should not be used for psoriasis during pregnancy.

Acitretin

Acitretin is an active metabolite of etretinate. It has an elimination half-life of approximately 60 h, as opposed to 100–120 days for etretinate. Eight cases of acitretin exposure during pregnancy have been published, and there was one infant with multiple congenital anomalies that were consistent with the retinoic acid embryopathy, and one case of congenital hearing deficit (Geiger et al., 1994). One case report of an infant born with features of the retinoic acid embryopathy was published. At 18 months' follow-up, the infants had microcephaly and significant neurodevelopmental delay (Barbero et al., 2004). Notably, the dose of acitretin that the mother took from conception to the 10th week of pregnancy was low (10 mg/day) compared to other reports (e.g., Geiger et al., 1994). Among 52 pregnancies where exposure to acitretin occurred after 6 weeks postconception, no congenital anomalies were observed (Geiger et al., 1994). Animal models of acitretin teratogenicity have produced anomalies consistent with the retinoic acid embryopathy (Lofberg et al., 1990; Turton et al., 1992).

Caution: Acitretin can be metabolized back to etretinate through re-esterification. Therefore, it would be prudent to test serum for etretinate in addition to acitretin (Almond-Roesler and Orfanos, 1996).

Tretinoin

Tretinoin (Retin-A) or retinoic acid is prepared as a liquid, gel, or cream for local application in the treatment of acne vulgaris. Minimal amounts of this topical agent are absorbed systemically, and the theoretical teratogenic risk of tretinoin appears quite low (Kligman, 1988). The drug is poorly absorbed topically, and skin is capable of metabolizing this agent, resulting in none to minimal amounts accumulating in maternal serum (DeWals et al., 1991; Kalivas, 1992; Nau, 1993; Nau et al., 1994).

Major congenital anomalies occurred among 2 percent of 212 pregnancies exposed to tretinoin during the first trimester, compared to 3 percent of controls (Jick et al., 1993). In another study of 112 infants born to women who received prescriptions for tretinoin, there was no increased frequency of major anomalies (Rosa, personal communication, cited in Briggs et al., 2005). In contrast, Johnson and colleagues (1994) reported 45 pregnancies in which tretinoin was used, and one infant had features of the retinoid embryopathy. However, the mother of the affected infant had also taken Accutane during pregnancy.

Major structural malformations in 106 infants and minor anomalies in a subset of 62 infants were examined by an experienced dysmorphologist to test the hypothesis that topical tretinoin during the first trimester might pose a risk for birth defects similar to those associated with the retinoic acid embryopathy. No differences in major or minor anomaly frequencies between the tretinoin and control groups were found (Loureiro *et al.*, 2005), offering reassurance for patients exposed to the drug during the first trimester.

Tretinoin administered to pregnant animals during embryogenesis in doses up to 50 times those used in humans was not associated with congenital anomalies or adverse fetal effects. In summary, tretinoin does not appear to be associated with an increased risk of congenital anomalies in infants born to women who used the drug *as directed* during pregnancy. ('As directed' is inserted here because we have encountered patients who ate – took orally – tretinoin cream.)

ANTIBIOTICS

Topical antibiotics are adjunct therapy for acne and for other skin infections (Box 13.2) and include: clindamycin, erythromycin, meclocycline, tetracycline, sulfa-drug creams, and lotions. It is unlikely that absorption of topical antibiotics through the skin results in significant serum concentration, or would be associated with an increased risk of congenital anomalies. Unlike oral or parenteral tetracycline, topical preparations are not associated with yellow-brown discoloration of the teeth.

Other topical antimicrobial agents are used to treat minor skin infections and include neomycin (usually in combination with polymixin B, bacitracin, gramicidin, and/or hydrocortisone). Some combinations of these agents are used to treat ophthalmic infections. No adequate human reproduction studies of polymixin B are available. The frequency of congenital anomalies was not increased among 30 or 61 infants whose mothers took neomycin or gramicidin, respectively, during early pregnancy (Heinonen *et al.*, 1977).

Other topical antimicrobials used to treat local skin infections include chloramphenicol, gentamicin, and metronidazole. When applied topically, physiologically significant amounts of these agents are not likely to be absorbed systemically. These agents are discussed in other chapters, and do not increase the risk of congenital anomalies.

Mupirocin (Bactroban) is a topical antibacterial used to treat skin infections and folliculitis. Mupirocin was not teratogenic in several animal studies, but no human studies of this drug have been published.

Box 13.2 Topical antibacterial agents to treat of acne and minor skin infections

Chloramphenicol	Mupirocin
Clindamycin	Neomycin
Clioquinol	Neomycin plus polymixin B, bacitracin,
Erythromycin	gramicidin, and hydrocortisone
Gentamicin	Silver sulfadiazine
Meclocycline	Sulfur
Metronidazole	Tetracycline

Clioquinol is an antibacterial and antifungal agent. No studies are published of the use of this drug during human or animal pregnancy.

Mafenide (Sulfamylon) and silver sulfadiazine (Silvadene, Thermazene, Flint SSD, Sildimac) are topical antibacterial and antifungal agents used to treat infections secondary to skin burns. No human studies have been published on mafenide or silver sulfadiazine. No animal teratology studies of mafenide are available. According to its manufacturer, silver sulfadiazine was not teratogenic in animal studies (unpublished).

ANTIFUNGALS

Several topical antifungal agents are used to treat vaginitis (butoconazole, clotrimazole, econazole, miconazole, nystatin, and terconazole). Some systemic preparations are also used for vaginitis: amphotericin B, griseofulvin, and ketoconazole. These agents are discussed in Chapter 2. Systemic antifungals are not associated with an increased risk of birth defects, except for griseofulvin (conjoined twinning is hypothesized with griseofulvin; see Chapter 2). Topical application of these agents on parts of the body is not associated with an increased frequency of congenital anomalies or other medical complications.

Ciclopirox, haloprogin, naftifine, and tolnaftate are antifungals used to treat tinea corpus, cruris, pedis, and versicolor. No human studies of these drugs during pregnancy have been published, but their manufacturers report that these antifungal agents were not teratogenic in several animal studies.

Tolnaftate (Aftate, Genaspore, NP27, Tinactin, Ting, Zeasorb-AF) is another topical antifungal, available as a powder, aerosol solution, spray solution, gel, or cream. Applied topically, it is used to treat tinea captis, corporis, cruris, versicolor, pedis, and barbae. No human or animal reproduction studies are available.

ANTIPARASITICS

Topical antiparasitics are discussed in detail in Chapter 2.

KERATOLYTICS, ASTRINGENTS, AND DEFATTING AGENTS

Nearly all of the large number of agents in this category may be purchased over the counter and are used to treat acne and related dermatologic conditions (Box 13.3). No human reproduction studies for any of these agents have been published and the same is true for animal data. Benzoyl peroxide, resorcinol, and salicylic acid have significant potential for systemic absorption, but no cases of adverse fetal effects are documented related to the topical route of delivery. Salicylates are discussed in detail in Chapter 8, Analgesics during pregnancy. Manufacturer data on salicylic acid was reported to be teratogenic in animals when used in large doses, several times that used in humans.

ANTISEBORRHEIC AGENTS

Antiseborrheic agents are used primarily in the treatment of dandruff or seborrheic dermatitis (Box 13.4). The mechanism of action is unknown. No animal or human repro-

Box 13.3 Ketatolytic, defatting, and astringent agents

Alcohol and sulfur (Liquimat, Transact, Xerac)

Alcohol and acetone (Seba-Nil, Tyrosum)

Benzoyl peroxide (Clearasil, Oxy-10, Acne-10, Benoxyl, Del-Aqua, Desquam, Dry & Clear,
   Fostex, Neutrogena, Acne Mask, Zeroxin-10)

Resorcinol (RA)

Resorcinol and sulfur (Acnomel, Clearsil, Rezamid, Sulforcin)

Salicylic acid (numerous brand names)

Salicylic acid and sulfur (numerous brand names)

Salicylic acid, sulfur and coal tar (Sebex-T, Sebutone, Vanseb-T)

Box 13.4 Antiseborrheic agents

Chloroxine (Capitrol)

Coal tar (numerous brands)

Pyrithione (Danex, Head & Shoulders, Sebex, Sebulon, Zinolon)

Salicylic acid (numerous brands)

Selenium sulfide (Episel, Exsel, Glo-Sel, Selsun)

duction studies have been published. It is very unlikely that these agents have any effect on prenatal development because they are not absorbed systemically. Coal tar and salicylic acid are often used in combination with other agents, such as sulfa, and in combination with one another to treat seborrhea and seborrheic dermatitis.

ADRENOCORTICOSTEROIDS

Numerous topical adrenocorticosteroids are used to treat dermatologic disorders (Box 13.5) and are usually used to treat localized dermatitis with associated inflammation and pruritis.

No studies in pregnant women using topical steroids have been published. According to the manufacturer, however, several of these agents may be teratogenic in laboratory animals. Topical steroids are very unlikely to be associated with significant risk to the human fetus, except triamcinolone (see below).

Systemic adrenocorticosteroids are sometimes indicated to treat dermatologic diseases and there is a small collection of these agents (Box 13.6). Prednisone and prednisolone

Box 13.5 Topical adrenocorticoids for dermatological conditions

Alclometasone	Desoximetasone	Flurandrenolide
Amcinonide	Dexamethasone	Halcinonide
Betamethasone	Diflurasone	Hydrocortisone
Clobetasol	Flumethasone	Methylprednisolone
Clocortolone	Fluocinolone	Mometasone
Desonide	Fluocionide	Triamcinolone

Box 13.6 Commonly used systemic adrenocorticoids

Betamethasone	Methylprednisolone
Cortisone	Prednisone
Dexamethasone	Prednisolone
Hydrocortisone	Triamcinolone

are the two most commonly used systemically of this drug class. The frequency of congenital anomalies was not increased among 43 infants born to women who took prednisone during early pregnancy (Heinonen *et al.*, 1977). Perinatal deaths were increased in frequency among infants born to women who took this steroid throughout pregnancy, but the disease being treated (e.g., lupus) may in itself be etiologic, rather than prednisone *per se* (Warrell and Taylor, 1968). Fetal growth retardation was associated with prednisone use during gestation by one research group (Reinisch *et al.*, 1978), but not several others (Lee *et al.*, 1982; Walsh and Clark, 1967).

Prednisone and prednisolone

Prednisone and prednisolone are active adrenoglucocorticoids. Prednisolone is an active metabolite of prednisone. Numerous animal studies reported an increase in the frequency of cleft palate with prednisolone (as well as other steroids) when given in large doses (e.g., Ballard *et al.*, 1977; Pinsky and DiGeorge, 1965; Shah and Killistoff, 1976; Walker, 1967).

The association between oral clefts and prednisone exposure was assessed among humans using data from well-regarded case–control studies (Carmichael and Shaw, 1999; Rodriguez-Pinilla and Martinez-Frias, 1998) and it was concluded that the risk of nonsyndromic cleft palate may be associated with prednisone/prednisolone and other glucocorticoid exposure during embryogenesis. However, if such a risk exists it is less than 1 percent (Shepard *et al.*, 2002). Note that most oral clefts can be surgically corrected and this isolated defect is not associated with other physical or mental abnormalities.

Hydrocortisone

Hydrocortisone, another glucocorticoid, is the main steroid produced by the adrenal glands. The frequency of congenital anomalies was not increased among infants whose mothers took hydrocortisone during early pregnancy, including the first trimester (Heinonen *et al.*, 1977). As with prednisone/prednisolone, an increased frequency of cleft palate was found among the offspring of experimental animals whose mothers were given hydrocortisone during embryogenesis (Chaudhry and Shah, 1973; Harris *et al.*, 1980). This is similar to experimental findings with other glucocorticoids. It is possible that a small risk for cleft palate in humans exists with hydrocortisone use during embryogenesis, but it is likely that the risk is small at less than 1 percent (Shepard *et al.*, 2002).

Dexamethasone and betamethasone

These agents (dexamethasone and betamethasone) are glucocorticoids that are closely related to prednisone (see Prednisone and prednisolone above). No human teratology studies of dexamethasone or betamethasone have been published. These drugs are commonly used in the late second and early third trimesters to promote fetal lung maturity, preventing respiratory distress syndrome (Collaborative Group on Antenatal Steroid Therapy, 1984; Liggins, 1976; Liggins and Howie, 1974). Consistent with other corticosteroids, dexamethasone and betamethasone are reported to be associated with an increased frequency of cleft palate in the offspring of pregnant animals that received these agents during embryogenesis (Mosier et al., 1982; Pinsky and DiGeorge, 1965). Fetal body and organ weight were decreased in several animal studies with exposure to these glucocorticoids during pregnancy (Barrada et al., 1980; Epstein et al., 1977; Johnson et al., 1981; Mosier et al., 1982). As with other glucocorticoids, it is possible that a small risk for cleft palate in humans exists with dexamethasone and betamethasone use during early pregnancy. However, the risk is very likely small at less than 1 percent (Shepard et al., 2002).

Triamcinolone

No human epidemiological studies of triamcinolone use during early pregnancy have been published. The published case–control studies are confounded and it is not possible to interpret them for triamcinolone exposures. The cause of concern for triamcinolone exposure during embryogenesis is an increased frequency of congenital anomalies found in offspring of three species of nonhuman primates that received this corticosteroid during embryogenesis (Bacher and Michejda, 1988; Hendrickx and Tarara, 1990; Hendrickx et al., 1980; Jerome and Hendrickx, 1988; Parker and Hendrickx, 1983). The collection of congenital anomalies included neural tube defects, craniofacial malformations, and skeletal anomalies. Therefore, triamcinolone should be avoided during pregnancy, especially during the first trimester (Friedman and Polifka, 2006). Triamcinolone will most probably be associated with an increased risk of birth defects in humans when these studies are reported. This warning is issued to attempt a reduction of the number of infants who will be damaged, i.e., exposed to this drug, before official warnings are issued.

Cortisone

The risk of congenital anomalies among women who used cortisone during pregnancy and its possible adverse fetal effects cannot be assessed with the available published data. Among only 34 infants exposed to cortisone during early pregnancy, the frequency of congenital anomalies was not increased (Heinonen et al., 1977). Cortisone is in the drug class (glucocorticoids) noted above to be associated with an increased frequency of cleft palate in several animal models, including nonhuman primates (Biddle and Fraser, 1976; Walker, 1971). The nonhuman primate association, even with small sample sizes, is an ominous indicator. Based mostly on primate data, these agents will predictably be shown to be associated with an increased frequency of isolated cleft palate in human infants exposed to glucocorticoids during embryogenesis. However, the risk will be small at less than 1 percent (Shepard *et al.*, 2002).

Glucocorticoids summary

In summary, limited human data are published of adrenocorticosteroid use during early human pregnancy and possible association with congenital anomalies or other possible adverse fetal effects. Although these agents were used for many years in pregnant women without apparent adverse effects, no systematic studies are available. Recent analyses based upon reputable case–control studies indicate that a low risk (< 1 percent) for cleft palate may be associated with glucocorticoid exposure during the first trimester.

Triamcinolone effects are possibly more severe, suggesting that it would be prudent to avoid this drug during pregnancy – especially during early gestation. However, the consequence of not treating certain conditions during pregnancy, such as systemic lupus erythematosus and asthma, generally outweigh any theoretical risk of these medications. Failure to treat lupus and asthma during pregnancy may result in congenital heart block or maternal death, respectively.

Follow-up studies of children whose mothers received betamethasone and dexamethasone are reassuring because they show no growth and development deficits. Emphasis should be placed on the <1 percent of infants born following exposure during the first trimester who may have isolated cleft palate. Among infants exposed to triamcinolone during the first trimester, a cluster of congenital anomalies may occur given the evidence from nonhuman primate studies. These data suggest that a 'fetal triamcinolone syndrome' will be discovered that comprises debilitating congenital anomalies such as neural tube defects, characteristic facies, and skeletal dysplasias.

Therefore, triamcinolone – and other glucocorticoids – should be avoided in early pregnancy (first trimester) if possible.

OTHER AGENTS

Anthralin

Anthralin (Anthra-Derm, Drithocreme, Lisan) is a topical antipsoriatic agent. It is also used as a hair growth stimulant. No animal or human reproduction studies have been published. Based upon related medication and the assumption of topical administration, a panel of experts inferred that if there is any risk of congenital anomalies associated with first-trimester exposure to anthralin, it must be very small (Friedman and Polifka, 2006). This may be interpreted to mean that the risk may be so small that it is indiscernible from the background risk of congenital anomalies (3.5–5 percent).

Methotrexate

Methotrexate, a folate antagonist, is used most frequently as an antineoplastic agent, but is effective in the treatment of psoriasis. It is similar to the well-known teratogen, aminopterin (see Chapter 7, Antineoplastic drugs during pregnancy). Anomalies associated with methotrexate and aminopterin include ossification and skeletal anomalies, hydrocephalus, and cleft palate (Milunsky *et al.*, 1968; Reich *et al.*, 1977; Warkany, 1978). Methotrexate should not be used to treat psoriasis during pregnancy, but its benefits in the treatment of leukemia and other neoplastic diseases may outweigh its risk (especially after the first trimester). For dermatologic maladies, other less potentially dangerous therapies are available.

Podophyllin

The topical chemical compound, podophyllin, is used primarily to treat condyloma acuminata. The formulation used to treat condyloma is a solution of 20 percent podophyllin solution in tincture of benzoin. Use of podophyllin during pregnancy has been associated with significant edema, skin irritation, and discomfort. The frequency of birth defects was not increased in frequency among 14 infants whose mothers used podophyllin during the first trimester (Heinonen *et al.*, 1977), but this sample was too small to interpret. Several anecdotal reports of maternal and fetal toxicity include a case of fetal demise in a mother who experienced systemic toxicity following the topical application of podophyllin (Gorthey and Krebs, 1954) and others that reported similar adverse effects (Chamberlain *et al.*, 1972; Slater *et al.*, 1978).

One case report of major congenital anomalies associated with podophyllin has been published (Karol *et al.*, 1980), but a causal link cannot be inferred from a case report. Nonetheless, it seems prudent to avoid use of this agent during pregnancy because safer therapies (e.g., laser removal of warts) are of equal efficacy (see Condyloma under Special Considerations below).

Trichloroacetic acid

Trichloroacetic acid (TCA) is another topical chemical compound used to treat condyloma acuminata. It is a caustic and astringent agent that primarily causes sloughing of the skin. Among rats fed TCA during embryogenesis, the rate of congenital heart defects was increased in one study (Smith *et al.*, 1989) and replicated in another (Johnson *et al.*, 1998).

SPECIAL CONSIDERATIONS

Dermatologic diseases in most pregnant women rarely require emergency or extensive therapy during the first trimester. Most conditions can be treated with topical agents with little systemic effects.

Acne and psoriasis

Acne is common in young women and young gravidas. In contrast, psoriasis occurs infrequently during pregnancy (fewer than 1 percent of gravidas), and may actually improve during pregnancy. Three vitamin A congeners, isotretinoin (for acne), acitretin (for psoriasis), and etretinate (for psoriasis) are contraindicated for use during pregnancy (Table 13.1). Women inadvertently exposed to these agents during early pregnancy should be counseled regarding the serious risk of major congenital anomalies in

Table 13.1 Teratogen Information System (TERIS) risk for congenital anomalies and Food and Drug Administration (FDA) pregnancy risk category

Drugs	TERIS risk	FDA pregnancy risk category rating
Acitretin	High	X_m
Aminopterin	Moderate to high	X
Amphotericin B	Undetermined	B_m
Anthralin	Undetermined	NA
Bacitracin	Undetermined	C
Betamethasone	Undetermined	C*
Butoconazole	Undetermined	C_m
Ciclopirox	Undetermined	B_m
Chloramphenicol	Unlikely	C
Clindamycin	Undetermined	B_m
Clioquinol	Undetermined	NA
Clotrimazole	Unlikely	B
Dexamethasone	Minimal	C*
Econazole	Undetermined	NA
Erythromycin	None	B_m
Etretinate	High	X_m
Gentamicin	Undetermined	C
Gramicidin	None	NA
Griseofulvin	Undetermined	C
Haloprogin	Undetermined	NA
Hydrocortisone	Unlikely	C*
Isotretinoin	High	X_m
Ketoconazole	Undetermined	C_m
Mafenide	Undetermined	NA
Meclocycline	Undetermined	NA
Methotrexate	Moderate to high	X_m
Metronidazole	None	B_m
Miconazole	Undetermined	C_m
Mupirocin	Undetermined	NA
Naftifine	Undetermined	NA
Neomycin	None	C
Nystatin	None	C_m
Podophyllum	Undetermined	C
Prednisone/prednisolone	Oral clefts: small	C*
	Other congenital anomalies: unlikely	
Terconazole	Undetermined	C_m
Tetracycline	Unlikely	D
Tolnaftate	Undetermined	NA
Tretinoin	Topical use: unlikely	D_m
	Systemic administration: undetermined	
Triamcinolone	Undetermined	C_m *

NA, not available.

Compiled from: Friedman *et al.*, *Obstet Gynecol* 1990; **75**: 594; Briggs *et al.*, 2005; Friedman and Polifka, 2006.

their babies. The patient should also be informed that even if the child does not have a major congenital anomaly at birth, intellectual development would most likely be impaired. The best counseling option is to contact TERIS (see Chapter 1, Introduction to drugs in pregnancy) and purchase the comprehensive summary on isotretinoin to (1) use in counseling, (2) place in the medical record, and (3) share with the patient. The option of pregnancy termination should be discussed. On the other hand, topical tretinoin (Retin-A) poses no known risk to the developing conceptus.

A variety of topical agents, including antibiotics (such as topical erythromycin), keratolytics, and astringents, can be used to treat acne during pregnancy. Topical steroids can generally be used safely for the treatment of psoriasis during pregnancy, except for triamcinolone.

Abnormalities of pigmentation and striae gravidarum

Striae and abnormal pigmentation can be especially worrisome to the pregnant patient. Chloasma (increased pigmentation along the linea nigra or areola of the nipple) and melasma (brownish discoloration of areas of the face) are the two most common forms of abnormal pigmentation. No specific therapy is available or required for these conditions, other than possibly cosmetic make-up. Importantly, striae and pigmentation usually regress and spontaneously disappear following delivery.

Stretch marks or striae gravidarum may be especially disconcerting to pregnant women. Numerous creams and ointments (including 'mink oil') are available in the over-the-counter market to treat stretch marks. However, no known medical therapy has been shown to be effective. Most striae, which are hyperemic during pregnancy, will diminish in appearance (often becoming small, silvery lines). Most patients simply require reassurance.

Condyloma acuminata

Wart-like growths, condyloma acuminata, may proliferate rapidly during pregnancy. A common therapy in the nonpregnant patient is local application of a 20 percent solution of podophyllin in benzoin. Podophyllin is contraindicated in pregnancy because of the potential for maternal and fetal toxicity. Another local agent, when applied topically, TCA is associated with no known serious maternal or fetal side effects. Unfortunately, TCA is not very effective in the eradication of condyloma, especially during pregnancy. Use of 5-fluorouracil is not recommended because it is an antineoplastic agent and there are no human studies of the topical administration of this agent during pregnancy.

For small, isolated lesions, surgical excision, electrocoagulation, and cryotherapy generally produce satisfactory results. A CO_2 laser is a very effective tool in the treatment of large or massive vulvar condyloma acuminata (Ferenczy, 1984; Hankins *et al.*, 1989; Malfetano *et al.*, 1981).

Atopic/allergic dermatitis

This condition is characterized by a pruritic rash and is secondary to a variety of inciting factors, such as stress, soap (especially with aroma additives), and irritants.

Atopic/allergic dermatitis is usually treated by (1) removal of the inciting factors and (2) topical or systemic steroids. Topical steroids are recommended during pregnancy and generally prove satisfactory.

Erythema multiforme

The etiology of erythema multiforme, another dermatitis, is virtually unknown. It is characterized by erythematous 'target lesions.' An increased frequency of outbreaks occurs during pregnancy among women with this condition. The condition can be treated with antihistamines during pregnancy. If antihistamines are not sufficient, steroids may be effective in some cases. Triamcinolone should not be used.

Papular dermatitis of pregnancy

Papular dermatitis is very rare (< 1 percent) and is limited to pregnancy (Spangler et al., 1962). Recurrence in subsequent pregnancies is known and it is associated with an increased frequency of pregnancy loss. Papular dermatitis is characterized by small, erythematous papules that usually involve all of the skin. High-dose systemic steroids, such as prednisone, are used to treat this dermatitis. Triamcinolone should not be used.

Pruritic urticarial papules and plaques of pregnancy

Pruritic urticarial papules and plaques of pregnancy, also known as PUPPP, are common during pregnancy. Papular dermatitis of pregnancy can occur any time during gestation, but PUPPP tends to occur in late pregnancy. Recurrence of PUPPP in subsequent pregnancies is rare. Pruritis and erythematous papules and plaques characterize PUPPP. Unlike papular dermatitis, PUPP is not associated with an increase in pregnancy loss. The rash usually starts on the abdomen and spreads to the extremities, with facial sparing (Alcalay et al., 1988; Yancy et al., 1984). Treatment consists primarily of topical steroids, although oral prednisone may be required for severe cases. Triamcinolone should not be used.

Herpes gestationis

Another rare dermatologic disease of unknown etiology is herpes gestationis. Contrary to what might be implied from the name, herpes gestationis is not a viral infection but an autoimmune disease. It is peculiar to pregnancy and may recur in subsequent gestations. Erythematous papules and large, tense bullae, usually on the abdomen and extremities characterize this disease. Some investigators have reported that an increased frequency of pregnancy loss is associated with this condition in some studies (Lawley et al., 1978), but not in others (Katz et al., 1976). Treatment consists primarily of oral prednisone (30–50 mg daily). Triamcinolone should not be used.

Key references

Almond-Roesler B, Orfanos CE. Tran-acitretin is metabolized back into etretinate. Importance for oral retinoid therapy. *Hautarzt* 1996; **47**: 173.

Barbero P, Lotersztein V, Bronberg R, Perez M, Alba L. Acitretin embryopathy. A case report. *Birth Defects Res A Clin Mol Teratol* 2004; **70**: 831.

Carmichael SL, Shaw GM. Maternal corticosteroid use and risk of selected congenital anomalies. *Am J Med Genet* 1999; **86**: 242.

Coberly S, Lammer E, Alashari M. Retinoic acid embryopathy. Case report and review of literature. *Pediatr Pathol Lab Med* 1996; **16**: 823.

Johnson, PD, Dawson BV, Goldberg, SJ. Cardiac teratogenicity of trichloroethylene metabolites. *J Am Coll Cardiol* 1998; **32**: 540.

Loureiro KD, Kao KK, Jones KL *et al.* Minor malformations characteristic of the retinoic acid embryopathy and other birth outcomes in children of women exposed to topical tretinoin during early pregnancy. *Am J Med Genet* 2005; **136A**: 117.

Rodriguez-Pinilla E, Martinez-Frias ML. Corticosteroids during pregnancy and oral clefts. A case–control study. *Teratology* 1998; **58**: 2.

Shepard TH, Brent RL, Friedman JM *et al.* Update on new developments in the study of human teratogens. *Teratology* 2002; **65**: 153.

Further references are available on the book's website at http://www.drugsandpregnancy.com

14

Drug overdoses during pregnancy

Usually, drug overdoses during pregnancy are a suicide gesture or, less often, an attempt to induce abortion. Accidental overdoses are rare. Quinine overdoses are associated with an attempt to induce abortion over 90 percent of the time, but most other overdoses of the drug are also attempted suicide. Successful suicide during pregnancy occurs among one in every 88 000–400 000 live births (Table 14.1) (Rayburn *et al.*, 1984). Among 162 pregnant women who presented with an indication of poisoning, 86 percent were overdoses (78 percent suicide attempts and 8 percent induced abortion attempts (Czeizel *et al.*, 1984)). Maternal death associated with suicide gestures occurs in approximately 1 percent of gravid women and more than 95 percent of suicide gestures involve ingestion of a combination of drugs (Rayburn *et al.*, 1984). In New York city, suicide was identified as the cause of 13 percent of maternal deaths (Dannenberg *et al.*, 1995).

Use of drug megadoses that are potentially lethal in pregnant women involves two patients: mother and fetus. Assessment of the pregnant woman who has potentially toxic (megadoses) amounts of drugs must begin with laboratory evaluation of the substance(s) ingested (i.e., serum levels). The top three substances used in suicide gestures in the USA in the late 1970s–early 1980s were nonnarcotic analgesics, nutritional supplements, and antiaxiolytics (Table 14.1). In Finland in the late 1990s, the pattern was similar with the top three substances used in suicide attempts being benzodiazepines, analgesics, and psychotropics (antipsychotics/antidepressants) (Table 14.2).

The data in Tables 14.1 and 14.2 only provide a best guess, given that there is no history for assessing a pregnant woman who has made a suicide gesture. If the patient is

Table 14.1 Drugs used in suicide gestures among 111 pregnant women in the USA

Drug class	Percent
Nonnarcotic analgesics (acetaminophen, aspirin, ibuprofen)	26
Nutritional supplements (prenatal vitamins, iron)	12
Antianxiolytics (diazepam, hydroxyzine, other benzodiazepines)	11
Hypnotics and sedatives (phenobarbital, flurazepam, and others)	10
Narcotic analgesics (codeine, propoxyphene, and others)	8
Antibiotics (cephalexin, amoxicillin, trimethoprim sulfamethoxazole)	7
Antihistamines (diphenhydramine, others)	6
Antipsychotics (thioridazine, trifluoperazine)	3
Anorectics (sympathomimetics, phenylpropanolamine)	2
Hormonal agents (corticosteroids, oral contraceptives)	2
Antidepressants (doxepin, amitriptyline)	2
Anticonvulsants (phenytoin, carbamazepine)	2
Other drugs (miscellaneous drugs from other classes)	6
Nondrug chemicals (turpentine, camphorated oil, ammonia)	2

Compiled from Rayburn et al., 1984.

Table 14.2 Suicide attempts by pregnant women in Finland: 1977 to 1999[a]

	n	Percentage
Analgesics	21/43	49
Acetaminophen (paracetamol)	6	
Acetylsalicylic acid (aspirin)	5	
Carsioprodol	1	
Codeine	1	
Ibuprofen	2	
Indomethacin	1	
Phenobarbital	2	
Salicylamide	3	
Benzodiazepines	15/43	35
Diazepam	8	
Estrazolam	1	
Flinitrazepam	2	
Nitrazepam	2	
Oxazepam	1	
Triazolam	1	
Antipsychotic	2/43	5
Flupentixol	1	
Fluphenazine	1	
Antidepressants	2/43	5
Doxepin	1	
Nomifensine	1	
Iron supplement	1/43	2.3
Appetite suppressant	1/43	2.3

[a]272 attempted suicides; 177 excluded for complicating factors (e.g., carbon monoxide), 43 of 122 were suicide gestures during pregnancy; the remainder were suicide attempts in the months preconception.
Compiled from Flint et al., 2002.

still conscious she will likely provide the most accurate information on what drugs were taken because drug overdoses are largely premeditated. The patient will usually recall approximately how much she took of which substances. If family members or significant others are present, they may be able to provide corroborative information, such as presence of medicine bottles, known prescriptions, etc. Toxicology screens with samples every hour or two (for serial evaluation) should be ordered as soon as possible to determine exactly what substances are involved and whether or not levels are rising or falling, or toxic or approaching toxic. However, a generalized treatment plan may be undertaken before toxicology results are available.

CLINICAL MANAGEMENT

Blood and/or urine samples are obtained for toxicological analysis as soon as possible. If the patient still has a gag reflex, orogastric lavage with normal saline should be begun. Following lavage, administer an activated charcoal slurry regimen (the nonspecific antidote regimen). Whole-bowel irrigation has been used successfully in some cases of drug overdose and has a clinically significant effect on lowering serum drug levels.

Evaluation of the fetal heart rate should begin as soon as possible, especially in cases in which the fetus is viable. Supportive therapy should begin immediately. When toxicological screens are available to document what drugs and/or chemicals have been ingested and may be in potentially toxic doses, information on antidote regimens for given substances may be obtained from several sources. The authoritative source consulted by certified poison control centers (listed in the *Physician's Desk Reference*) is PoisIndex, which includes specific data on pregnancy from Teratogen Information System (TERIS). PoisIndex contains a detailed specific management plan for each sub-

---

Box 14.1 Management plan for the pregnant patient with an acute overdose

Acute stabilization
Establishment of an open airway
Assisted ventilation, if needed
Circulatory assistance, if needed
Fetal monitoring
Fetal heart rate
Ultrasound of target organs
Supportive care
As needed to maintain stabilization

Obtaining toxicological samples (serial measurements)
Blood, once per hour
Urine, once per hour
Amniotic fluid. twice in 48 h

Medical history
This suicide gesture
Past history of suicide gestures
Other medical history
Physical examination
Special attention to central nervous system function
Special attention to cardiac function
Nonspecific antidote therapy
Prevent absorption
Orogastric lavage
Whole-bowel irrigation
Activated charcoal PO
Enhance elimination
Increase liquid intake
Increase plasma volume
Balance electrolytes

Table 14.3 Selected antidotes available (see Appendix)

Antidote	Overdose of drug/toxin
Acetylcysteine	Acetaminophen
Activated charcoal	Nonspecific substance(s)
Amyl nitrate	Cyanide
Cholestyramine	Specific for negatively charged medications
Cholinesterase inhibitors	Atropine
Deferoxamine	Iron
Edrophonium	Curare
Fab antidigoxin antibody fragments	
(Digoxin immune Fab)	Digoxin/digitalis
Flumazenil	Benzodiazepines
Glucagon	Beta-blockers
Hyoscyamine	Cholinesterase inhibitors
Leucororin	Folic acid antagonists
	(methotrexate, pyrimethamine, others)
Muscarine	Organophosphate poisoning
Naloxone: Nalmefene	Opioids
Neostigmine	Curare
Penicillamine	Heavy metals (except iron)
Physostigmine	Anticholinergics
Prazosin[a]	Ergot alkaloids
Protamine	Heparin
Pyridostigmine	Curare
Pyridoxine	Cycloserine
Pyridoxine	Isoniazid
Quinidine	None

[a]Nitroprusside is another antidote to ergot alkaloid overdoses, but it conjugates to cyanide in fetal liver and should not be used in pregnancy.

stance. A general plan for the management of the drug-overdosed gravida includes stabilization, monitoring, supportive care, and toxicology screens (Box 14.1).

Specific management plans should be formulated in consultation with the regional certified poison control center, which is available 24 h per day, and handles international calls.

Maternal and fetal sequelae for specific antidote regimens are provided below for the 14 drug classes most frequently taken in suicide gestures by pregnant women (Table 14.3).

NONNARCOTIC ANALGESIC OVERDOSES

Acetaminophen

Acetaminophen is the most frequently used drug in suicide gestures during pregnancy (Czeizel *et al.*, 1984; Rayburn *et al.*, 1984). Sixty-nine cases of acetaminophen overdose in suicide gestures during pregnancy have been reported (Table 14.4). The salient clinical features of these cases are that early administration of the specific antidote (N-acetylcysteine) can prevent maternal hepatotoxicity if the antidote is tolerated and fetal hepatotoxicity is uncommon.

Table 14.4 Case reports of acetaminophen overdose during pregnancy

Amount Ingested (g)	EGA (weeks)	Treatment	Outcome	Maternal	Fetal	Authors
< 20		Nonspecific	Hepatotoxicity	Elective abortion[a]		Silverman and Carithess, 1978
32.5	36	N-acetylcysteine	Uncomplicated	Normal		Byer et al., 1982
32.5	29	Nonspecific	Hepatotoxicity	Normal[b]		Lederman et al., 1983
26	38	N-acetylcysteine	Uncomplicated	Normal		Ruthnum and Goel, 1984
25	18	N-acetylcysteine	Hepatotoxicity	Normal		Stokes, 1984
20	36	N-acetylcysteine	Uncomplicated	Normal		Roberts et al., 1984
29.5	28	N-acetylcysteine[d]	Hepatotoxicity[c]		Fetal death	Haibach et al., 1984
36	16	N-acetylcysteine	Uncomplicated	Normal		Robertson et al., 1986
64	15	N-acetylcysteine	Hepatotoxicity	Normal		Ludmir et al., 1986
50	32	N-acetylcysteine	Uncomplicated	Normal		Rosevear and Hope, 1989
35	31	None	Hepatorenal failure	Death	Death	Wang et al., 1997
19	40	N-acetylcysteine	Uncomplicated	Normal	Normal	Sancewicz-Pach et al., 1999

EGA, estimated gestation age.

[a]Not autopsied.

[b]Hyaline membrane disease pursuant to preterm delivery.

[c]Maternal outcomes were not listed.

[d]Antidote not tolerated.

Table 14.5 Outcome of 300 acetaminophen overdoses during pregnancy

	n		Outcome	Authors
Toxic	33 (11%)	*N*-acetylcysteine	24 normal, 1 malformed, 3 sp ab, 5 el ab	McElhatton *et al.*, 1997
Toxic	16 (5%)	Methionine	11 normal, 5 el ab	
Toxic	52 (17%)	Ipecacuanha	42 normal, 1 malformed, 2 sp ab, 7 el ab	
Toxic	16 (5%)	Charcoal	13 normal, 1 sp ab, 2 el ab	
Toxic	42 (14%)	Gastric lavage	28 normal, 4 malformed, 2 sp ab, 8 el ab	
Toxic	3 (1%)	Miscellaneous	1 normal, 1 malformed, 1 el ab	
Subtoxic	81 (27%)	No treatment	62 normal, 1 malformed, 5 sp ab, 14 el ab	
Unknown	59 (20%)	Treatment not recommended	40 normal, 3 malformed, 5 sp ab, 12 el ab	

sp ab, spontaneous abortion; el ab, elective abortion.

In a case series of 60 acetaminophen overdoses during pregnancy from a multicenter study in which 24 mothers had serum acetaminophen levels in the toxic range (Riggs *et al.*, 1989), only one case of fetal hepatotoxicity and maternal death occurred. In addition, there were four spontaneous abortions. The distribution of these cases across trimesters of pregnancy is given in Table 14.4. No evidence of teratogenicity of acetylcysteine (or paracetan) was found in one study (Janes and Routledge, 1992). However, the investigators concluded that delays in the administration of the antidotal treatment might increase the risk of spontaneous abortions, fetal death, and serious maternal liver damage.

Published case reports (Table 14.4) suggest that treatment of acetaminophen overdose during pregnancy has the best outcome when the antidote is given as early as possible. Of the available antidote regimens, N-acetylcysteine is the most effective (Table 14.5). Acetaminophen overdose during pregnancy should be treated with either oral or intravenous N-acetylcysteine without delay according to the protocols provided in the manufacturer's insert. Delay in administering the antidote increases the risk of maternal and fetal toxicity, hepatorenal failure, and death (Kozer and Koren, 2001).

Measured levels of acetaminophen at time postingestion can broadly predict whether or not hepatotoxicity should be expected (Fig. 14.1). However, acetaminophen *per se* is not the toxic agent in overdoses. Acetaminophen's metabolic pathways (sulfation and glucuronidation) become saturated, causing an increased metabolic load to cytochrome P-450 oxidases. The P-450 system oxidizes the drug and produces a highly reactive intracellular metabolite that complexes with hepatic glutathione. The P-450-produced metabolite binds to hepatocellular macromolecules when glutathione is depleted and hepatotoxicity ensues (Andrews *et al.*, 1976; Davis *et al.*, 1976). Fetal P-450 has 10 percent or less of adult activity and produces negligible amounts of the toxic metabolite. Some authorities speculate that the increased risk of maternal hepatotoxicity compared to fetal hepatotoxicity may be related to the largely inactive fetal enzyme complement, i.e., a protective effect of not being able to metabolize the drug to toxic intermediate. It was also speculated that fetuses of more advanced gestational age may be at greater risk

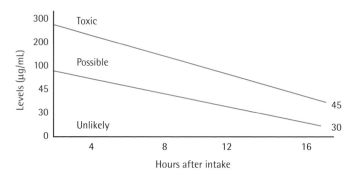

Figure 14.1 *Acetaminophen levels plotted against hours after intake and likelihood of liver damage. (Adapted from Zimmerman HJ.* Clin Liver Dis *1998; **2**: 529, with permission.)*

for acetaminophen toxicity than fetuses early in gestation. However, in the largest series studied, this relationship was not readily apparent (Table 14.6). The critical determinant of maternal–fetal outcome following acetaminophen overdose is the expediency in administering the antidote.

The most critical aspect of treating acetaminophen overdoses is administering the antidote as early as possible. Those gravidas given N-acetylcysteine within 10 h of ingesting large doses of acetaminophen have the best pregnancy outcomes (Table 14.6).

Aspirin

Aspirin is the second most frequently used drug in attempted suicide or gestures among pregnant women (Rayburn *et al.*, 1984). Clinical details have been reported of several cases of aspirin overdose during pregnancy as part of a suicide gesture (Table 14.7). The mean salicylate half-life has been shown to be approximately 20 h, and disappearance of salicylate from the circulation in the post-absorptive period (approximately 6 h after ingestion) is a first-order reaction (Done, 1968). Unfortunately, there is no specific antidote to aspirin, and nonspecific antidote treatment (i.e., activated charcoal) and supportive therapy are the mainstays of management. Alkalinization of the urine by intravenous administration of bicarbonate greatly increases the renal excretion of salicylic acid, as well as enhancing ionization of salicylate in plasma, which facilitates movement of the drug out of the central nervous system (Done, 1968). Both of these factors may contribute to shortening the duration of toxicity.

The risk of congenital anomalies does not seem to be higher among children of women who used aspirin during pregnancy. Among 41 infants born to women who had taken significant amounts of aspirin at various times during pregnancy, one infant was born with congenital anomalies (McElhatton *et al.*, 1991b). One fetal death was reported in the study. Notably, aspirin overdose during pregnancy poses a greater risk for fetal death than acetaminophen. Aspirin is the toxic agent, and not a metabolite; it is transferred across the placenta and reaches concentrations in the fetus that are higher than those in the mother (Garrettson *et al.*, 1975; Levy *et al.*, 1975). The cases of salicylate poisoning in pregnancy that have been reported support the same basic

Table 14.6 Acetaminophen toxicity in one large series

Time of treatment	n	Maternal deaths	Maternal hepatotoxic	Infant/fetal hepatotoxic	Stillbirths/ spontaneous abortion	Elective abortions	Viable infants	Viable preterm
Less than 10 h after overdose	10	0	0	0	0	2	7	1
10–16 h after overdose	10	0	2	0	3	2	4	1
16–24 h after overdose	4	1	3	1	2	1	1	0
Total	24	1	5	1	5	5	12	2

Adapted from Riggs *et al.*, 1989.

Table 14.7 Case reports of aspirin overdose during pregnancy

Amount ingested	EGA (weeks)	Treatment	Outcome Maternal	Fetal	Author
100 × 5 grain	24	300 ml mg citrate	Tinnitus, hyperventilated state	Stillborn, anomalies	Rejent and Baik, 1985
8 × 365 mg daily for several days up to delivery	37	Not mentioned	Not mentioned	Tachypnea, compensated metabolic acidosis	Ahlfors et al., 1982
Megadose	First trimester	Not mentioned	Not mentioned	Metanephric adenoma	Bove et al., 1979
Unknown	32	Not mentioned	Uncomplicated	Generalized hypertonia, increased reflex, irritability	Lynd, 1976
5–6 g daily	0–40	Not mentioned	Abruptio placenta; C-section	Unremarkable	Levy et al., 1975
15–18 g	40	Exchange	Not mentioned	Hyperpnoea, intercostal and suprasternal retractions present	Earle, 1961

EGA, estimated gestation age.

Table 14.8 Recommended treatment of aspirin overdose

Management

Early management
Adult: >120 mg/kg: give 50 g activated charcoal.

Child: for >120 mg/kg give activated charcoal.

Consider charcoal even for late-presenting patients; peak absorption may be delayed up to 12 h postingestion especially with enteric coated tablets.

Adults only: > 500 mg/kg.

Consider gastric lavage followed by 50 g activated charcoal, if patient presents within 1 h. Contact National Poison Information Service (NPIS) in the UK on 0870 600 6266 and in the US on 1-800-222-1222

Maintenance management
Check salicylate concentration 4 h postingestion, then every 2–3 h until peak concentration achieved and is falling consistently. If history is reliable for an ingestion >120 mg/kg and tablets are enteric coated, consider measuring levels for minimum 12 h postingestion even if no salicylate is detected initially. Monitor and correct urine and electrolytes, arterial blood gases and pH, blood sugar, prothrombin time.

Rehydrate with oral or IV fluids; large volumes may be necessary to correct dehydration (care required with the elderly or those with cardiac disease). Moderate or severe cases may require central venous pressure monitoring particularly patients with cardiac disease or elderly people Repeat doses of activated charcoal (RAC) (adult, 25–50 g; child, 1 g/kg) every 4 h until salicylate level has peaked and is consistently falling. RAC is effective in preventing excessive delayed absorption.

Urinary alkalinisation
For salicylate level 500–700 mg/L in adults or salicylate level 350–600 mg/L in children/elderly where patients have moderate clinical effects. In the presence of alkaline urine (optimum pH 7.5–8.5), renal elimination of salicylate is enhanced (10- to 20-fold with an increase from a urine pH of 5 to 8). Forced alkaline diuresis is not recommended.

Adult: 1 L of 1.26 percent sodium bicarbonate (isotonic) + 40 mmol potassium IV over 4 h and/or 50 mL boluses of 8.4 percent sodium bicarbonate IV (ideally via a central line).

Child: 1 ml/kg 8.4 percent sodium bicarbonate saline infused at 2–3 mL/kg.h 1 mmol/kg potassium diluted in 10 mL/kg hypokalemia prevents urinary excretion of alkali so must be corrected. Check urinary pH hourly aiming for pH 7.5–8.5, the rate of bicarbonate administration alone (avoiding hyperkalemia) may need to be increased if pH remains <7.5.

Check urine and electrolytes every 2–4 h and keep potassium between 4.0 and 4.5.

From Kamanyire, 2002.

conclusion as acetaminophen overdoses: early therapy antidote (activated charcoal, lavage, bowel irrigation) is associated with better outcomes (Table 14.8).

Naproxen

One case of naproxen overdose during pregnancy was published in detail. An estimated 8 h after maternal ingestion of 5 g of naproxen at 35 weeks of gestation, nonspecific and supportive antidote therapy was initiated because no specific antidote is available.

Following nonspecific therapy, spontaneous labor ensued and a preterm infant was delivered. The newborn had severe hyponatremia and water retention. Subsequently the infant recovered with no apparent sequelae at follow-up. The mother recovered with no evidence of hepatotoxicity or other adverse effects (Alon-Jones and Williams, 1986).

In contrast to the pharmacokinetics of salicylate elimination, high doses of naproxen (1–4 g) result in a disproportionate increase in renal excretion of the drug without apparent saturation of the excretory mechanism or metabolic pathway (Erling and Strand, 1977; Runkel et al., 1976). Increase in renal elimination may contribute to a lower incidence of acute toxicity compared with salicylate overdose.

Ibuprofen

Ibuprofen overdose during pregnancy has not been described in case studies and no specific antidote exists. Therefore, nonspecific antidote and supportive therapy should be given. Symptoms of ibuprofen toxicity include nausea, epigastric pain, diarrhea, vomiting, dizziness, blurred vision, and edema. The half-life of ibuprofen is 0.9–2.5 h in the post-absorptive period (Baselt, 1978). Among 67 cases of ibuprofen overdose, 36 percent occurred among children. Fifty reports of ibuprofen overdose during pregnancy have been reported, with mothers and infants suffering no untoward effects (i.e., hepatorenal failure, etc.) among those followed prospectively (Barry et al., 1984).

NUTRITIONAL SUPPLEMENT OVERDOSES

Prenatal vitamins

The course of pregnancy and infant outcome following prenatal vitamin overdoses has not been published. Since there is no specific antidote to prenatal vitamins, nonspecific and supportive antidote therapy should be given. It is reasonable to think that most cases of vitamin overdose would probably result in little, if any, risk to either mother or fetus. However, the retinoic acid content of the vitamins should be determined to estimate the total exposure. It is possible that megadose vitamin A may be involved, in which case Chapter 13, Use of dermatologics during pregnancy, should be consulted.

Iron

The clinical course following iron overdose during pregnancy has been reported for six cases (Table 14.9). Notably, adverse outcomes were associated with nonspecific treatment. The dangers of iron overdose vary according to the amount ingested. Iron poisoning is associated with gastrointestinal hemorrhage, physiological shock, acidosis, hepatic failure, and coagulopathies (Table 14.10). Death is usually the result of liver failure or cardiac collapse. The highest serum iron concentrations are likely to occur within 4 h of ingestion, with serum levels in excess of 500 µg/100 mL being more likely to be associated with severe poisoning (James, 1970). Thus, these patients should be treated aggressively.

The specific antidote to iron overdose is deferoxamine. From clinical experience, it is clear that early administration of the antidote is essential if therapy is to be efficacious.

Table 14.9 Cases of iron overdose during pregnancy

Amount	EGA (weeks)	Treatment	Outcome Maternal	Fetus	Author
50 Ferrous gluconate tablets	27	Lavage, Deferoxamine	Uncomplicated	Uncomplicated	Tran et al., 1998
40 Ferrous sulfate tablets	25	Deferoxamine	Uncomplicated	Uncomplicated	Schauben et al., 1990
5 g Elemental iron (25 g ferrous sulfate)	36	Deferoxamine	Hepatic necrosis, coma and subsequent expiration in cardiac failure	Uncomplicated	Olenmark et al., 1987
50 300 mg Ferrous sulfate (30–50 mg/kg Elemental iron)	15	Deferoxamine	Temporary abdominal tenderness and mild metabolic acidosis	Uncomplicated	Blanc et al., 1984
Unknown amount, along with prenatal vitamins	34	Deferoxamine	Brief episodes of vomiting and mild pain	Uncomplicated	Rayburn et al., 1983
Unknown amount	34	Deferoxamine	?	Uncomplicated	Rayburn et al., 1983
95 tablets of Fer-In-Sol	14	Deferoxamine	Died on the third day; pulmonary edema and hypotension	Spontaneous abortion	Strom et al., 1976
90 325 mg Ferrous sulfate capsules	16	Deferoxamine	Metabolic acidosis, depressed mental status; subsequent death 80 h postadmission	Spontaneous abortion	Manoguerra, 1976
4–6 g Elemental iron with 1–5 Sodium amytal, 6 g Aspirin	10	DPTA	Brief episode of abdominal pain, drowsiness, a systolic BP fall to 60 mmHg	Uncomplicated	Dugdale and Powell, 1964

EGA, estimated gestation age; DPTA, diethylenetriaminepentaacetic acid.

Table 14.10 Time course of iron overdose

Phase	Time to onset	Symptoms
I	0–3 h	Vomiting, hemetemesis, abdominal pain, diarrhea, lethargy, restlessness
II	up to 12 h	Quiescent period, symptoms subside
III	12–48 h	Shock, acidosis, hepatic necrosis, renal tubular necrosis, increasing lethargy, coma, seizures, hypotension, cyanosis, pulmonary edema, hypoglycemia, coagulopathies
IV	2–4 weeks	Gastric scarring, gastric/pyloric strictures

Adapted from Friedman, 1987.

Total iron-binding capacity and liver function should be routinely monitored in the patient with an iron overdose, as should thrombin and prothrombin times. Essentially, the gravida with an iron overdose should be managed similarly to the nonpregnant adult, as is described in detail elsewhere (Friedman, 1987). Guidelines for treatment according to ingested dose (if known) are given in Table 14.11. In a report of 49 pregnancies in which iron overdose occurred, there were 43 live births. Three infants had congenital anomalies, but they were exposed to the iron overdose and deferoxamine after the first trimester. Hence, the relationship appears not to be causal. The authors urge aggressive treatment of iron overdose with the specific antidote to prevent maternal death or organ toxicity (McElhatton *et al.*, 1991a). Review of 61 pregnancies indicated that in iron poisoning during pregnancy (1) peak maternal serum iron levels are associated with iron toxicity, and (2) deferoxamine should be administered without hesitation (Tran *et al.*, 2000).

Table 14.11 Sequelae of iron overdose based on amount ingested

Amount	Risk of toxicity
Less than 20 mg/kg	Minimal risk, no action required
20–60 mg/kg	Moderate risk, monitor for symptoms, induce vomiting
More than 60 mg/kg	High risk, requires treatment, gastrointestinal decontamination, chelation

Adapted from Friedman, 1987.

Following unpublished animal studies that suggest deferoxamine may cause significant fetal effects in animals, clinical experience has not shown this to be true in the human. Iron-overdose-associated pathophysiological effects on the mother seem to be the cause of adverse fetal outcomes, and not the direct result of iron overdose or antidote. No abnormalities have been reported among infants whose mothers consumed high doses of iron during pregnancy (Lacoste *et al.*, 1992; Tenenbein, 1989). It appears as though the placenta acts as a partial barrier to iron (Olenmark *et al.*, 1987; Rayburn *et al.*, 1983; Richards and Brooks, 1966). Chemical properties of the deferoxamine molecule strongly suggest that it would not cross the placenta in large amounts because it is a large molecule (molecular weight, 657) and is highly polarized.

ANTIANXIOLYTIC OVERDOSES

Benzodiazepines

Benzodiazepines are the most frequently used psychotropic medication in suicide gestures. The US Food and Drug Administration (FDA) approved a benzodiazepine receptor antagonist, flumazenil, in 1992 for the management of benzodiazepine overdose (The Flumazenil in Benzodiazepine Intoxication Multicentre Study Group, 1992; J Clin Pharmacol, 1992). Several investigators have shown the efficacy of flumazenil in reversing the clinical signs and symptoms of a benzodiazepine overdose (Krisanda, 1993; L'Heureux et al., 1992; Spivey et al., 1993). Flumazenil can cause complications (e.g., seizures) among patients with clinically high, but subtoxic, antidepressant poisoning or those who are taking benzodiazepines to therapeutically control seizures (The Flumazenil in Benzodiazepine Intoxication Multicentre Study Group, 1992; L'Heureux et al., 1992). One case study reported on the reversal of fetal benzodiazepine intoxication using flumazenil (Stahl et al., 1993). A 36-weeks, 22-year-old primipara ingested between 50 and 60 5 mg diazepam tablets. The patient was intravenously given two small doses (0.3 mg) of flumazenil. No adverse effects or withdrawal symptoms were noted in the patient or in the infant, who was born spontaneously 2 weeks later. The 'floppy infant syndrome' has been described, showing that benzodiazepines (1) cross the placenta and (2) have a depressive effect on the fetus. Warnings signs of complications in benzodiazepine overdoses in pregnancy are bradycardia and other symptoms of the drugs' depressive physiologic effects on mother and fetus.

Hydroxyzine

The clinical courses of pregnancies after hydroxyzine overdoses have not been published. Hypersedation and hypotension are the most frequently observed abnormalities with hydroxyzine overdose in nonpregnant adults. Hydroxyzine counteracts epinephrine's pressor effect. Therefore, hydroxyzine overdose-associated hypotension should not be treated with epinephrine. Intravenous fluids and other pressor agents (levarterenol or metaraminol) should be used instead to treat hypotension. Between 1 and 2 g of hydroxyzine pamoate commonly produces drowsiness and lethargy that may progress to a coma (Magera et al., 1981). Elimination half-life of hydroxyzine is 2.5–3.4 h, with a single dose of the drug and given that no more is taken (Baselt, 1978). No specific antidote to hydroxyzine is available. Therefore, nonspecific and supportive antidote therapy should be given.

HYPNOTIC AND SEDATIVE OVERDOSES

Phenobarbital and secobarbital

The course of pregnancy following barbituric-acid-derivative overdoses during gestation has not been published. Barbituric acid derivatives have no specific antidote. Therefore, nonspecific and supportive antidote therapy is indicated. Barbituric acids cross the placenta and these drugs may induce fetal hepatic enzymes. No congenital anomalies have

Box 14.2 Phenobarbital overdose stages

Stage I: Awake, competent, and mildly sedated. Average blood level of 3.5 mg/100 mL.

Stage II: Sedated, deep tendon reflexes (DTRs) present, prefers sleep, answers questions when aroused, does not cerebrate properly. Average blood level of 4.4 mg/100 mL.

Stage III: Comatose, DTRs present. Average blood level of 6.5 mg/100 mL.

Stage IV: Comatose, no DTRs obtainable. Average blood level of 10.0 mg/100 mL.

Stage V: Comatose, no DTRs obtainable, and with circulatory and/or respiratory difficulty. Half-lives of phenobarbital and secobarbital range from 2 to 6 days and 22 to 29 h, respectively (Baselt, 1978).

been observed in several studies of children born to women treated with phenobarbital during pregnancy (Bertollini *et al.*, 1987; Heinonen *et al.*, 1977). Five clinical stages of intoxication have been described in adults with acutely toxic (i.e., in nontolerant individuals) levels of phenobarbital (Sunshine, 1957), as shown in Box 14.2.

Pyrilamine

No reports of pregnancy following pyrilamine overdoses have been published. No specific antidote to pyrilamine is available. Therefore, nonspecific and supportive antidote therapy should be given.

NARCOTIC ANALGESIC OVERDOSES

Opioid narcotics

Opioid narcotics are either derived from opium or are synthetics, and include morphine, codeine, oxycodone, and hydromorphone. These drugs are metabolized to monoacetyl-morphine. Approximately 6 percent of suicide gestures in one study involved opioid analgesic preparations (Rayburn *et al.*, 1984) and 2.5 percent in another (Flint *et al.*, 2002). An opioid-specific antidote, naloxone, is available. It competitively binds to opioid receptors and opioid analgesics and blocks uptake. Opioid analgesics are eventually excreted.

If the patient is addicted to opioids, naloxone will cause an almost immediate onset of withdrawal symptoms. Most narcotic analgesic preparations also contain other substances, such as acetaminophen and aspirin. When an opioid overdose is documented, naloxone should be given according to directions in the *Physicians' Desk Reference* (PDR). Opioids cross the placenta freely and affect the fetus, as will the antidote. Therefore, it follows that treatment of maternal overdose will also treat the fetal overdose. Nalmefene has an 11-h half-life and was found to have potential benefits over naloxone (Kaplan and Marx, 1993), which has a shorter duration of action (1–2 h half-life). Nalmefene produces a longer period of withdrawal in opioid-dependent patients because of its long half-life (Anonymous, 1995; Kaplan and Marx, 1993). Importantly, overdose of other nonopioid constituents (e.g., acetaminophen) must be considered in devising the antidote regimen and treatment plan because they may have serious hepatic and renal toxicities that need immediate attention. Half-lives in the post-absorptive period are: morphine, 1.3–6.7 h; codeine, 1.9–3.9 h; oxycodone, 4.0–5.0 h; and hydromorphone, 1.5–3.8 h (Baselt, 1978).

Propoxyphene and pentazocine

Propoxyphene and pentazocine are synthetic narcotic preparations; however, naloxone and nalmefene are not antidotes to either of them. The minimum lethal dose of propoxyphene has been estimated at 500–800 mg (Baselt, 1978). Whole-blood concentrations of 1 mg/L indicate serious toxicity and 2 mg/L or more of propoxyphene are associated with death (Baselt, 1978). Fatalities due to pentazocine overdose generally occur with blood concentrations in the 1–5 mg/L range, with brain concentrations often exceeding blood levels except in cases of intravenous administration (Baselt, 1978).

The course of pregnancy following propoxyphene or pentazocine overdose has not been published. Nonspecific and supportive antidote therapy should be given because the effectiveness and safety of nalmefene for narcotic overdose have been demonstrated only in a pilot study. It is known that significant amounts of these synthetic narcotic drugs cross the placenta to reach the fetus. Narcotics may stimulate fetal hepatic maturation, inducing enzymatic activity, but effects of a potentially toxic dose are unknown. Among adult males, the half-lives of propoxyphene and pentazocine in the post-absorptive period are 8–24 h and 2.1–3.5 h, respectively (Baselt, 1978).

ANTIBIOTIC OVERDOSES

Cephalexin, amoxicillin, and trimethoprim sulfamethoxazole

In one study two decades ago, antibiotics were used in 7 percent of suicide gestures during pregnancy. The course of pregnancy following antibiotic overdoses has not been published. Nonspecific and supportive antidote therapy should be given because no specific antidote to antibiotic overdoses is available. Appreciable amounts of these drugs cross the placenta and expose the fetus to high drug doses, but the effects of potentially toxic doses on the fetus are unknown.

ANTIHISTAMINE AND DECONGESTANT OVERDOSES

Six percent of attempted suicides by pregnant women included large doses of antihistamines and/or decongestants in one study (Table 14.1), but not another (Table 14.2). One pregnancy following antihistamine overdose, diphenhydramine (35 Benadryl pills), in a suicide gesture at 26 weeks estimated gestation age (EGA) has been published. In the emergency room with palpable contractions, preterm labor was successfully treated with intravenous magnesium as tocolysis. Diphenhydramine overdose was treated with activated charcoal slurry because no specific antidotes are available. After 3 days the patient was released from the hospital in good health.

Preterm labor was attributed to the oxytocin-like effects of diphenhydramine (not listed in the *Physicians' Desk Reference*) (Brost *et al.*, 1996).

Hence, nonspecific and supportive antidote therapy should be given. It is known that considerable amounts of these drugs cross the placenta to reach the fetus. However, the effects of a potentially toxic dose are unknown.

ANTIPSYCHOTIC OVERDOSES

Thioridazine and trifluoperazine

Approximately 3 percent of pregnant women who attempted suicide during pregnancy used antipsychotic preparations (Flint et al., 2002; Rayburn et al., 1984). One case report is published regarding overdose of trifluoperazine (including misoprostol) during pregnancy (Bond and Van Zee, 1994). Fetal death was the final outcome, but the authors noted misoprostol as the probable cause of fetal death.

Antipsychotic overdose therapy includes nonspecific supportive therapy because there is no specific antidote. These drugs cross the placenta and achieve a near-therapeutic fetal concentration. Large doses of these drugs cause hypersedation in the nonpregnant adult and would be expected to have the same effect on the gravid woman and fetus. The effects of a potentially toxic dose during pregnancy have not been published. Thioridazine and trifluoperazine half-lives in the post-absorptive period are 26–36 h and 7–18 h, respectively (Baselt, 1978).

ANORECTIC OVERDOSES

Sympathomimetic amines, phenylpropanolamine

In one study, anorectic agents were used by approximately 2 percent of pregnant women in suicide gestures (Table 14.1). The course of pregnancy following anorectic agent overdoses has not been published. Therapy consists of nonspecific antidote and supportive therapy. The drugs cross the placenta and reach near therapeutic levels in the fetus. Oral doses of 50–75 mg produce anxiety, agitation, dizziness, and hallucinations (Dietz, 1981). Higher doses (85–400 mg) are associated with severe headaches, hypertensive crisis, and occasionally vomiting (Frewin et al., 1978; Horowitz et al., 1979; Ostern, 1965; Salmon, 1965; Teh, 1979).

Potentially toxic dose effects on the fetus are unknown. The half-life of phenylpropanolamine is unknown.

HORMONAL AGENT OVERDOSES

Corticosteroids and oral contraceptives

An estimated 2 percent of pregnant women used large doses of hormonal agents in their suicide attempt (Rayburn et al., 1984). The course of pregnancy following hormonal agent overdoses has not been published. Nonspecific supportive therapy should be given because no specific antidote to hormonal agents is available. Near-therapeutic amounts of these drugs cross the placenta and can be detected in the fetus. The effects of a potentially toxic dose of hormonal agents are unknown, but fetal adrenal suppression should be anticipated based upon known pharmacology and physiology.

One overdose of misoprostol and trifluoperazine has been reported (Bond and Van Zaa, 1994). Signs of toxicity included hypertonic uterine contraction with fetal death, hyperthermia, rhabdomyolysis, hypoxemia, respiratory alkalosis, and metabolic acidosis. The clinical impression was that misoprostol was being used as an illegal abortifacient.

ANTIDEPRESSANT OVERDOSES

Doxepin and amitriptyline

Approximately 2 percent of pregnant women used antidepressants in suicide gestures in two studies (Flint *et al.*, 2002; Rayburn *et al.*, 1984). The clinical details of the course of pregnancy following antidepressant agent overdoses have not been reported and therapy is mostly supportive. The toxic systemic effects (tachycardia, dry mouth, dilated pupils, and urinary retention) as well as the central nervous system effects (agitation, hallucinations, and hyperpyrexia) are anticholinergic in nature (Burks *et al.*, 1974). For this reason, physostigmine (an anticholinesterase) has been used in the diagnosis and antidotal therapy of poisoning with amitriptyline and other tricyclic antidepressants (Burks *et al.*, 1974; Slovis *et al.*, 1971). Large doses of antidepressants are associated with coma in nonpregnant adults and cardiac toxicity has been reported with acute ingestion of high doses of these drugs. Although these drugs cross the placenta to reach the fetus, the effects of a potentially toxic dose are unknown. Half-lives in the post-absorptive period for doxepin and amitriptyline are 8–25 h and 8–51 h, respectively (Baselt, 1978).

ANTICONVULSANT OVERDOSES

Phenytoin and carbamazepine

An estimated 2 percent of pregnant women who attempted suicide used large doses of anticonvulsants (Rayburn *et al.*, 1984). Pregnancy outcome following anticonvulsant agent overdoses has been published in one isolated case report. A case of carbamazepine megadose in attempted suicide with more than 10 g of carbamazepine during early pregnancy resulted in a fetus with a large meningomyelocele and frontal lobe necrosis that was electively aborted. The mother recovered without complication following nonspecific therapy and coma for 5 days (Little *et al.*, 1993). This is a cautionary anecdote regarding overdoses of anticonvulsants. Damage to the embryo or fetus is probable because the two anticonvulsants listed (phenytoin, carbamazepine) are known human teratogens. Anticonvulsant agents have no specific antidote, and supportive therapy should be given.

Near-therapeutic amounts of these drugs cross the placenta and achieve significant concentrations in the fetus. It is known that phenytoin may induce fetal hepatic enzymes, but the effects of a potentially toxic dose are unknown. Phenytoin's half-life ranges from 8–60 h and is dose dependent because each individual has a threshold plasma concentration beyond which the drug exhibits zero-order kinetics (Arnold and

Gerber, 1970; Kostenbauder *et al.*, 1975). Carbamazepine half-life after a single dose is 18–65 h (Baselt, 1978).

OVERDOSES OF OTHER DRUGS

Miscellaneous other drugs (Bendectin, docusate, cimetidine, methyldopa) were used by about 6 percent of pregnant women in their suicide gestures (Table 14.1). Details of the clinical course of pregnancy after overdoses of any of these agents have not been published. No specific antidotes to any of these agents are available. It is known that significant amounts of these drugs cross the placenta to reach near-therapeutic levels in the fetus. Megadose effects on mother or fetus are unknown.

OVERDOSES OF NONDRUG CHEMICALS

An estimated 2 percent of pregnant women who attempted suicide used nondrug chemicals in one study (Rayburn *et al.*, 1984).

Camphorated oil

Camphor, a gastrointestinal irritant and central nervous system stimulant, was used in four suicide attempts during pregnancy that have been published (Blackmon and Curry, 1957; Jacobziner and Raybin, 1962; Riggs *et al.*, 1965; Weiss and Catalano, 1973). Uniformly, maternal seizures occurred and should apparently be expected with camphor ingestion. Three of the four infants survived with no obvious abnormalities. The fourth pregnancy was compromised by preeclampsia, abruptio placenta, and other serious complications, and the infant died less than 1 h after delivery. Clearly, the death cannot be directly attributed to megadose camphor oil.

Clinical experience with camphor overdose is very limited and no specific antidote is available. Therefore, the nonspecific antidote regimen should be given and supportive therapy provided. Even limited experience with gravid women who have ingested camphor is sufficient to begin antiseizure medication as a component of the antidote regimen in anticipation that seizures may ensue.

Turpentine and ammonia

No details of the course of pregnancy following poisoning with these nondrug chemicals have been reported. No specific antidote to these poisons is available and nonspecific antidote regimens and supportive therapy should be given.

Quinine overdose

An attempt to induce abortion should be suspected when quinine overdose is encountered in pregnant women. Quinine has not been used in suicide attempts based upon published experience. Among 70 published cases of pregnant women taking quinine at high doses in an attempt to induce abortion suggest the drug may be teratogenic (Dannenberg *et al.*, 1983). At least 11 women died as a result of quinine overdose and many who did not expire experienced toxic effects of the drug. No fewer than 41 infants with major congenital anomalies were born to women who took large doses of quinine during pregnancy. Causality cannot be proven using these data because the information comprised of only case reports. Nonetheless, large doses of quinine appear to pose an increased risk of some specific abnormalities that parallel toxicity from the drug often seen in adults. Eighteen of 60 infants (30 percent) born to women who ingested large amounts of quinine during pregnancy were congenitally deaf (Dannenberg *et al.*, 1983). Ototoxicity is a common and well-documented complication of quinine therapy in adults.

Large doses of quinine during the first trimester of pregnancy are anecdotally associated with major congenital anomalies, including central nervous system anomalies (especially hydrocephalus or otolithic damage), limb defects, cardiac defects, and gastrointestinal tract anomalies (Nishimura and Tanimura, 1976). No characteristic pattern of anomalies or syndrome was identified, and the association of these anomalies with maternal quinine ingestion remains empirically uncertain, but seems plausible.

Nonspecific antidote treatment and supportive therapy should be given because no specific antidote for quinine overdose is available.

Ergotamine overdose

Overdose of ergotamine during pregnancy was published in a case report of a woman at 35 weeks' gestation who took 10 tablets of ergotamine tartrate in a suicide gesture. Two hours later uterine contractions began with no relaxation between contractions. Fetal death occurred approximately 8 h after the overdose. Two weeks after the overdose, a macerated stillbirth with no gross abnormality was delivered. Impaired placental perfusion and fetal anoxia associated with ergotamine was speculated to have caused the fetal death (Au *et al.*, 1985).

Spontaneous onset of preterm labor following ingestion of ergot also occurred with therapeutic levels of the drugs, but at usual therapeutic levels prematurity was the only complication, and there were no fetal deaths. Two antidotes to ergot alkaloid overdose (prazosin and nitroprusside) are now available that were unavailable to patients described above (Au *et al.*, 1985). Nitroprusside should be avoided during pregnancy because it conjugates to cyanide and accumulates in the fetal liver. Therefore, prazosin is the preferred antidote for use during pregnancy.

SUMMARY

Early aggressive treatment of attempted suicide during pregnancy is associated with better outcomes than late or passive treatment. Fetal monitoring should begin as early as possible. If a specific antidote exists, it should be given as soon as possible. If there is no specific antidote, a nonspecific aggressive treatment should be instituted as early as possible (see Appendix).

Key References

Anonymous. Nalmefene, a long-acting injectiable opioid antagonist. *Med Lett Drugs Ther* 1995; **37**: 97.

Brost BC, Scardo JA, Newman RB. Diphenhydramine overdose during pregnancy. Lessons from the past. *Am J Obstet Gynecol* 1996; **175**: 1376.

Dannenberg AL, Carter DM, Lawson HW, Ashton DM, Dorfman SF, Graham EH. Homicide and other injuries as causes of maternal death in New York City, 1987 through 1991. *Am J Obstet Gynecol* 1995; **172**: 1557.

Flint C, Larsen H, Nielsen GL, Olsen J, Sørensen HT. Pregnancy outcome after suicide attempt by drug use. A Danish population-based study. *Acta Obstet Gynecol Scand* 2002; **81**: 516.

Kamanyire R. Aspirin overdose. *Emerg Nurse* 2002; **10**: 17.

Kozer E, Koren G. Management of paracetamol overdose. current controversies. *Drug Safety* 2001; **24**: 503.

Sancewicz-Pach K, Chmiest W, Lichota E. Suicidal paracetamol poisoning of a pregnant woman just before a delivery. *Przegl Lek* 1999; **56**: 459.

Tran T, Wax JR, Philput C, Steinfeld JD, Ingardia CJ. Intentional iron overdose in pregnancy – management and outcome. *J Emerg Med* 2000; **18**: 225.

Tran T, Wax JR, Steinfeld JD, Ingardia CJ. Acute intentional iron overdose in pregnancy. *Obstet Gynecol* 1998; **92**: 678.

Wang PH, Yang MJ, Lee WL, Chao HT, Yang ML, Hung JH. Acetaminophen poisoning in late pregnancy. A case report. *J Reprod Med* 1997; **42**: 367.

Wilkes JM, Clark LE, Herrera JL. Acetaminophen overdose in pregnancy. *South Med J* 2005; **98**: 1118.

Zimmerman HJ. Acetaminophen toxicity. *Clin Liver Dis* 1998; **2**: 529.

Further references are available on the book's website at http://www.drugsandpregnancy.com

Appendix to Chapter 14: 2005 List of antidotes available

Antidote	Used for drug overdose, poison, or toxin
N-Acetylcysteine (Mucomyst\reg;, Acetadolte\reg;)	Acetaminophen
	Carbon tetrachloride
	Other hepatotoxins
Amyl nitrite, sodium nitrite, and sodium thiosulfate (Cyanide antidote kit)	Acetonitrile
	Acrylonitrile
	Bromates (thiosulfate only)
	Chlorates (thiosulfate only)
	Cyanide (e.g., HCN, KCN, and NaCN)
	Cyanogen chloride
	Cyanogenic glycoside natural sources (e.g., apricot pits and peach pits)
	Hydrogen sulfide (nitrites only)
	Laetrile
	Mustard agents (thiosulfate only)
	Nitroprusside (thiosulfate only)
	Smoke inhalation (combustion of synthetic materials)

Appendix to Chapter 14: 2005 List of antidotes available – *continued*

Antidote	Used for drug overdose, poison, or toxin
Antivenin, Crotalidae Polyvalent (equine origin)	Pit viper envenomation (e.g., rattlesnakes, cottonmouths, timber rattlers, and copperheads)
Antivenin, Crotalidae Polyvalent Immune Fab – Ovine (CroFab)	Pit viper envenomation (e.g., rattlesnakes, cottonmouths, timber rattlers, and copperheads)
Antivenin, *Latrodectus mactans* (Black widow spider)	Black widow spider envenomation
Atropine sulfate	Alpha$_2$ agonists (e.g., clonidine, guanabenz, and guanfacine)
	Alzheimer drugs (e.g., donepezil, galantamine, rivastigmine, tacrine)
Antimyesthenic agents (e.g. pyridostigmine)	Bradyarrhythmia-producing agents (e.g., beta blockers, calcium channel blockers, and digitalis glycosides)
	Cholinergic agonists (e.g., bethanechol)
	Muscarine-containing mushrooms (e.g., *Clitocybe* and *Inocybe*)
	Nerve agents (e.g., sarin, soman, tabun, and VX)
	Organophosphate and carbamate insecticides
Calcium disodium	Lead
EDTA (Versenate)	Zinc salts (e.g., zinc chloride)
Calcium chloride and Calcium gluconate	Beta blockers
	Calcium channel blockers
	Fluoride salts (e.g., NaF)
	Hydrofluoric acid (HF)
	Hyperkalemia (not digoxin-induced)
	Hypermagnesemia
Deferoxamine mesylate (Desferal)	Iron
Digoxin immune Fab (Digibind, Digifab)	Cardiac glycoside-containing plants (e.g., foxglove and oleander)
	Digitoxin
	Digoxin
Dimercaprol (BAL in oil)	Arsenic
	Copper
	Gold
	Lead
	Lewsite
	Mercury
Ethanol	Ethylene glycol
	Methanol
Flumazenil (Romazicon)	Benzodiazepines
	Zalepion
	Zolpidem
Folic acid and Folinic acid (Leucovorin)	Methanol
	Methotrexate trimetrexate
	Pyrimethamine
	Trimethoprim
Fomepizole (Antizol)	Ethylene glycol
	Methanol

Appendix to Chapter 14: 2005 List of antidotes available – *continued*

Antidote	Used for drug overdose, poison, or toxin
Glucagon	Beta blockers
	Calcium channel blockers
	Hypoglycemia
	Hypoglycemic agents
Hyperbaric oxygen (HBO)	Carbon monoxide
	Carbon tetrachloride
	Cyanide
	Hydrogen sulfide
	Methemoglobinemia
Methylene blue	Methomoglobin-inducing agents including
	aniline dyes
	Dapsone
	Dinitrophenol
	Local anesthetics (e.g., benzocaine)
	Metoclopramide
	Monomethylhydrazine-containing mushrooms (e.g., *Gyromitra*)
	Naphthalene
	Nitrates and nitrites
	Nitrobenzene
	Phenazopyridine
Nalmefene (Revex) and Naloxone (Narcan)	ACE inhibitors
	Alpha$_2$ agonists (e.g., clonidine, guanabenz and guanfacine)
	Coma of unknown cause
	Imidazoline decongestants (e.g., oxymetazoline and tetrahydrozoline)
	Loperamide
	Opioids (e.g., codeine, dextromethorphan, diphenoxylate, fentanyl, heroin, meperidine, morphine, and propoxyphene)
D-Penicillamine (Cuprimine)	Arsenic
	Copper
	Lead
	Mercury
Physostigmine salicylate (Antilirium)	Anticholinergic alkaloid-containing plants (e.g., deadly nightshade and jimson weed)
	Antihistamines
	Atropine and other anticholinergic agents
	Intrathecal baclofen
Phytonadione	Indandione derivatives
(Vitamin K$_1$)	Long-acting anticoagulant rodenticides (e.g., brodifacoum and bromadiolone)
(AquaMEPHYTON, Mephyton)	Warfarin
Pralidoxime chloride	Antimyesthenic agents (e.g., pyridostigmine)
(2-PAM)	Nerve agents (e.g., sarin, soman, tabun and VX)
(Protopam)	Organophosphate insecticides
	Tacrine

Appendix to Chapter 14: 2005 List of antidotes available – *continued*

Antidote	Used for drug overdose, poison, or toxin
Protamine sulfate	Enoxaparin
	Heparin
Pyridoxine hydrochloride	Acrylamide
(Vitamin B$_6$)	Ethylene glycol
	Hydrazine
	Isoniazid (INH)
	Monomethylhydrazine-containing mushrooms (e.g., *Gyromitra*)
Sodium bicarbonate	Chlorine gas
	Hyperkalemia
	Serum alkalinization:
	agents producing a quinidine-like effect as noted by widened QRS complex on EKG (e.g., amantadine, carbamazepine, chloroquine, cocaine, diphenhydramine, fecainide, propagenone, propoxyphene, tricyclic antidepressants, quinidine and related agents)
	Urine alkalinization:
	Weakly acidic agents (e.g., chlorophenoxy herbicides), chlorpropamide, phenobarbital, and salicylates)
Succimer (Chemet)	Arsenic
	Lead
	Lewisite
	Mercury
Benztropine mesylate (Cogentin)	Medications causing a dystonic reaction
Bromocriptine mesylate (Parlodel)	Medications causing neuroleptic malignant syndrome (NMS)
L-Carnitine (Camitor)	Valproic acid
Cyproheptadine HCL (Periactin)	Medications causing serotonin syndrome
Dantrolene sodium (Dantrium)	Medications causing NMS
	Medications causing malignant hyperthermia
Diazepam (Valium)	Chloroquine and related antimalarial drugs
	NMS
	Serotoninc syndrome
Diphenhydramine HCL (Benadryl)	Medications causing a dystonic reaction
Insulin and dextrose	Beta blockers
	Calcium channel blockers (diltiazem, nifedipine, verapamil)
Octreotide acetate (Sandostatin)	Sulfonylurea hypoglycemic agents (e.g., glipizide, glyburide)
Phentolamine mesylate (Regitine)	Catecholamine extravasation
	Intradigital epinephrine injection
Thiamine	Ethanol
	Ethanol glycol

Appendix to Chapter 14: 2005 List of antidotes available – *continued*

Antidote	Used for drug overdose, poison, or toxin
Calcium-diethylenetriamine penaacetic acid (Ca-DTPA; Pentetate calcium trisodium injection) Zinc-diethylenetriamine pentaacetic acid (Zn-DTPA: pentetate zinc trisodium injection)	Internal contamination with transuranium elements: americium, curium, plutonium
Potassium Iodide, KI tablets (Iostate, Thyro-Block, Thyrosafe) KI liquid (Thyroshield)	Prevents thyroid uptake of radioactive iodine (I-131)
Prussian blue, ferric hexacyanoferrate (Radiogardase)	Radioactive cesium (Cs-137), radioactive thallium (TI-201), and nonradioactive thallium)

ACE, angiotensin-converting enzyme; DTPA, diethylenetriaminepentaacetic acid; EDTA, ethylenediaminetetraacetic acid.

Compiled from Illinois Poison Center Antidote List, 2005, with permission.

15

Miscellaneous drugs during pregnancy: tocolytics and immunosuppressants

TOCOLYTICS

Of an estimated 4 million women in the USA who give birth annually, approximately 11 percent of women deliver prematurely (less than 36 weeks). No tocolytic agent is universally effective, although more than 100 000 pregnancies will receive tocolysis therapy. Efficacy of most tocolytic agents is not universally accepted by physicians. Pregnant women treated with tocolytics are at increased risk for serious cardiopulmonary complications that are directly attributed to the tocolytic drug. Tocolytic therapy invariably occurs outside embryogenesis, so congenital anomalies are not an issue. The primary concern is for adverse maternal, fetal, and neonatal effects (Sanchez-Ramos *et al.*, 2000). The three principal indications that guide the use of tocolysis in the treatment of preterm labor are: (1) prophylaxis, (2) acute therapy, and (3) maintenance.

Instances do exist when exposure to tocolytic agents occurs during organogenesis, and is used for other indications: terbutaline (asthma), indomethacin (pain), and nifedipine (hypertension). Use for these indications is discussed in the chapters on antiasthma (Chapter 5), analgesic (Chapter 8), and cardiovascular drugs (Chapter 3), respectively.

Pharmacokinetics of tocolytic drugs

Pharmacokinetic data on tocolytic drugs in pregnancy are limited to five studies of four drugs (Table 15.1). Half-life and steady-state concentrations are generally not different between pregnant and nonpregnant states.

Beta-adrenergic receptor agonists

Ritodrine and terbutaline are beta-agonist drugs, structurally related to epinephrine, and are used as tocolytics. Fenoterol is another drug in this class which has been popular in Europe.

Table 15.1 Pharmacokinetics of tocolytic agents during pregnancy

Agent	n	EGA (weeks)	Route	AUC	V_d	C_{max}	C_{ss}	$t_{1/2}$	Cl	PPB	Control group[a]	Authors
Fenoteral	4	30–32	IV	↑		=	=	=			No	Mandach et al. (1995)
Ritodrine	91	28–36	IV, IM, PO	→		=	=	=			Yes (1)	Van Lierde et al. (1984)
Ritodrine	10	20–34	IV	→		→	=	=			Yes (1)	Caritis et al. (1989)
Salbutamol	7	16–33	IV, PO	→		=	=	=	=		Yes (3,4)	Hutchings et al. (1987)
Terbutaline	8	27–35	IV	→		=	→	=	↑		Yes (4)	Berg et al. (1984)

Source: Little BB. *Obstet Gynecol* 1999; **93**: 858.

EGA, estimated gestational age; AUC, area under the curve; V_d, volume of distribution; C_{max}, peak plasma concentration; C_{ss}, steady-state concentration; $t_{1/2}$, half-life; Cl, clearance; PPB, plasma protein binding; PO, by mouth; ↓ denotes a decrease during pregnancy compared with nonpregnant values; ↑ denotes an increase during pregnancy compared with nonpregnant values; = denotes no difference between pregnant and nonpregnant values; IV = intravenous; IM = intramuscular.

[a]Control groups: 1, nonpregnant women; 2, same individuals studied postpartum; 3, historic adult controls (sex not given); 4, adult male controls; 5, adult male and female controls combined.

Box 15.1 Tocolytic agents

Beta-sympathomimetic agents	Sulindac
Fenoterol	*Calcium channel blockers*
Hexoprenaline	Atosiban
Ritodrine	Nifedipine
Solbutanol[a]	Nitric oxide donor drugs
Terbutaline	Nitroglycerin
Magnesium sulfate	Oxytocin analog
Indomethacin	Verapamil
Prostaglandin synthetase inhibitors	

[a]Not available in the USA.

There are several other beta-agonists that have been utilized for tocolysis that are currently either not approved for tocolysis or not available in the USA (Box 15.1). This type of tocolytic binds to beta-adrenergic receptors on the outer myometrial cell membrane and activates adenylate cyclase. Adenylate cyclase catalyzes conversion of ATP to cAMP. Increased intracellular cAMP activates cAMPase-dependent protein kinase, decreasing intracellular calcium, resulting in reduced myometrial contractility (Caritis *et al.*, 1988; Roberts, 1984). Another pathway is the phosphorylation of myosin light chain kinase which inactivates the enzyme, thus inhibiting subsequent phosphorylation of the myosin light chain.

Maternal metabolic abnormalities (gluconeogenesis, hypokalemia, and hyperglycemia), as well as cardiopulmonary complications (tachycardia, hypotension, arrhythmias, myocardial ischemia, pulmonary edema) are associated with beta-agonist tocolytics (Box 15.2). Apprehension, electrocardiogram (EKG/ECG) changes (S-T segment depression) and maternal death are also associated with this class of tocolytic agents. Every beta-agonist is associated with pulmonary edema and occurs among as many as 5 percent of gravidas who took any of these drugs (Boyle, 1995; McCombs, 1995).

Maternal tocolytic therapy has been associated with neonatal hypoglycemia and tachycardia. Several fetal and neonatal cardiovascular adverse effects are associated with beta-sympathomimetic therapy (Katz and Seeds, 1989) (Box 15.3). Decreases in the systolic/diastolic ratios of the umbilical artery have been reported in patients using either terbutaline or ritodrine (Brar *et al.*, 1988; Wright *et al.*, 1990).

RITODRINE

Ritodrine is only drug approved by the US Food and Drug Administration (FDA) for obstetric use for tocolysis. After being developed specifically for tocolysis, it was

Box 15.2 Maternal adverse effects of beta-sympathomimetic therapy

Cardiac arrhythmia	Hypotension
Chest pain	Pulmonary edema
Hyperglycemia	Shortness of breath
Hypokalemia	Tachycardia

Box 15.3 Possible adverse fetal effects of maternal beta-sympathomimetic therapy

Hypoglycemia
Hypotension and tachycardia
Other cardiovascular effects[a]
    Cardiac dysrhythmia
    Decrease in umbilical artery systolic/diastolic ratios
    Heart failure
    Myocardial ischemia
    Neonatal death
    Ventricular hypertrophy

[a]From Brar et al., 1988; Hill, 1995; Katz and Seeds, 1989.

approved in 1980, in the USA. By 1979, ritodrine was available as a tocolytic agent in 23 foreign countries (Barden, et al., 1980). Ritodrine hydrochloride is a beta-adrenergic agonist with beta$_2$-receptor effects that relax smooth muscle in the arterioles, bronchi, and uterus. Although ritodrine use is in widespread use for the inhibition of preterm labor (Leveno et al., 1990), controversy remains concerning its clinical efficacy in prevention of preterm birth (Calder and Patel, 1985; Canadian Preterm Labor Investigation Group, 1992; Casparis et al., 1971; King et al., 1988; Larsen et al., 1980, 1986; Leveno et al., 1986; Merkatz et al., 1980).

Tocolytic agents may successfully inhibit labor for up to 48 h. No long-term beneficial effect of tocolytic therapy (decreased perinatal mortality or severe neonatal respiratory disorders) was found in meta-analysis of 890 pregnancies in which ritodrine or another beta-mimetic tocolytic agent was used to prevent premature delivery (King et al., 1988). Downregulation of beta$_2$-adrenergic receptors following the use of these drugs may explain their poor efficacy because uterine-relaxant effects are short lived (Berg et al., 1985; Fredholm et al., 1982; Harden, 1983; Hausdorff et al., 1990; Mickey et al., 1975; Ryden et al., 1982; Swillens et al., 1980; Wolfe et al., 1977). Ritodrine is also used to reverse 'fetal distress' and uterine hypertonus. For this indication, a dose of 1–3 mg is usually given over a 2-min period (Smith, 1991).

In the longer term, preterm labor is not effectively prevented by tocolysis. We analyzed national ritodrine sales over a 7-year period and found no evidence that treatment of preterm labor with ritodrine hydrochloride was associated with a decreased incidence of low birth weight (LBW) infants in the USA. Estimates of ritodrine usage suggest a lack of impact, even though as many as 40–50 percent of the preterm labors that resulted in LBW infants (approximately 116 000 annually) were probably managed with ritodrine therapy (Leveno et al., 1990). It is possible that a weak effect was present and the signal could not be separated from background noise.

Maternal effects

Acute maternal pulmonary edema, in addition to hypokalemia and hyperglycemia, has been reported among women given ritodrine. Steroids administered concomitantly to accelerate fetal lung maturity seem to increase the risk for this maternal complication (see Box 15.2). Severe maternal cardiovascular complications occurred among nearly 5 percent of women treated with terbutaline (Katz *et al.*, 1981). The risk of pulmonary edema among women receiving ritodrine or other beta-mimetics is increased with certain maternal complications: infection, excessive intravenous hydration, multifetal gestation, underlying cardiac disease increase (ACOG, 1995).

Beta-mimetics also alter glucose tolerance and have been associated with ketoacidosis among women with poorly controlled insulin-dependent diabetes. Maternal deaths have also been reported with the use of beta-mimetic therapy.

Fetal effects

Fetal tachycardia and arrhythmias are associated with beta-mimetic therapy, including ritodrine (Barden *et al.*, 1980; Hermansen and Johnson, 1984). Protracted ritodrine therapy has been associated with increased septal thickness in exposed neonates (Nuchpuckdee *et al.*, 1986). However, these do not appear to be frequent complications of ritodrine, or beta-mimetic, therapy in general.

Beta-sympathomimetic tocolytic therapy, including ritodrine, was associated with a 2.5-fold increased risk of periventricular-intraventricular hemorrhage (Groome *et al.*, 1992). However, grades 3 and 4 hemorrhages were not increased. In another investigation, no association of ritodrine with intraventricular–periventricular hemorrhage was found (Box 15.3) (Ozcan *et al.*, 1995).

Beta-mimetics are generally not used during the period of organogenesis, with the exception of terbutaline for asthma. No reports of teratogenic effects of ritodrine in the human have been published. An increased frequency of cardiovascular anomalies in chick embryos exposed to ritodrine and terbutaline was found in one study, and it was concluded that teratogenic effects were secondary to stimulation of beta-2-adrenergic receptors (Lenselink *et al.*, 1994). The significance of these findings to human pregnancies is unknown.

TERBUTALINE

Although terbutaline has not been approved by the FDA for the specific indication of premature labor, it is probably the most commonly used beta-mimetic for this purpose. Interestingly, according to its manufacturer, it should not be used for tocolysis. Terbutaline has also been utilized in the management of symptomatic placenta previa in pregnancies remote from term (Besinger *et al.*, 1995), for the management of uterine hypotonus, especially in the presence of a nonreassuring fetal heart rate pattern (Smith, 1991) and for inducing uterine relaxation prior to attempting external cephalic version (Fernandez *et al.*, 1996).

Neonatal myocardial dysfunction and necrosis have been associated with terbutaline tocolytic therapy (Fletcher *et al.*, 1991; Thorkelsson and Loughead, 1991), but the causal relationship to the maternal therapy is controversial (Bey *et al.*, 1992; Kast and Hermer, 1993). Neonatal hypoglycemia and fetal tachycardia were associated with terbutaline tocolytic therapy late in pregnancy (Peterson *et al.*, 1993; Roth *et al.*, 1990; Sharif *et al.*, 1990), but these effects were transient. Neonatal behavior was transiently altered among the infants of pregnant women who received terbutaline tocolysis (Thayer and Hupp, 1997).

Maternal effects

Terbutaline may be associated with maternal cardiovascular effects (including pulmonary edema) similar to those associated with ritodrine (Katz *et al.*, 1981). One review of cardiopulmonary effects of low-dose continuous terbutaline infusion in 8709 women found 47 women (0.5 percent) developed one or more adverse cardiopulmonary effects. Twenty-eight women (0.3 percent) developed pulmonary edema (Perry *et al.*, 1995). In another review of 1000 women given a combination of intravenous terbutaline and magnesium sulfate, the side effects of protracted therapy were negligible (Kosasa *et al.*, 1994). Two cases of terbutaline hepatitis in pregnancy have been reported (Quinn *et al.*, 1994).

ETHANOL

Alcohol is not recommended for use during pregnancy as it is associated with both teratogenic and fetal effects. This agent is reviewed in detail in Chapter 16, Substance abuse during pregnancy.

MAGNESIUM SULFATE

Magnesium sulfate inhibits uterine contractions by apparently antagonizing calcium flow into the myometrial cell. Magnesium sulfate has no proven efficacy in delaying delivery beyond 24–48 h (Cotton *et al.*, 1984; Cox *et al.*, 1990; Kimberlin *et al.*, 1996), as with other tocolytic agents.

Maternal effects

Hypermagnesemia (cutaneous flushing, nausea, vomiting, respiratory depression, intracardiac conduction delays) is the major maternal adverse effect of magnesium sulfate therapy. Respiratory arrest is frequent when $MgSO_4$ levels reach 12 mEq/L or greater. Protracted therapy (many days) with magnesium sulfate for preterm labor increases calcium loss and may decrease bone mineralization (Smith *et al.*, 1992). Bleeding time during pregnancy may be prolonged with magnesium sulfate therapy, but this is not clinically significant (Fuentes *et al.*, 1995). Unlike ritodrine, magnesium sulfate is not associated with a 'peripheral vascular steal' syndrome and does not decrease placental perfusion (Dowell and Forsberg, 1995).

Fetal effects

Magnesium sulfate crosses the placenta and, in extremely large doses, may cause neonatal cardiorespiratory depression and transient loss of beat-to-beat variability (Hallak *et al.*, 1999; Hiett *et al.*, 1995; Idama and Lindow, 1998; Wright *et al.*, 1996). Calcium gluconate can reverse these symptoms if they become severe.

Osseous lesions (metaphyses, costochondral junctions, skull) have been reported among infants born to women treated with magnesium sulfate for more than a week prior to delivery (Malaeb *et al.*, 2004; Tsukahara *et al.*, 2004), but they are resorbed within months of life (Santi *et al.*, 1994; Tsukahara *et al.*, 2004).

Nonsteroidal antiinflammatory agents

INDOMETHACIN

Indomethacin is a prostaglandin synthetase inhibitor that has been used to delay labor (Carlan *et al.*, 1992; Niebyl *et al.*, 1980; Zuckerman *et al.*, 1974). Indomethacin is efficacious as a tocolytic for short periods of time (Niebyl *et al.*, 1980), but it may be associated with significant adverse fetal effects: oligohydramnios, ductus arteriosus constriction, persistent fetal circulation, neonatal hypertension, intracranial hemorrhage, necrotizing enterocolitis, anemia, cystic renal changes, neonatal death (Csapo *et al.*, 1978; Goldenberg *et al.*, 1989; Manchester *et al.*, 1976; Moise *et al.*, 1988; Norton *et al.*, 1993; Rubattelli *et al.*, 1979; Rudolph, 1981; van der Heijden *et al.*, 1994).

Maternal effects

Indomethacin resulted in few maternal side effects when used as a tocolytic. Potential adverse effects include: interstitial nephritis, acute renal failure, peptic ulcer disease, decrease in platelets, prolonged bleeding time (Clive and Stoff, 1984; Lunt *et al.*, 1994; Norton *et al.*, 1993). It may exacerbate hypertension (Gordon and Samuels, 1995).

Among 83 women who received indomethacin during pregnancy, no adverse maternal or fetal effects were noted, except for oligohydramnios, which resolved spontaneously (Sibony *et al.*, 1994).

Fetal effects

In a review of 28 studies including 1621 infants exposed to indomethacin for tocolysis, the risk for adverse neonatal outcomes was not increased (Loe *et al.*, 2005). However, there were only three randomized clinical trials included and one of them did find an increased risk for adverse neonatal outcomes associated with indomethacin tocolysis.

SULINDAC

Sulindac is another prostaglandin synthetase inhibitor, similar to indomethacin. It has been used to treat preterm labor. Sulindac was as effective as indomethacin, but with fewer adverse fetal effects in a randomized prospective study of 36 women in preterm labor (Carlan *et al.*, 1992). No epidemiological studies of sulindac during pregnancy have been published, but it is probably associated with potential adverse effects similar to indomethacin.

Calcium channel blockers

NIFEDIPINE

Nifedipine is a calcium channel blocker which promotes smooth muscle relaxation by reducing intracellular calcium. It is also a cardiovascular agent because of its vasodilating effects. Owing to smooth muscle relaxation, there may be maternal hypotension and subsequent decreased uteroplacental perfusion, although in human studies there has been no evidence that nifedipine compromises the fetus (Ray and Dyson, 1995).

In a preliminary study of nifedipine versus ritodrine, it was suggested that nifedipine was associated with fewer maternal and fetal side effects (van Dijk *et al.*, 1995). A recent case report of severe hypotension and fetal death associated with nifedipine, tocolysis-ascribed causality (van Veen *et al.*, 2005) has led to the suggestion that the association may not be causal (Johnson and Mason, 2005; Kandysamy and Thomson, 2005; Papatsonis *et al.*, 2005).

VERAPAMIL

As discussed in Chapter 3, verapamil is used as an antiarrhythmic, antihypertensive, and tocolytic agent. No epidemiologic studies on the safety of this agent during pregnancy have been published. Maternal hypotension and resultant decreased uterine blood flow are the major risks from the use of this agent.

OXYTOCIN ANTAGONISTS

Atosiban inhibits oxytocin-induced uterine contractions. It is a nonapeptide oxytocin analog with competitive oxytocin antagonist actions. Consistent reduction in uterine activity during the infusion of atosiban has been observed (Goodwin *et al.*, 1995). No studies regarding the safety of this agent have been published, but a review is available (Shubert, 1995).

NITRIC OXIDE DONOR DRUGS

Among 13 women given nitroglycerin patches, the drug was effective in preventing preterm birth, but maternal side effects involved hypotension and sedation (Lees *et al.*, 1994).

No difference in tocolytic efficacy was noted in a randomized investigation comparing intravenous nitroglycerin with magnesium sulfate (Clavin *et al.*, 1996). Parenteral nitroglycerin is associated with severe maternal hypotension, which suggests that placental hypoperfusion may be a serious risk.

Special considerations

Tocolytic therapy is controversial. Concern includes efficacy of specific agents and whether these agents can effectively delay labor for greater than 48 h, i.e., for 1 week or longer. Tocolytics do appear to be effective for delaying labor for short intervals (24–48 h) and possibly for relieving hypertonic contractions. This may be of benefit with regard to corticosteroid therapy in an attempt to accelerate fetal lung maturation.

PREMATURE LABOR

The most commonly used agents for treating premature labor are: ritodrine, terbutaline, and magnesium sulfate. The usual doses of ritodrine and terbutaline are shown in Boxes 15.4 and 15.5, respectively.

Magnesium sulfate treatment is an initial loading intravenous dose of 4 g of a 20 percent solution, followed by an infusion of 2–3 g/h until uterine contractions stop (Cox *et al.*, 1990). Infusions are usually continued for 12–24 h.

Box 15.4 Protocol for intravenous ritodrine[a]

Initial, 50–100 µg/min
Incremental increases, 50 µg/min every 20 min
Maximum dose, 350 µg/min

[a]See manufacturer's recommendations.

Box 15.5 Protocol for terbutaline

Intravenous	*Subcutaneous*
Initial, 2.5 mg/min	Dose, 250 µg every hour until contractions stop
Increases, 2.5 mg/min every 20 min	Oral
Maximum, 20 mg	Dose, 2.5–5 mg q 4–6 h

Indomethacin is given in an initial oral dose of 100 mg followed by 25 mg orally every 4 h for 48 h (Carlan *et al.*, 1992). Sulindac is given in an oral dose of 200 mg every 12 h for 48 h (Carlan *et al.*, 1992).

UTERINE HYPERTONUS OR 'FETAL DISTRESS'

The usual ritodrine dose in this clinical setting is an intravenous bolus of 1–3 mg over 2 min, and for terbutaline, 0.25 mg subcutaneously or intravenously (Smith, 1991). Magnesium sulfate can also be given in a 4 g intravenous bolus.

EXTERNAL VERSIONS OF BREECH PRESENTATION

Ritodrine and terbutaline may be used to relax the uterus prior to attempting external version of breech presentations. Preference has been to use terbutaline in a dose of 0.25 mg intravenously. If ritodrine is chosen, a dose of 1–3 mg intravenously over 2 min should be used (Fernandez *et al.*, 1996).

IMMUNOSUPPRESSANTS DURING PREGNANCY

Immunosuppressants are indicated for use during pregnancy only as therapy for specific life-threatening situations and the majority of cases have no other options. Three primary indications for immunosuppressant use during pregnancy are: (1) organ transplant maintenance; (2) treatment of autoimmune disease; and (3) systemic lupus. Most posttransplantation immunosuppressive regimens include prednisone with either azathioprine or cyclosporine. This raises the issue of the possible small risk of cleft palate associated with prednisone during pregnancy (see Chapter 13, Use of dermatologics during pregnancy). Virtually all the known immunosuppressants (Box 15.6), even proximate metabolites of the very large molecule cyclosporine, will cross the placenta (Little, 1997). Neonates are at high risk for a transiently compromised immune system when exposed to the effects of immunosuppressant drug(s). Hence, risk of opportunistic infection is a danger until the infant's immune system recovers following exposure to immunosuppressant therapy. Long-term effects on the infant's immune system are unknown.

Box 15.6 Immunosuppressant agents

Adrenocorticoids	Gold salts (Myochrysine, Ridaura, Solganol)
Azathioprine (Imuran)	Monoclonal antibody
Chloroquine (Aralen)	Muromonab-CD3 (Orthoclone OKT3)
Corticosteroids	Tacrolimus
Cyclosporine (Samdimmune)	

Immunosuppressant agents

Immunosuppressants reduce the immune response by toxicity action on, downregulation of, and/or decreased production of immune system components, especially T cells. Chronic long-term use of immunosuppressants has been associated with a higher incidence of neoplastic disease. Relevance of this observation to exposure *in utero* is unknown.

AZATHIOPRINE

Azathioprine is a 6-mercaptopurine derivative and a purine antimetabolite that acts by suppression of T-lymphocytes and cell-mediated immunity. *In vivo*, the drug is metabolized to mercaptopurine. It is used to treat autoimmune diseases and to prevent transplant rejection. Dose-dependent maternal side effects include bone marrow suppression, increased susceptibility to infection, alopecia, rash, gastrointestinal disturbances, arthralgias, hypersensitivity, pancreatitis, and toxic hepatitis (Berkowitz *et al.*, 1986).

Among 154 infants born to renal transplant recipients treated with azathioprine and prednisone throughout gestation, congenital anomalies occurred among 9 percent (four of 44) and 6.4 percent (seven of 110), respectively (Penn *et al.*, 1980; Registration Committee, 1980). No pattern of anomalies was present. It is not possible to determine whether this rate of congenital anomalies is higher than expected because these mothers took other drugs in addition to azathioprine, and were ill.

Prematurity and fetal growth retardation are increased in frequency among infants born to renal transplant recipients treated with azathioprine compared to infants born to healthy untreated women (Penn *et al.*, 1980; Pirson *et al.*, 1985; Registration Committee, 1980). The disease process itself (i.e., the need for renal transplantation) may be responsible in part for prematurity and growth retardation. Conditions resulting in chronic renal failure, such as hypertension, diabetes, and other vascular diseases, are also associated with an increased frequency of prematurity and/or growth retardation.

An increased frequency of congenital anomalies (limb defects, ocular anomalies, and cleft palate) occurred among the offspring of experimental animals born to mothers treated with azathioprine in doses similar to those used medically in humans (Davison, 1994; Rosenkrantz *et al.*, 1967; Tuchmann-Duplessis and Mercier-Parot, 1964; Williamson and Karp, 1981), but not in other studies (Fein *et al.*, 1983; Rosenkrantz *et al.*, 1967; Tuchmann-Duplessis and Mercier-Parot, 1964).

A case report of fatal neonatal pancytopenia was published of an infant born to a renal transplant recipient treated with azathioprine and prednisone during pregnancy (DeWitte *et al.*, 1984). Neonatal lymphopenia and thrombocytopenia were reported in several other children born to women who received similar therapy (Davidson *et al.*, 1985; Lower *et al.*, 1971; Penn *et al.*, 1980; Price *et al.*, 1976; Rudolf *et al.*, 1979). These disorders are similar to those reported among adults on these medications.

Frequencies of acquired chromosomal breaks and rearrangements were increased in somatic cells of renal transplant recipients receiving azathioprine therapy and, transiently, in the infants of women who were given such treatment during pregnancy (Price *et al.*, 1976; Sharon *et al.*, 1974). One child with two separate *de novo* constitutional chromosomal anomalies was born to a woman treated before and during pregnancy with azathioprine and prednisone (Ostrer et al., 1984). Relevance of either observation to clinical situations is unclear. Importantly, chromosome abnormalities in somatic cells cannot be extrapolated to interpret possible gonadal effects.

CYCLOSPORINE

Cyclosporine is a large molecule (cyclic polypeptide) of fungal origin that is used as an immunosuppressant in the prevention and treatment of allograft rejection. It acts on cell-mediated immunity and T-cell-dependent humoral immunity (Hou, 1989). Cyclosporine, > 1000 in molecular weight, metabolizes to several amino acids ranging from 300 to 500 in molecular weight, that easily cross the placenta, resulting in detectable fetal levels (Claris et al., 1993; Lewis et al., 1983). Maternal risks of cyclosporine use include hypertension, nephrotoxicity, hepatotoxicity, tremor, hirsutism, paresthesias, seizures, gout, and gingival hypertrophy (Berkowitz et al., 1986). Doses of cyclosporine need not be increased during pregnancy to maintain therapeutic levels although body weight and blood volume increase during pregnancy. One study found that cyclosporine doses needed to be lowered during the later stages of pregnancy (Flechner et al., 1985). Cyclosporine has been detected in breast milk, with breastfeeding contraindicated in patients who remain on cyclosporine (Flechner et al., 1985). Blood levels of cyclosporine decline to 50 percent at 48 h postpartum and should be undetectable at 1 week (Berkowitz et al., 1986). Thus, suppression of the infant's immune system should be short-lived (Rose et al., 1989). One report found persistent (1–3 months) hematologic abnormalities in newborns from renal transplant mothers receiving cyclosporine A, azathioprine, and methylprednisolone (Takahashi et al., 1994).

There have been no studies of the frequency of congenital anomalies among infants born to women treated with cyclosporine during pregnancy. The frequency of abortions (spontaneous and induced) and preterm deliveries was higher among cyclosporine-exposed pregnancies (Haugen et al., 1994).

The frequency of malformations was not increased among rats and rabbits whose mothers were treated with doses within several multiples of the usual human therapeutic doses of cyclosporine. Maternal toxicity, fetal growth retardation, and intrauterine death were increased in frequency in both species at doses at or just above the maximum used therapeutically in humans (Brown et al., 1985; Mason et al., 1985; Ryffel et al., 1983).

TACROLIMUS

Tacrolimus is a cyclosporine-like immunosuppressant. It decreases T-cell production by inhibiting enzymes essential to T-cell proliferation. Several small case series or case reports of the use of tacrolimus during pregnancies of transplant patients have been published (Jain et al., 1993; Laifer et al., 1994; Yoshimura et al., 1996). There were no malformations and pregnancy outcome was uneventful except for slightly reduced birth weight and transient immunocompromise.

Among 100 pregnancies in women treated with tacrolimus, 71 infants were born and four (5.6 percent) had congenital anomalies (Kainz et al., 2000). Another clinical series reported favorable outcomes in pregnancies maintained on tacrolimus (Garcia-Donaire et al., 2005). This is no different from the rate in the general population. The frequency of congenital anomalies was not increased among mice exposed to the drug during embryogenesis, although litter weights were slightly reduced (Farley et al., 1991).

PREDNISONE AND PREDNISOLONE

Corticosteroids are among the most commonly used immunosuppressants. Use of both prednisone, which is metabolized to prednisolone, and prednisolone during pregnancy has been studied intensively (see Chapter 13, Use of dermatologics during pregnancy).

MONOCLONAL ANTIBODY

T-lymphocyte monoclonal antibodies can eradicate circulating T cells within hours of administration. Acute rejection reactions to organ transplantation can be treated acutely and prophylactically with monoclonal antibodies. Untoward maternal effects include increased vulnerability to infection and neoplasm. Other side effects include tremor, headache, anaphylactic shock, chest pain, hypotension, neurospasm, pulmonary edema, gastrointestinal upset, rash, and allograft vascular thrombosis.

No studies or case reports have been published of congenital anomalies in infants born to mothers treated with this type of agent. According to its manufacturer, it is unknown if muromonab-CD3 is excreted in breast milk.

GOLD COMPOUNDS

Gold salts act as immunosuppressants via both the humoral and cell-mediated mechanisms, are antirheumatic agents, and cross the placenta (Gimovsky and Montoro, 1991). Patients taking gold compounds should delay conception for 1–2 months after cessation of therapy. Fetal exposure to gold compounds has adverse neonatal renal and hemolytic effects.

The frequency of congenital anomalies was not increased among more than 100 infants born to women treated with gold salts during the first trimester (Miyamoto *et al.*, 1974). According to the manufacturers, gold compounds were shown to be teratogenic in some but not all animal studies.

CHLOROQUINE

This antimalarial agent also has some immunosuppressant properties and has been utilized for the treatment of rheumatoid arthritis. It should be avoided in pregnancy if possible (see Chapter 2, Antimicrobials during pregnancy).

SPECIAL CONSIDERATIONS

Autoimmune disorders

'All autoimmune disorders occur more frequently in women' (Gimovsky and Montoro, 1991). Many women of reproductive age have disorders that require immunosuppressant therapy and clinicians providing care for pregnant women can expect to encounter gravid patients who are receiving immunosuppressant therapy.

Systemic lupus erythematosus

Systemic lupus erythematosus (SLE) is rare during pregnancy, ranging from approximately one in 2952 deliveries (Gimovsky and Montoro, 1991; Gimovsky *et al.*, 1984) to one in 5000 pregnancies (Tozman *et al.*, 1982). It is sometimes first manifested during pregnancy and can adversely affect pregnancy with increases in abortion, prematurity,

Box 15.7 Indications for steroid therapy in pregnant women with systemic lupus erythematosus (SLE)

Central nervous system involvement	Nephritis
Hemolytic anemia	Pericarditis
Leukopenia	Pleuritis
Myocarditis	Thrombocytopenia

From Gimovsky and Montoro, 1991.

intrauterine death, and congenital heart block (Gimovsky and Montoro, 1991; Gimovsky *et al.*, 1984). Among an estimated 20–60 percent of gravid SLE, the disease is exacerbated during pregnancy (Gimovsky *et al.*, 1984; Mintz *et al.*, 1986; Mor-Yosef *et al.*, 1984). Newborns whose mothers had SLE during pregnancy may manifest a transient lupus-like picture and congenital heart block (Scott *et al.*, 1983; Watson *et al.*, 1984).

Glucocorticoids are the agents most commonly used to treat SLE during pregnancy (Dombroski, 1989; Gimovsky and Montoro, 1991). It would seem reasonable to continue the patient on steroids if she was on such therapy when the pregnancy was recognized, or if steroids are required during pregnancy (Box 15.7).

Prednisone is the adrenocorticoid most often used to treat patients with SLE. The usual starting dose is 60 mg/day and this can be increased or decreased as needed to control symptoms of the disease (Gimovsky and Montoro, 1991).

It is controversial whether patients should be treated with large-dose steroid therapy at the time of delivery and early postpartum period (Dombroski, 1989). Asymptomatic gravid patients who were not on steroid therapy before the pregnancy will not necessarily require such therapy during pregnancy and postpartum. Steroid dose should be increased during pregnancy for women who are maintained on steroid therapy and who have active disease during gestation. Intravenous hydrocortisone (100 mg) can be given every 6–8 h during labor and the first 24 h postpartum. Beyond 24 h postpartum, the patient can be returned to her usual maintenance dose of steroids. Low-dose aspirin may be used as necessary throughout pregnancy in patients with lupus anticoagulant.

Other immunosuppressants (e.g., azathioprine, cyclophosphamide – an alkylating agent) may be used in pregnant women with SLE exacerbations who are refractory to high-dose steroids. According to the manufacturer, the dose of azathioprine is lower for patients with SLE than for patients with organ transplants. Notably, it is recommended that alkylating agents be avoided in early pregnancy if possible, but they can be used during the second and third trimesters of pregnancy (Glantz, 1994). The antimalarial agent chloroquine has been used to treat SLE and in usual doses (for malaria) carry little risk to the fetus (Dombroski, 1989).

Etiology, pathogenesis, and diagnosis of SLE have been expertly reviewed elsewhere (Gimovsky and Montoro, 1991).

Rheumatoid arthritis

Rheumatoid arthritis affects women more frequently than men. It seems common among women of childbearing age, although the prevalence of this disease during

Box 15.8 Agents utilized for the treatment of rheumatoid arthritis

Salicylates	Chloroquine[a]
Nonsteroidal anti-inflammatory agents (NSAIDs)	Gold salts
Steroids	Penicillamine[a]

[a]Not recommended for use during pregnancy.
Adapted from Gimovsky and Montoro, 1991.

pregnancy is unknown. Up to two-thirds of the patients with rheumatoid arthritis experience marked improvement during pregnancy (Neely and Persellin, 1977; Ostensen and Husby, 1983; Unger et al., 1983), suggesting that pregnancy may improve the symptoms of rheumatoid arthritis.

The mainstay of therapy for both pregnant and nonpregnant women with rheumatoid arthritis is aspirin (Box 15.8). To achieve therapeutic blood levels of 15–25 mg/dL, patients may require up to 4 g of salicylates daily (Thurnau, 1983). However, during pregnancy lower doses of salicylates (up to 3 g per day) are recommended. Large-dose salicylate therapy during pregnancy could cause hemorrhagic complications in the fetus, because salicylates cross the placenta. These complications may also occur in newborns and/or mothers.

Nonsteroidal antiinflammatory agents (NSAIDs) can be used in pregnant women with rheumatoid arthritis. These agents can be associated with mild to moderate oligohydramnios, premature closure of the ductus arteriosus and persistent fetal circulation, as well as intracranial hemorrhage in the neonate (Chapter 8, Analgesics during pregnancy). Chloroquine, as a mild immunosuppressant, has been used to treat rheumatoid arthritis and SLE, but because of low efficacy it is generally not recommended to treat pregnant women who have rheumatoid arthritis.

Penicillamine (Cuprimine) is used for rheumatoid arthritis, but should not be used during pregnancy. It is a chelating agent used in lead poisoning. However, its mechanism of action as an antirheumatoid agent is not understood. It crosses the placenta and is contraindicated for use during pregnancy because it interrupts fetal collagen formation (Gimovsky and Montoro, 1991) and is considered a human teratogen (Shepard, 1989).

Immunosuppressant drugs such as cyclosporine and azathioprine are used to treat rheumatoid arthritis in nonpregnant patients (Kerstens et al., 1995; Kruger and Schattenkirchner, 1994). These agents should be reserved to treat pregnant women with severe disease refractory to more commonly used agents with which there is greater clinical experience and published data.

Organ transplantation

Progress in organ transplantation and pharmacological therapy over the past three decades is significant. Occurrence of renal transplantation and subsequent pregnancy is increasing, and the literature on the subject is growing.

Renal transplantation

Among more than 800 pregnancies (from seven reports) after renal transplantation, there were 0.5 percent maternal deaths, 6–8 percent miscarriages, 12–20 percent therapeutic abortions, 1 percent stillbirths, and 2 percent neonatal deaths (Hou, 1989; Radomski *et al.*, 1995). Three first-line medications are used to prevent rejection following renal transplantation: corticosteroids, azathioprine, and cyclosporine. Corticosteroid, cyclosporine, azathioprine, and tacrolimus therapy have been discussed above.

Cyclosporine is key to decreasing the frequency of renal transplant rejection, especially of cadaver kidneys (Hou, 1989). This immunosuppressant agent's metabolites cross the placenta. If the situation is life threatening, the benefits of its use clearly outweigh any risks. Fetal growth retardation was reported in infants whose mothers used cyclosporine (Hou, 1989; Pickrell *et al.*, 1988; Radomski *et al.*, 1995), but it is not possible to differentiate drug effects from the renal disease being treated (e.g., chronic hypertension is a concomitant complication).

Pregnant women should be counseled for the increased risks of both maternal and fetal infection, and the possible increased risk of genital carcinoma associated with immunosuppressant therapy (Kossay *et al.*, 1988). Notably, women who have symptoms of rejection within 3 months of delivery usually progress to loss of the renal transplant within the next 24 months. The medical significance of the correct immunosuppressant therapy during pregnancy is emphasized by these sequelae.

Other organ transplantation

Several reports of pregnancies following liver, heart and heart–lung, and bone marrow transplants have been published (Deeg *et al.*, 1983; Kallen *et al.*, 2005; Key *et al.*, 1989; Kossay *et al.*, 1988; Lowenstein *et al.*, 1988; Miniero *et al.*, 2004; Newton *et al.*, 1988; Rose *et al.*, 1989; Walcott *et al.*, 1978). Immunosuppressant therapy, especially with regard to cyclosporine, is utilized similarly with other organ transplants as with renal transplantation. Among 152 infants born after transplantation, a high frequency of preeclampsia (22 percent), preterm birth (46 percent), low birthweight (41 percent), infants small for gestational age (16 percent), and infant death were found for deliveries after transplantation. Congenital anomalies were not increased in frequency (Kallen *et al.*, 2005).

Heart transplantation

More than 40 infants have been born to women with heart transplants (Miniero *et al.*, 2004; Radomski *et al.*, 1995; Scott *et al.*, 1993). Mothers were treated with cyclosporine or azathioprine throughout gestation. Signs of organ rejection occurred in about one-quarter of mothers, and about one-third of infants were of low birthweight and premature. The pregnancies, mothers' postpartum, and neonatal course were complicated by infection.

Liver transplantation

Among 38 pregnancies to 29 women with liver transplants, 13 percent of mothers had signs of organ rejection (Radomski *et al.*, 1995). There were 31 live births (eight abortions) and 32 percent were of low birthweight, with 39 percent premature. Slightly more than one-quarter of the pregnancies were complicated by infection. Among 15 infants born after liver transplantation, two were malformed (Kallen *et al.*, 2005).

Box 15.9 Agents utilized for the treatment of inflammatory bowel disease

Ulcerative colitis	Crohn's disease
5-aminosalicylic acid	6-mercaptopurine
6-mercaptopurine	Azathioprine
Azathioprine	Cyclosporine
Prednisone	Prednisone
Sulfasalazine	

Inflammatory bowel disease

Two of the most common forms of inflammatory bowel disease are ulcerative colitis and Crohn's disease (regional enteritis). The etiology of these diseases is unknown. Corticosteroids (i.e., prednisone) have been used for the active stages of both diseases (Box 15.9). Sulfasalazine and 5-aminosalicylic acid have also been used successfully for the treatment of ulcerative colitis during pregnancy (Cunningham, 1994; Habal *et al.*, 1993).

Refractory cases of ulcerative colitis and Crohn's disease during pregnancy are an indication for immunosuppressive drugs, such as azathioprine and 6-mercaptopurine (Cunningham, 1994). In a meta-analysis of azathioprine and 6-mercaptopurine to treat Crohn's disease, both drugs were effective in treating active disease and for maintaining remission (Pearson *et al.*, 1995), but efficacy during pregnancy was not studied. Agents utilized for the treatment of inflammatory bowel disease (Box 15.9) include cyclosporine for the treatment of Crohn's disease (Brynskov *et al.*, 1989). It seems reasonable to reserve these more potent immunosuppressants for pregnant women refractory to steroid therapy.

Multiple sclerosis

Immunosuppressants are used to treat secondary, progressive, and relapsing multiple sclerosis. The agents currently used are azathioprine, cyclophosphamide, cyclosporine, and methotrexate. Treatment of multiple sclerosis relapse with immunosuppressants is controversial. Treatment of multiple sclerosis with these drugs during pregnancy carries a risk of birth defects similar to use of the drug for other purposes. However, it should be noted that potential for adverse effects decreases as the dose is lowered (e.g., cyclophosphamide 'booster' doses).

SUMMARY

Immunosuppressant agents are used in pregnant women to treat a variety of diseases, including collagen-vascular disease and organ transplantation. Steroids, azathioprine, and cyclosporine are the agents most frequently used to treat collagen-vascular disease and organ transplantation, and apparently can be used in pregnant women with minimal risk to the fetus. Steroids seem to pose little or no risk to intrauterine development after the first trimester or to the mothers. Azathioprine and cyclosporine have not been studied adequately, and exposure in the first trimester has not been adequately assessed. However, organ transplant rejection is life-threatening and any risk is outweighed by the benefit.

Key references

Garcia-Donaire JA, Acevedo M, Gutierrez MJ *et al*. Tacrolimus as basic immunosuppression in pregnancy after renal transplantation. A single-center experience. *Transplant Proc* 2005; **37**: 3754.

Idama TO, Lindow SW. Magnesium sulphate. A review of clinical pharmacology applied to obstetrics. *Br J Obstet Gynaecol* 1998; **105**: 260.

Johnson KA, Mason GC. Severe hypotension and fetal death due to tocolysis with nifedipine. *BJOG* 2005; **112**: 1583.

Kainz A, Harabacz I, Cowlrick IS *et al*. Review of the course and outcome of 100 pregnancies in 84 women treated with tacrolimus. *Transplantation* 2000; **70**: 1718.

Kallen B, Westgren M, Aberg A, Olausson PO. Pregnancy outcome after maternal organ transplantation in Sweden. *BJOG* 2005; **112**: 904.

Kandysamy V, Thomson AJ. Severe hypotension and fetal death due to tocolysis with nifedipine. *BJOG* 2005; **112**: 1583.

Leveno KL, Little BB, Cunningham FG. National impact of tocolytic therapy on low birth weight. *Obstet Gynecol* 1990; **76**: 12.

Little BB. Immunosuppressant therapy during gestation. *Semin Perinatol* 1997; **21**: 143.

Miniero R, Tardivo I, Centofanti P *et al*. Pregnancy in heart transplant recipients. *J Heart Lung Transplant* 2004; **23**: 898.

Tsukahara H, Kobata R, Tamura S, Mayumi M. Neonatal bone abnormalities attributable to maternal administration of magnesium sulphate. *Pediatr Radiol* 2004; **34**: 673.

van Veen AJ, Pelinck MJ, van Pampus MG, Erwich JJ. Severe hypotension and fetal death due to tocolysis with nifedipine. *BJOG* 2005; **112**: 509.

Yoshimura N, Oka T, Fujiwara Y, Ohmori Y, Yasumura T, Honjo H. A case report of pregnancy in renal transplant recipient treated with FK506 (tacrolimus). *Transplantation* 1996; **61**: 1552.

Further references are available on the book's website at http://www.drugsandpregnancy.com

16

Substance abuse during pregnancy

Pregnant substance abusers are frequently (>50 percent) unmarried, have no prenatal care, or began using prenatal care late in pregnancy, and are dependent upon public health care resources. The substances most frequently used during pregnancy include: alcohol, cocaine, heroin, methamphetamine, and tobacco. Alcohol use with tobacco is frequently part of a polydrug use, but a small percentage of women use only alcohol. Typically, pregnant substance abusers are dependent on public assistance for medical care (Slutsker *et al.*, 1993). Use of mood-altering chemicals without medical supervision is widely prevalent in the USA today. According to some sources (Rouse, 1996), prevalence is as high as 70–90 percent of the population and women between 15 and 40 years of age use such substances and often conceive while using them (Finnegan, 1994). There are substantial health risks for pregnant women and their unborn children because of social and illicit substance use during gestation. The most critical period for the induction of congenital anomalies is the first trimester (specifically the first 58 days postconception) (see Chapter 1, Introduction to drugs in pregnancy). Importantly, most women do not know that they are pregnant during early gestation. Their usual life style practices are thus superimposed on the critical period of pregnancy, embryogenesis. Fetal development in the second and third trimesters of pregnancy is also a time of great vulnerability, and continued substance use during this period also carries the risk of atypical development (i.e., some congenital anomalies, but mainly growth retardation). Virtually every substance of abuse for which there is information crosses the placenta (Box 16.1) (Little and Vanbeveren, 1996).

Box 16.1 Substances of abuse that are known to cros placenta

Alcohol	Heroin	Methadone
Amphetamine	Inhalants (toluene)	Methamphe
Barbiturate	LSD (lysergic acid	Morphine
Benzodiazepines	diethylamide)	PCP (phencyclidine)
Cocaine	Marijuana	Tobacco (nicotine)
Codeine	Mescaline	Ts and Blues (pentazocine)

From Little and VanBeveren, 1996.

CLINICAL EVALUATION

Medicolegal considerations

Physician knowledge of patient use of social and illicit substances during pregnancy places certain legal obligations on the care providers. The intake interview and medical history-taking process should be sufficiently thorough to discover information regarding the use of potentially dangerous substances. Upon discovery of an exposure, the important second step is to determine timing of exposures during pregnancy, and the nature and extent of the social or illicit substance use. If the exposure actually occurred during gestation, the obstetrician needs to know as much as possible about the teratogenic and toxic potentials of the substance or combinations of substances. The physician may have his or her own resources for researching the topic or may refer the patient to a specialist. Medicolegally, the physician must disclose fully to the patient medically known risks that are posed by maternal substance abuse. This disclosure should also be documented in the medical record in a clear and concise manner. It is extremely important that the physician emphasizes to the patient that the use of social or illicit substances is totally contraindicated during the course of pregnancy.

These are not theoretical concerns because we have assisted in the defense of physicians sued for adverse pregnancy outcomes caused by substance abuse, despite the physician's appropriate counseling that the patient chose to ignore. The risk–benefit ratio for substance abuse during pregnancy is easily explained to be increased risk with no benefit. The patient consultation, particularly this aspect, must be documented in the medical record to show that the risk was recognized and patient appropriately advised. Patients have been asked to initial or sign counseling notes regarding substance abuse during pregnancy to acknowledge that they received and understood counseling. The sections that follow document the maternal and fetal medical risks for specific substances including: alcohol, amphetamine, cocaine, heroin, inhalants, lysergic acid diethylamide (LSD), marijuana, methadone, mushrooms, methamphetamine, morphine, phencyclidine (PCP), tobacco, and T's and blues.

Patient consultation

Pregnant women usually admit to some use of a substance, but rarely do they admit that they have a 'problem' with social or illicit substance. Once some substance use is admit-

., two tandem approaches to the history-taking process are suggested. Differences in substance use between weekdays and weekends are important to ascertain, because it is common for the user's pattern of use to differ greatly between these two time periods. The patient should describe her daily activities, including any substances used, from awakening to going to sleep at night on a normal weekday. Weekend activities and substance use should be assessed similarly. The second approach is to ask about substance use in particular. The patient should be asked when she begins drinking or using drugs during the course of a day and the duration of such use. For example, does the patient use the substance as an 'eye-opener' in the morning (Sokol et al., 1989) and is it what she uses to go to sleep. The patient should be asked to disclose how much of the substance is used in an average day and approximately how much would be consumed in an hour. Combined with information about the weekly pattern (weekend versus weekday), a semiquantitative estimate of the amount and frequency of substance use can be made.

Alcohol use during pregnancy is well studied and crude risks of fetal alcohol syndrome can actually be made by estimating the average daily dose. With other less well-researched substances used during pregnancy, daily dose information can be used only to assess the severity of maternal addiction. Very serious dependencies are, of course, associated with more severe adverse effects. At the outset, the physician should explain to the patient that the purpose of obtaining this personal and private information is to better manage the pregnancy, i.e., to give medical care more suited to the patient's specific needs. The patient should also be reassured that this information is

Table 16.1 Summary of embryo-fetal effects of social and illicit substance use during pregnancy

Substance	FGR	Congenital anomalies	Withdrawal syndrome	Perinatal morbidity	Documented syndrome
Alcohol	+	+	+	+	+
Amphetamines	+	?(−)	+	+	−
Barbituates	+	?(−)	+	+	+
Benzodiazepines	?(+)	?(−)	?(+)	+	−
Cocaine	+	+	+	+	−
Codeine	+	(−)	+	+	−
Heroin	+	−	+	+	−
Inhalants	+	+	?(−)	+	+
LSD	?	(−)	?(−)	?	?
Marijuana	+	−	−	+	−
Methadone	+	−	+	+	−
Methamphetamine	+	−	+	+	−
Morphine	+	(−)	+	+	−
PCP	+	?	+	+	?
Tobacco	+	−	−	+	−
Ts and Blues	+	(−)	+	+	−

FGR, fetal growth restriction; LSD, lysergic acid diethylamide; PCP, phencyclidine. +, Documented, positive; −, documented, negative; (−) data inconclusive but suggestive of a negative finding; (+) data inconclusive but suggestive of a positive finding; ?, unknown.
Modified from Little et al., 1990b.

Table 16.2 Summary of maternal effects of social and illicit substance use during pregnancy

Substance	Abruption	CNS Damage	ICH	Metabolic acidosis	Anorexia	Hepatorenal damage	Endocarditis (parenteral use)
Alcohol	+	+	−	+	+	+	NA
Amphetamines	(+)	+	+	?	+	?	+
Barbituates	−	+	+	?	+	?	?
Benzodiazepines	−	+	−	?	+	?	?
Cocaine[a]	+	+	+	?	+	+	+
Codeine	−	+	−	?	+	?	+
Heroin	+	+	+	+	+	+	+
Inhalants	?	+	−	+	+	+	NA
LSD	?	+	−	?	+	?	NA
Marijuana	−	(−)	−	?	−	−	−
Methadone	+	+	−	?	+	+	+
Methamphetamine	(+)	+	?	?	+	?	+
Morphine	(+)	+	−	?	+	+	+
PCP	?	(+)	(+)	?	+	+	?
Tobacco	+	(−)	−	?	+	+	NA
Ts and Blues[a]	(+)	(+)	(+)	?	+	+	+

CNS, central nervous system; ICH, intracranial hemorrhage; LSD, lysergic acid diethylamide; PCP, phencyclidine.

+, Documented, positive; (−), documented, negative; (−) data inconclusive but suggestive of a negative finding; (+) data inconclusive but suggestive of a positive finding; ? unknown; NA, not applicable/not available.

[a]Infarction/embolism.

Modified from Little et al., 1990b.

confidential. In the USA, these records are protected by Federal Law (CFR 37). The author's spouse is an attorney, and states that no release should ever be signed and that each person must protect their individual rights to privacy assertively.

Another important aspect of patient consultation is to provide information regarding specific risks from substance use (Tables 16.1 and 16.2). It is important that this information be as accurate as possible. 'Scare' tactics or exaggeration-type deterrents should be avoided because substance users are aware of this commonly employed approach and trust in the physician and his/her credibility will be eroded. The most ethical and legally sound approach is to provide information that may be verified directly with the medical literature. We currently use a standardized summary generated from a computerized database [Teratogen Information System (TERIS), see Chapter 1] for this information. The TERIS summaries are more detailed than this book's chapters and are very well documented. Ultimately, the clinical conclusion/treatment is that social and illicit substance use during pregnancy is contraindicated because of the associated maternal and embryo fetal risks.

The need for services to assist pregnant substance users is being recognized, and programs exist in most areas. For assistance in locating such a treatment program, the physician can contact their local substance abuse service, or their state's commission on substance abuse that accredits treatment facilities. Ideally, the pregnant substance user should be managed by the obstetrician in conjunction with a program designed to promote abstinence or at least to reduce the substance use during pregnancy. The medical positions of abstinence and treatment are the only appropriate ones clinically and legally.

Patient evaluation

Note: Use of 'legal, legally, etc.' is not intended as a substitution for legal advice and the reader is cautioned to contact a licenced attorney when confronted with questions concerning issues of the law and its application in the situation confronted, as noted in Chapter 1. Laws vary from state to state and from nation to nation. One's medical malpractice insurance provider is often the most economical and efficient source of legal information as this service is often included as a provision of a medical malpractice policy.

The pregnant substance user should be considered a high-risk obstetric patient. Pregnant substance users are at increased risk for a number of complications, including sexually transmitted diseases (STDs), hepatitis, poor nutrition, and bacterial endocarditis. With the exception of tobacco and marijuana, chronic use of the substances reviewed in this chapters is an indication for syphilis, gonorrhea, herpes, chlamydia, HIV, and hepatitis testing. Women who use drugs administered by the parenteral route are at greatest risk not only for HIV but also for other STDs, including hepatitis. Drug injection sites on the upper forearm ('track marks') are strong evidence of a serious substance use problem, but this is not frequently observed. Among 122 gravid parenteral substance users (intravenous drug abusers, IVDAs), only one woman presented with track marks on the forearm. The other 121 IVDA women used hidden sites of injection (veins in breasts, thighs, calves, and ankles) (Little *et al.*, 1990b).

Substances of abuse usually have an anorectic effect and often result in poor weight gain during pregnancy. Other possible signs of substance use during pregnancy include new-onset 'spontaneously arising' heart murmur and hypertension not associated with preeclampsia. Heart murmurs occur with increased frequency among women who are chronic substance users. Heart murmurs also occur in association with bacterial endocarditis or a history of this disease. Chronic substance use can induce hypertension in the nonpregnant adult, although not all have been studied for hypertensive effects during pregnancy. Cocaine, heroin, and tobacco use is known to be associated with hypertension during pregnancy (Abel, 1980a,b; Little et al., 1989b, 1990a; Stillman et al., 1986). In addition, abruptio placentae or a history of this serious complication is also an indication that substance use may be a factor. Risk of abruptio placentae may be as high as 1–2 percent among substance abusers compared to 0.1 percent (one in 830) in the general population (Cunningham et al., 1997). Stillbirths are increased in frequency with substance use during pregnancy. A history of stillbirths may, along with other risk factors, be a clue to the obstetrician that substance abuse is a complicating factor.

Hidden risks of substance abuse: impurities

All substances of abuse, even alcohol, may be contaminated by certain impurities. 'Moonshine' (illegally distilled alcohol) can contain significant amounts of lead and cause heavy metal poisoning in the mother and fetus. Amphetamine and methamphetamines may contain impurities, such as lead oxides (Allcott et al., 1987). Leaded gasoline is sometimes used as the solvent, resulting in lead contamination in the extraction of cocaine paste from cocoa leaves. Production of illicit drugs, such as PCP, involve cyanohydrin intermediate reactions. If not fully reacted, cyanide may be contained in the final product because illicit laboratories are usually crudely equipped for purification, with no quality control. Lead and cyanide poisoning have resulted from the use of illicitly manufactured substances and are associated with significant maternal–fetal morbidity and mortality. In the manufacture of LSD, incomplete amination of lysergic acid or failure to purify the product, will result in lysergic acid toxicity (peripheral neuropathy and progressive necrosis) in humans and animals (Rall and Schleifer, 1985). Drugs available as tablets or capsules (for example, codeine, methadone, morphine, benzodiazepines, pentazocine) contain a significant amount of the tablet/capsule vehicle agent (usually more than 97 percent), typically microcrystalline cellulose. When prepared for parenteral use by the IVDA, the substance is frequently dissolved in water with no attempt to separate the drug from the vehicle, resulting in a very high potential for pulmonary emboli, placental infarcts, and other maternal vascular blockages.

Inhalants are aromatic (benzene ring-containing) substances, such as toluene or gasoline, that may also contain lead or nitriles that can cause toxicity. Even marijuana may contain dangerous vegetable contaminants such as nightshade, poison sumac, poison ivy, and poison oak, all of which may cause serious pulmonary-cardiac morbidity or even death when smoked. In addition, herbicides (e.g., paraquat) and/or pesticides (i.e., chlordane) may be contained in the marijuana itself as a result of treatment during the plant's growth, since there is no quality control of production practices (Klaassen, 1985). Death may also be associated with smoking marijuana contaminated with herbicides.

Other drugs and chemicals as dilutants

Other substances are used by dealers to 'cut' or dilute illicit drugs to increase their profits. Sometimes the dilutant is more dangerous than the illicit drug. Cocaine is cut with lidocaine, amphetamines, and sometimes fine glass beads. Amphetamines are diluted, sometimes heavily, with certain antihistamines or ephedrine. Heroin is known to have been cut with diverse compounds: talcum, confectioner's sugar, and even finely ground sawdust. Perhaps the most notorious case of the dilutant being more dangerous than the substance of abuse is cutting heroin with warfarin, leading to a cluster of warfarin embryopathy cases that were never published. Some of these dilutants were teratogenic and these and others may cause serious maternal and/or placental complications, especially when used parenterally. Strychnine and arsenic have been intentionally added to amphetamine, methamphetamine, cocaine, heroin, and LSD to intensify their effects, although the 'intensification' is actually due to subclinical strychnine/arsenic toxicity.

TREATMENT OF SUBSTANCE USE DURING PREGNANCY

Treatment of nonpregnant adults who have problems with substance use normally includes withdrawal from the substance. Opiates are the exception because methadone replacement/maintenance therapy is available for such drugs as heroin. Regimens used as an adjunct to assist in withdrawal include a benzodiazepine plus an antidepressant (e.g., diazepam and amitriptyline). Others have used diazepam and fluoxetine. A different pharmacological strategy is suppression of alpha-adrenergic action with drugs, such as clonidine, and to alleviate withdrawal symptoms, frequently with a benzodiazepine or barbiturate (nembutal) adjunct. Such regimens are given in doses adjusted to the individual case to facilitate asymptomatic withdrawal, and the dose is gradually decreased over periods ranging from 10 days to 3–6 months.

Substance addiction is a psychological phenomenon as well as a physical one, and both aspects must be addressed adequately in treatment protocols. Specialists in addiction psychology/psychiatry should be involved in the treatment plan early. Their recommendations may include private and/or group counseling, such as Narcotics Anonymous (NA) or Alcoholics Anonymous (AA). Physicians support these programs because they increase patient success rate.

We reported that in patient substance abuse treatment during pregnancy was associated with increased birth weight and head circumference, and fewer perinatal complications compared to untreated matched substance-abusing pregnant controls (Little *et al.*, 2003). Prenatal care and routine substance abuse screening was part of the program.

Obstetrical goals of substance abuse treatment

Minimization of maternal and fetal/infant morbidity and mortality is the obstetrical goal of substance abuse treatment during pregnancy. In one study, prenatal care was the main determinant of pregnancy outcome among substance abusers, not attaining abstinence (MacGregor *et al.*, 1989). Regardless of continued substance use, regular prenatal care was associated with better pregnancy outcomes than those who did not have prenatal care. This observation is important to obstetrical goals in the treatment of the gravid substance user (risks to both the mother and the fetus) because it implies that the single most important intervention in the pregnancy of a substance abuser is to provide prenatal care early and regularly.

When considering treatment for the pregnant substance abuser, the risks from continued substance use (for example, maintenance) versus risk of withdrawal, and the benefits of withdrawal, i.e., improved fetal growth, must be evaluated. Based upon anecdotal data from the 1970s (Rementeria and Nunag, 1973), it was recommended that withdrawal from heroin or methadone not be attempted after 32 weeks of gestation because of the possible risk of abruptio placentae, preterm labor, premature rupture of membranes (PROM), or fetal death in more advanced pregnancies. However, recent clinical experience does not support these increased risks with withdrawal (Luty *et al.*, 2003). Currently, withdrawal of the gravid patient from substances of abuse is generally advocated, although no generally accepted regimen is recommended for use during pregnancy. As with nonpregnant adults, a benzodiazepine and antidepressant or a benzodiazepine and a low-dose alpha-blocker (e.g., clonidine) regimen has been used to assist pregnant women withdrawing from a wide variety of substances, such as alcohol, cocaine, methamphetamine, and amphetamine. The primary danger of the alpha-blockers is maternal hypotension, which may impede placental perfusion. In France, buprenorphine has been used, and the incidence of adverse pregnancy outcomes was no different from controls (Auriacombe *et al.*, 2004). However, a neonatal withdrawal was reported with buprenorphine (Marquet *et al.*, 1997). Therefore, only minimal effective dose levels are used. Blood pressure and fetal heart rate should be monitored closely with this regimen. Doppler flow studies may prove useful for monitoring umbilical blood flow in these patients.

Naltrexone has been used to treat several substance dependencies during pregnancy without apparent untoward effects, but no long-term follow-up studies have been published (Hulse *et al.*, 2001). An alternative therapy with little or no potential for abuse is buprenorphine/naloxone (Suboxone), but there are no studies of its use during pregnancy. Disulfiram (Anabuse), a deterrent for alcohol abuse, should not be used at any time during pregnancy because of its strong copper-chelating properties. Copper is essential to normal fetal neuronal formation and migration, and any impediment in these processes may result in fetal brain malformations. Notably, this is a theoretical risk.

ALTERNATIVES TO TRADITIONAL TREATMENT FOR SUBSTANCE DEPENDENCE DURING PREGNANCY

Substance abuse during pregnancy can be treated without the use of substances that are addicting. New approaches for detoxification have included drug combinations, such as clonidine and naltrexone, and other drug regimens (Hulse *et al.*, 2001; Rayburn and Bogenschutz, 2004). A combined regimen of these two drugs has been successfully employed for rapid opioid withdrawal for outpatient treatment. The combination of naloxone with midazolam or methohexitone can be used for inpatient settings. Investigators also found that this treatment can be used by using the partial opioid-receptor agonist buprenorphine for either heroin or methadone addiction. Limited experience with clonidine transdermal patches has shown that these can be successfully applied in suppressing symptoms of withdrawal (MacGregor *et al.*, 1985). Low-dose nembutal as an adjunct may assist in sleep. Importantly, the use of low-dose clonidine does not seem to be associated with adverse effects on the course of pregnancy (Boutroy, 1989). Moreover, limited experience with this regimen seems to indicate that it is effective and does not pose serious risks to advanced pregnancies (beyond 32 weeks). However, these results come from uncontrolled, anecdotal studies and the ability to extrapolate is very limited. In 1993, the US Food and Drug Administration (FDA) approved a drug for the treatment of opioid dependence: levo-alpha-acetyl-methadol (LAAM). This drug has a slower onset and a longer half-life than methadone, and because it is a prodrug, its onset is slower when administered intravenously than when given orally. This reduces its potential for abuse (Rowe, 1993).

Risks of withdrawal

Data from the 1970s suggested an increased frequency of fetal deaths and maternal morbidity associated with opiate withdrawal, especially later in pregnancy (Finnegan *et al.*, 1977; Rementeria and Nunag, 1973). Pregnancies reported in these case reports and series were complicated by several other factors in addition to heroin addiction (i.e., hypertension, syphilis, and chorioamnionitis).

Risks of maintenance

The most common maintenance protocol for heroin-addicted gravidas involves the use of methadone. The efficacy of this regimen in such pregnancies is somewhat controversial (Edelin *et al.*, 1988). Babies born to mothers on methadone, as with heroin, may experience withdrawal symptoms. Methadone withdrawal symptoms occur much later (i.e., at or after 1 week after the birth) because of methadone's much longer half-life (30–40 h) compared to heroin (8–10 h). Furthermore, withdrawal symptoms of methadone-exposed infants are more severe than those of heroin-exposed infants, with more seizures and a greater number of days of displaying withdrawal symptoms in the maintained group (Blinick *et al.*, 1973). In addition, it was found that fetal growth retardation is more severe among methadone-exposed infants than among heroin-exposed infants (Blinick, 1973), a finding that was not supported by other studies (Lifschitz *et al.*, 1983; Soepatimi, 1986). Methadone withdrawal using dose tapering employing adjuvants such as numbutal were not associated with adverse pregnancy outcomes in a more recent study in a large public hospital where a number of studies of substance abuse were undertaken (Dashe *et al.*, 1998, 2002).

SPECIFIC SOCIAL AND ILLICIT SUBSTANCES USED DURING PREGNANCY

Substance use during pregnancy has not been studied as extensively as it should be to assess fully the risks to the embryo/fetus and to the mother. The available information is often confounded by many factors, including poor maternal health, lack of prenatal care, malnutrition, presence of infectious diseases, and the use of a myriad of substances. It is rare that a gravid substance user takes only one substance. The sections that follow are a summary of the known maternal-fetal effects of the 16 social and illicit substances most commonly used during pregnancy. This chapter concludes with a section that summarizes the complex issues that attend polydrug use during pregnancy. Each substance is described, highlights of human embryo-fetal risks are reviewed, and perinatal effects are defined. A summary of the embryo-fetal effects is given in Table 16.1 and a summary of the maternal effects in Table 16.2. Details underlying Tables 16.1 and 16.2 are discussed in the sections that follow.

Alcohol use during pregnancy and maternal alcoholism

Alcohol is a central nervous system depressant and its abuse during pregnancy has adverse effects on both the mother and the fetus. It is now a well known human and animal teratogen, a fact that was discovered in the USA in 1973 (Jones et al., 1973) and in France in 1968 (Lemoine et al., 1968).

PREVALENCE AND EPIDEMIOLOGY

The actual rate of alcohol use during pregnancy is not known, but up to 70 percent of the adult population in the USA use alcohol socially. Alcohol use during pregnancy ranges from less than 2 percent to more than 70 percent (Abel and Sokol, 1987; NIAAA, 1983). We found that the prevalence of drinking four or more drinks [2 ounces (59 ml) of absolute alcohol] per day was 1.4 percent in a large urban public hospital in Texas (Little et al., 1989a).

It is estimated that 30–50 percent of infants born to alcoholic women (those who consume eight or more drinks per day) have fetal alcohol syndrome (FAS) (Jones, 1989). We observed an 80 percent rate for FAS in the offspring of frankly alcoholic women – those who consumed eight or more drinks per day (Little et al., 1990a). The prevalence of fetal alcohol syndrome varies widely among countries and is estimated at one per 100 live births in northern France (Daehaene et al., 1977), one per 600 in Sweden (Olegard et al., 1979), and one per 750 in Seattle (Hanson et al., 1978). It averages 1.9 per 1000 live births worldwide (Abel and Sokol, 1987). In the USA, FAS is generally estimated to occur in 1.95 per 1000 live births (Abel, 1995). An estimated FAS prevalence of about one per 1000 live births was seen in Dallas, Texas (Little et al., 1990b).

Approximately 2–3 percent of pregnant women drink heavily (Abel and Sokol, 1987; NIAAA, 1983). The rate of infants born with FAS in 1993 is estimated to be 6.7 per 1000 births (MMWR, 1995). It is estimated that as many as 5 percent of congenital anomalies may be due to maternal alcohol intake during pregnancy (Sokol, 1981), although precise estimates of alcohol-induced birth defects are difficult to ascertain. Alcohol abuse during pregnancy appears to be the most frequent known teratogenic cause of mental retardation (Abel and Sokol, 1987; Clarren and Smith, 1978).

Maternal effects

Alcohol abuse during pregnancy generally affects the course of pregnancy negatively and reported adverse pregnancy outcomes related to alcohol consumption include stillbirths, premature deliveries, decreased placental weight, and spontaneous abortion (Parazzini et al., 1994). Such outcomes may occur even at low levels of alcohol consumption – less than four drinks per day (Little, 1977; Plant, 1984; Sokol et al., 1980; Streissguth et al., 1981).

'Binge' drinking during pregnancy carries significant risks of congenital anomalies and development abnormalities. Some studies on the effects of alcohol use of various durations during pregnancy has shown that occasional binge drinking by moderate drinkers did not negatively affect birth outcome (Autti-Ramo et al., 1992; Tolo and Little, 1993), but prenatal exposure to alcohol throughout gestation has been found to be associated with an increased rate of alcohol-related birth defects (Autti-Ramo and Granstrom, 1991; Coles et al., 1991). Continuous drinking throughout pregnancy appears to cause fetal damage in a dose-dependent manner (Halmesmaki, 1988). In addition, the frequency of sexually transmitted diseases and other infections is higher among women who abuse alcohol during pregnancy.

Effects on intrauterine development

A constellation of congenital anomalies called the fetal alcohol syndrome (FAS) was delineated in 1973 by Jones *et al.*, who described eight children born to mothers with chronic alcoholism. These anomalies repeatedly occurred among infants born to women who were chronic alcoholics, drinking eight or more such beverages every day (Clarren and Smith, 1978; Larroque, 1992; Sokol *et al.*, 1986; Streissguth *et al.*, 1980, 1981, 1985).

The diagnostic features of FAS are: (1) prenatal and postnatal growth deficiency (Faden and Graubard, 1994; Greene *et al.*, 1991; Larroque *et al.*, 1993); (2) mental retardation (Autti-Ramo *et al.*, 1992a; Jacobson *et al.*, 1993); (3) behavioral disturbances (Coles *et al.*, 1987); and (4) typical recognizable facial appearance (Box 16.2) (Autti-Ramo *et al.*, 1992b; Lewis and Woods, 1994). The most frequent congenital anomalies are heart defects (Loser *et al.*, 1992) and brain anomalies (Mattson *et al.*, 1992), but other major congenital anomalies (e.g., spina bifida, limb defects, genitourinary defects, eye anomalies, airway obstructions, renal hypoplasia) also occur (Carones *et al.*, 1992; Froster and Baird, 1992; Hinzpeter *et al.*, 1992; Lewis and Woods, 1994; Taylor *et al.*, 1994; Usowicz *et al.*, 1986). Absence of the full syndrome but presence of mild to moderate mental and physical growth retardation, and are known collectively as fetal alcohol effects (FAE) (Jones, 1989).

Box 16.2 Features of fetal alcohol syndrome

Craniofacial anomalies	*Major anomalies*
Absent-to-hypoplastic philtrum	Brain defects
Broad upper lip	Cardiac defects
Flattened nasal bridge	Spinal defects
Hypoplastic upper lip vermillion	Limb defects
Micrognathia	Genitourinary defects
Microphthalmia	
Short nose	
Short palpebral fissures	

Effects on postnatal development

In one study, children born to women who abused alcohol during pregnancy had physical growth delays of 2 years or more reported as the long-term consequences of intrauterine alcohol exposure on the child's physical and cognitive development. The investigators found that at 5 years of age the children whose mothers had continued drinking during pregnancy showed more alcohol-related deficits than non-alcohol-exposed children or children whose mothers stopped drinking in the second trimester of pregnancy. Transient withdrawal symptoms, including tremors, hypertonia, and irritability, were reported among infants born to women who chronically drank alcohol late in pregnancy (Coles *et al.*, 1984), and we have also observed similar findings at Parkland Memorial Hospital (Little *et al.*, 1990a).

Children continually exposed to alcohol had smaller heads, lower IQs, other deficits in intellectual functioning (short-term memory and encoding), problems in preacademic skills, including abstraction, arithmetic, and speech (Autti-Ramo and Granstrom, 1991; Becker *et al.*, 1990; Caruso and ten Bensel; 1993; Coles *et al.*, 1991; Spohr *et al.*, 1993; Streissguth *et al.*, 1985, 1991a, 1991b).

Factors other than alcohol abuse that may have an etiologic role in FAS include poor protein-calorie nutrition, vitamin deficiencies, and alcohol contaminants (e.g., lead). In addition, there is genetic polymorphism for alcohol dehydrogenase, implying a pharmacogenetic etiologic role in the severity of effects.

COUNSELING

It is clear that women who abuse alcohol during pregnancy should be counseled to stop drinking completely. Importantly, medical and psychological support for cessation of drinking should be offered. Since many of these women may also abuse other substances, they should also be advised to stop using these agents.

Alcohol summary

Fetal alcohol syndrome is one of the three leading causes of mental retardation. Importantly, FAS is the only one that is potentially preventable. In addition, this syndrome is a leading cause of poor pregnancy outcome and childhood morbidity (congenital anomalies, including mental retardation). Advice against any use of alcohol during pregnancy cannot be overemphasized. Even maternal consumption of less than three drinks per day has been associated with mild to moderate lowering of IQs among infants (Streissguth *et al.*, 1981) and with prenatal growth retardation (Larroque, 1992; Larroque *et al.*, 1993).

AMPHETAMINE ABUSE DURING PREGNANCY

Dextroamphetamines (D-amphetamine, amphetamine) and methamphetamines are sympathomimetic agents used medically during pregnancy to treat narcolepsy. They are also used illicitly as stimulants and have a number of street names. Approximately 6 percent of pregnant women tested positive for methamphetamines at delivery in one study (Little *et al.*, 1988a; Ramin *et al.*, 1994) and the majority of such women were White (Little *et al.*, 1988a, 1988b). No studies are available regarding the illicit use of amphetamines during pregnancy. Several factors complicate extrapolation of these results to illicit use or abuse: (1) dose regimens in illicit use are not controlled; (2) they likely involve amounts much greater than those used therapeutically; and (3) harmful impurities (e.g., dilutants) may be present in illicit amphetamines or methamphetamines. Methylphenidate (Ritalin), dextroemphetamine (Dexedrine) and a cocktail of amphetamine salts (Adderall) are stimulants with potential for abuse that are often represented as amphetamine or methamphetamine by those who distribute illegal drugs.

Amphetamines

HUMAN CONGENITAL ANOMALIES

The frequency of congenital anomalies was not increased among 69 infants whose mothers abused amphetamines during the first trimester. However, preterm delivery and perinatal mortality were increased in frequency (Eriksson *et al.*, 1981). Follow-up of these children found that 15 percent were delayed in academic achievement in school, but other adverse effects were not reported (Eriksson *et al.*, 2000).

Medically supervised use of amphetamines during pregnancy is not convincingly associated with an increased frequency of congenital anomalies among several thousand infants exposed during the first trimester (Heinonen *et al.*, 1977; Milkovich and van den Berg, 1977; Nelson and Forfar, 1971; Nora *et al.*, 1967, 1970)

ANIMAL STUDIES OF AMPHETAMINES

Cardiac, eye, and a variety of other congenital anomalies were increased in frequency at maternally lethal doses among mice whose mothers were treated with massive doses of amphetamines during pregnancy (Nora *et al.*, 1965). The relevance of these findings to human amphetamine use is unknown.

Methamphetamines

HUMAN CONGENITAL ANOMALIES

Methamphetamines are sympathomimetics and are potent central nervous system stimulants. They are prescribed medically to treat obesity and narcolepsy. Illegal methamphetamines are known as 'designer drugs' because they are synthesized by methylating novel sites along the carbon chain and ring in a one-step reduction process. This 'design' creates molecules so different from pharmaceutical forms of the drug that they were technically legal in the USA for several years in the mid-1980s. They are a popular class of recreational drug. Sometimes methamphetamines are used to 'cut' or dilute other illicit drugs (cocaine). In 2006, they are called 'club drugs' because they are available in night clubs, and are used in parties called 'raves' that may last 24 hours or longer. The stimulant effects of methamphetamines keep the party-goers awake, although some varieties of this drug may cause hallucinations or other altered states of consciousness.

The prevalence of methamphetamine use during pregnancy was 5.2 percent in one large cohort in a public hospital and was used predominately by White women who were single, had fewer prenatal visits than the general obstetric population, and were dependent on public health care (Arria *et al.*, 2006), consistent with findings in other studies of pregnant methamphetamine abusers (Cantanzarite and Stein, 1995; Ho *et al.*, 2001; Little *et al.*, 1988b). Notably, the prevalence of methamphetamine use has not decreased over the past decade (Buchi *et al.*, 2003), or 15 years (unpublished data from Dallas, Texas).

We reported 52 pregnancies complicated by methamphetamines finding that symmetric fetal growth retardation was increased above controls. The frequency of congenital anomalies was not significantly increased (Little *et al.*, 1988b). Perinatal infant abnormalities and maternal pregnancy complications were not increased in frequency. The small sample size of the metamphetamine-exposed groups limits the ability to extrapolate these findings. Methamphetamines and cocaine use in pregnancy were associated with lower birth weight but not with anomalies (Oro and Dixon, 1987; Chomchai *et al.*, 2004), as we found in another study of 863 infants (Ramin *et al.*, 1994). Fetal growth retardation was associated with methamphetamine use throughout pregnancy, but when drug use was discontinued after the second trimester no difference in birth weight was found (Smith *et al.*, 2003).

Lower birth weight was associated with maternal methamphetamine use during pregnancy among 47 infants in a study from Thailand (Chomchai *et al.*, 2004).

Medically supervised use of methamphetamines among 89 infants born to women who took the drug during the first trimester reported a frequency of congenital anomalies no different from controls. Among 320 infants born to women who used the drug after the first trimester there were no abnormalities (Heinonen *et al.*, 1977). The relevance of medically supervised use of methamphetamines to abuse employing much higher doses is not possible to assess.

INTRACEREBRAL HEMORRHAGE

Intracerebral hemorrhage and other cardiovascular accidents are markedly increased in frequency among methamphetamine abusers and their fetuses/infants (Catanzarite and Stein, 1995; Dixon and Bejar, 1989; Keogh and Baron, 1985; Sachdeva and Woodward, 1989), often resulting in maternal and/or infant death (Perez *et al.*, 1999; Stewart and Meeker, 1997).

LONG-TERM EFFECTS OF PRENATAL AMPHETAMINE EXPOSURE ON CHILD DEVELOPMENT

Children whose mothers took amphetamines during pregnancy followed postnatally had slightly lower IQ scores, were more aggressive, and were delayed in academic achievement (Billing *et al.*, 1985; Cernerud *et al.*, 1996; Eriksson and Zetterstrom, 1994; Eriksson *et al.*, 2000).

ANIMAL STUDIES

At doses of methamphetamine similar to those prescribed for narcolepsy, no congenital anomalies were found among nonhuman primates (macaque monkeys) (Courtney and Valerio, 1968). Frequencies of congenital anomalies (brain, anencephaly, eye, cleft palate) were increased among mice and rabbits whose mothers were given methamphetamines during pregnancy at doses up to 20 times the therapeutic adult human dose (Kasirsky and Tansy, 1971; Martin *et al.*, 1976; Yamamoto *et al.*, 1992).

Summary of amphetamine/methamphetamine use

Medically supervised use of amphetamines and methamphetamines during pregnancy does not seem to pose significant risks for increased frequencies of congenital anomalies or maternal–fetal complications. Risks for congenital anomalies and pregnancy complications for those who abuse this class of drugs may exist and probably involve serious complications secondary to vascular disruption and other cardiovascular accidents.

CANNABINOID USE DURING PREGNANCY

More than 12 million people in the USA use marijuana or its derivatives [hash, hash oil, Thai sticks, tetrahydrocannabinol (THC)] regularly. Fifty percent or more of users are women of reproductive age. An estimated 3 percent of the population uses marijuana daily and as many as 10–15 percent of Americans use the drug on a monthly basis (NIDA, 2004). Estimated prevalence rates of cannabinoid use during pregnancy vary widely, ranging from 3 to more than 20 percent of gravidas.

Maternal effects

Preterm labor was increased in frequency among women who smoked marijuana during pregnancy in several investigations (Fried *et al.*, 1984; Gibson *et al.*, 1983; Hatch and Bracken, 1986), but other investigators have failed to confirm this observation (Fried, 1980; Hingson *et al.*, 1982; Shiono *et al.*, 1995; Tennes, *et al.*, 1985; Zuckerman *et al.*, 1989). Prolonged labor and meconium-stained amniotic fluid apparently increased in frequency in one uncontrolled study of 35 women who smoked marijuana late in pregnancy (Greenland *et al.*, 1982), but not replicated in several other controlled studies with large sample sizes (Fried *et al.*, 1983; Greenland *et al.*, 1983; Witter and Niebyl, 1990).

Perinatal infant effects

Significantly lowered birth weights have been reported among infants whose mothers used marijuana during pregnancy in three studies (Cornelius *et al.*, 1995; Hingson *et al.*, 1982; Zuckerman *et al.*, 1989), but not in others (Fried, 1980; Greenland *et al.*, 1983; Linn *et al.*, 1983; Shiono *et al.*, 1995; Witter and Niebyl, 1990). Among more than 1200 infants whose mothers smoked marijuana during pregnancy, 137 during the first trimester, the frequency of major congenital anomalies was not increased (Linn *et al.*, 1983).

Although not generally accepted, a syndrome (fetal growth retardation, craniofacial and other minor dysmorphologic features) was proposed in a clinical case series that included five infants born to women who used two to 14 joints (cigarettes) of marijuana daily throughout pregnancy (Qazi *et al.*, 1985). The infants probably had fetal alcohol syndrome and this finding has not been replicated.

Many studies of marijuana and THC have been performed in pregnant rats, mice, hamsters, and rabbits (Abel, 1980; Schardein, 1985). Most animal teratology studies of marijuana are negative, particularly if dosing (amount, route of intake) was comparable to the human situation.

Withdrawal symptoms

Among infants born to women who used marijuana near the time of delivery, certain neonatal neurobehavioral abnormalities (tremulousness, abnormal response stimuli) were found (Fried, 1980; Fried and Makin, 1987), but other studies found no differences (Tennes *et al.*, 1985).

Summary of cannabinoid use

Mild fetal growth retardation and maternal lung damage are the only untoward outcomes that can reasonably be attributed to marijuana use during pregnancy. Importantly, woman who use marijuana during pregnancy frequently use other substances know to be harmful substances (i.e., alcohol and/or cocaine) (Cornelius *et al.*, 1995; Shiono *et al.*, 1995) because illicit substance abuse is often a polydrug use (Little *et al.*, 1990c).

COCAINE ABUSE DURING PREGNANCY

Cocaine use is widespread, and not limited to Western society as it has been detected in the urine of people from around the world, and in areas as remote as the Arctic. It is an epidemic that began in the mid to late 1970s and has reached users of virtually every age, sex, ethnic, and socioeconomic subgroup. At least half of these users are women of reproductive age (GAO, 1990).

The use of cocaine is accepted to be dangerous to intrauterine development and can cause birth defects (not a syndrome), fetal growth retardation, and transient withdrawal symptoms. Postnatal intellectual development also seems to be adversely affected by the drug.

Cocaine use among pregnant women

We first estimated the prevalence of cocaine use during pregnancy at 9.8 percent in one of the nation's largest hospitals (Little *et al.*, 1988a). Survey results in public hospitals range from 11 to 31 percent (Brody, 1989; Nair *et al.*, 1994; Ostrea *et al.*, 1992) and an incredibly high rate of 48 percent was reported in a San Francisco public hospital (Osterloh and Lee, 1989). Much of the professional community was unprepared to deal with the large number of cocaine-exposed fetuses over the last decade (Landry and Whitney, 1996; Kuczkowski, 2005). In one study, approximately 77 percent of pregnant cocaine abusers at a large public hospital used other drugs of abuse and/or alcohol (Little *et al.*, 1990d) and in another study, 90 percent of female cocaine users were of reproductive age (Kuczkowski, 2005).

We found that cocaine crosses the placenta and is metabolized in the placenta through plasma cholinesterase to ecgonine methyl ester, a major active metabolite (Roe *et al.*, 1990). Actions of cocaine on the vasculature precipitate a number of serious effects. Coronary artery vasospasm and arrhythmias occur at even very low doses of cocaine (Lange *et al.*, 1989). Chronic cocaine use can lead to myocardial infarction, congestive heart failure, dilated cardiomyopathy, or severe ischemic events in the heart or brain (Box 16.3). In more severe situations, cocaine can aggravate vascular weakness and cause serious vascular accidents (intracerebral infarctions and hemorrhages, acute ischemic brain events). Death from cocaine toxicity is usually preceded by hyperpyrexia, shock, unconsciousness, respiratory/cardiac depression. Chronic cocaine use is associated with epileptogenic seizures and cerebral atrophy (Pascual-Leone *et al.*, 1990; Karch, 2005).

Box 16.3 Complications among pregnant women who use cocaine

Abruptio placentae
Hepatitis
Intracerebral hemorrhage
Placental vasculitis
Pregnancy-induced hypertension
Premature delivery (shortened gestation length)

Premature rupture of membranes
Preterm labor
Ruptured ectopic pregnancy
Sexually transmitted diseases
Spontaneous abortion

The literature is replete with reports regarding the increased frequency of abruptio placentae after intravenous or intranasal cocaine use (Acker *et al.*, 1983; Bingol *et al.*, 1987a, 1987b; Chasnoff and MacGregor, 1987; Chasnoff *et al.*, 1985, 1987, 1989a; Cherukuri *et al.*, 1988; Collins *et al.*, 1989; Cregler and Mark, 1986; Dixon and Oro, 1987; Dusick *et al.*, 1993; Hladky *et al.*, 2002; Keith *et al.*, 1989; Little *et al.*, 1988a; Miller *et al.*, 1995; Neerhof *et al.*, 1989; Oro and Dixon, 1987; Shiono *et al.*, 1995; Townsend *et al.*, 1988; Witlin and Sibai, 2001), although some investigators did not observe any cases (Chouteau *et al.*, 1988; Doberczak *et al.*, 1988).

Maternal cocaine use during pregnancy was associated with significantly shortened mean gestational periods and increased frequencies of preterm labor (Chasnoff *et al.*, 1985, 1989a; Chasnoff and MacGregor, 1987; Cherukuri *et al.*, 1988; Chouteau *et al.*, 1988; Cohen *et al.*, 1991; Dixon and Oro, 1987; Keith *et al.*, 1989; Kliegman *et al.*, 1994; Little *et al.*, 1989b, 1999; MacGregor *et al.*, 1987; Neerhof *et al.*, 1989; Oro and Dixon, 1987; Ryan *et al.*, 1986, 1987a, 1987b; Zuckerman *et al.*, 1989). This drug is significantly associated with an increased frequency of precipitous labor (Bateman *et al.*, 1993; Chasnoff *et al.*, 1987), but in a study of 1220 gravid women no decrease in duration of labor was associated with cocaine use (Wehbeh *et al.*, 1995). Gestation length and frequency of preterm delivery among women who used only cocaine during the first trimester were not found to be significantly different from women who did not use cocaine during pregnancy (Chasnoff *et al.*, 1989a). Others have found no association with preterm labor or low birth weight when other obstetric complications were controlled (Miller *et al.*, 1995; Shiono *et al.*, 1995).

In a meta-analysis, increased risks for abruptio placentae and premature rupture of membranes (PROM) were statistically related to cocaine use. However, other risks (birth defects, low birth weight, prematurity, decreased length, and lower head circumference) were said to be related to polydrug use, and could not be attributed to cocaine use (Addis *et al.*, 2001).

Cerebrovascular accidents and related cocaine toxicity

Fatalities following adult cocaine use have frequently been reported. However, only four cases have been documented that involve pregnant women (Burkett *et al.*, 1990; Greenland *et al.*, 1989; Henderson and Torbey, 1988), although many have occurred among pregnant women and have not been published. Of the published cases, two were due to subarachnoid hemorrhage resulting from ruptured aneurysms and a third case involved a pregnant woman admitted to the hospital in a comatose condition after about 1.5 g of cocaine had been placed in her vagina. She was maintained on life-support systems and eventually died approximately 4 months later, never having regained consciousness. The fourth maternal death was attributed to cardiac ischemia and arrhythmia (Burkett *et al.*, 1990). Among more than 4 million women studied in California, the risk of maternal mortality was more than doubled among women who used cocaine during pregnancy (Wolfe *et al.*, 2005). This is a large, reliable study whose findings are important.

Pregnancy-induced hypertension and cocaine

Two studies have reported an increased frequency of pregnancy-induced hypertension associated with cocaine use (Chouteau *et al.*, 1988; Little *et al.*, 1989b). Other factors, such as maternal age, race, and use of multiple substances of abuse, may have accounted for this difference, but a causal association seems likely. Finally, one study reported hepatic rupture during pregnancy as a result of severe pregnancy-induced hypertension associated with cocaine use (Moen *et al.*, 1993).

Cocaine and embryofetal development

INTRAUTERINE GROWTH

Fetal growth retardation, cerebrovascular accidents, and congenital anomalies are frequently observed in pregnancies complicated by maternal cocaine use (Box 16.4). A number of studies have found that *in utero* cocaine exposure adversely affects fetal growth parameters such as birth weight, length, and head circumference (Bateman *et al.*, 1993; Bauchner *et al.*, 1987, 1988; Bingol *et al.*, 1987a,b; Chasnoff and MacGregor, 1987; Chasnoff *et al.*, 1985, 1987, 1989b; Cherukuri *et al.*, 1988; Chouteau *et al.*, 1988; Dixon and Oro, 1987; Donvito, 1988; Eyler *et al.*, 1994; Fulroth *et al.*, 1989; Hadeed and Siegel, 1989; Keith *et al.*, 1989; Little *et al.*, 1988a; MacGregor *et al.*, 1987; Madden *et al.*, 1986; Neerhof *et al.*, 1989; Oro and Dixon, 1987; Petitti and Coleman, 1990; Ryan *et al.*, 1986, 1987a, 1987b; Zuckerman *et al.*, 1989).

Box 16.4 Fetal complications reported to be associated with antepartum cocaine exposure

Bradycardia	Fetal heart rate abnormalities
Brain cavitations	Growth retardation
Brain growth retardation	Intracerebral hemorrhage/infarction
Cardiac arrhythmias	Meconium staining
Cerebral ischemia	Prematurity
Congenital anomalies	Tachycardia

Importantly, head circumference is significantly reduced among infants exposed to cocaine prenatally (Chasnoff *et al.*, 1992; Bateman *et al.*, 1993; Bateman and Chrirboga, 2000). Head circumference was reduced proportionately more than birth weight among 80 infants whose mothers used only cocaine during pregnancy, exhibiting a pattern of brain growth similar to that observed in 67 infants whose mothers had used only alcohol during pregnancy (Little and Snell, 1991a). This is an ominous sign because head circumference is a rough indicator of brain growth, and this pattern of growth is statistically similar to that observed among infants with FAS, and infants exposed to other human teratogens.

Serial ultrasound examinations (two to four) were used to evaluate fetal growth, and reduced head circumference and biparietal diameter were found, although estimated birth weight was not significantly reduced (Mitchell *et al.*, 1988).

CONGENITAL ANOMALIES

Cocaine abuse during pregnancy has been associated with numerous congenital anomalies (Box 16.5). The most consistent association between cocaine use and fetal malformations involves the genitourinary tract (Buehler *et al.*, 1996). In publications from

Box 16.5 Congenital anomalies associated with cocaine use during pregnancy

Absent digits 3 and 4 on hand
Ambiguous genitalia, absent uterus and ovaries
Anal atresia
Atrial septal defect
Bilateral cryptorchidism
Blepharophimosis
Cardiomegaly
Cleft palate
Cleft palate[a]
Club foot
Complete heart block
Congenital hip dislocation
Cryptorchidism
Cutis aplasia
Duplex kidney
Esophageal atresia
Exencephaly[b]
Facial skin tags
Horse shoe kidney
Hydrocele
Hydrocephaly
Hydronephrosis, bilateral
Hydronephrosis, bilateral, prune belly syndrome, patent ductus arteriosus
Hydronephrosis, unilateral, contralateral renal infarct
Hydronephrosis, unilateral, incompetent ureteral orifices
Hydroureter
Hypertelorism, maxillary hypoplasia, high palate, holoprosencephaly with agenesis of corpus callosum
Hypoplastic right heart
Hypospadias
Hypospadias with accessory nipple
Hypospadias, one with chordee
Ileal and colonic infarction
Ileal atresia
Inguinal hernia
Intracranial hemorrhage
Intraparietal encephalocele
Limb reduction/amputation
Mid-colonic atresia
Multiple ventricular septal defects
Necrotizing enterocolitis
Oro-orbital cleft, unilateral
Parietal bone malformation
Patent ductus arteriosus   *continued*

Pierre–Robin anomaly[c]

Poland sequence,[d] ulnar ray deficiencies

Polydactyly

Prune belly syndrome with urethral obstruction

Ptosis and facial diplegia

Pulmonary atresia

Pulmonary stenosis

Renal agenesis

Renal and ureteral agenesis, unilateral, ambiguous genitalia, unilateral ectopic fallopian tube and ovary, gastroschisis, eventration of abdominal contents, hypoplastic gall bladder, spina bifida, hydrocephalus, postural scoliosis, asymmetric chest, congenital dislocation of a hip, clubfoot, flexion deformity of knee joints, arthrogryposis of a lower limb

Renal tract dilation

Sacral exostosis and capillary hemangiomas

Sirenomelia

Transposition of great vessels

Transverse limb reduction, unilateral

Unilateral hemimelia (absent right hand and right leg below the knee)

Ventricular septal defect

Bader and Lewis, 1990; Bingol *et al.*, 1987a, 1987b; Dominguez *et al.*, 1991; Hoyme *et al.*, 1988, 1990; Isenberg *et al.*, 1987; Kobori *et al.*, 1989; Little and Snell, 1991b; Little *et al.*, 1988; Little *et al.*, 1989; Madden *et al.*, 1986; Neerhof *et al.*, 1989; Oriol *et al.*, 1993; Porat and Brodsky, 1991; Puvabanditsin *et al.*, 2005; Ricci and Molle, 1987; Sarpong and Headings, 1992; Sehgal *et al.*, 1993; Shanske *et al.*, 1990; Telsey *et al.*, 1988; Teske and Trese, 1987

[a]Associated with Trisomy 13 and causation by cocaine is not plausible.

[b]Probably really encephalocele.

[c]Pierre–Robin anomaly is cleft palate and severe micrognathia.

[d]Poland sequence is defect of pectoralis muscle with syndactyly of hand.

1985 to 2006, numerous isolated congenital anomalies have been described (Box 16.6). These include ileal atresia in two infants (with bowel infarction in one) and genitourinary tract malformations in nine infants (Chasnoff *et al.*, 1985; 1987, 1988, 1989a; MacGregor *et al.*, 1987; Sarpong and Headings, 1992; Sheinbaum and Badell, 1992; Spinazzola *et al.*, 1992; Viscarello *et al.*, 1992), prune belly syndrome with urethral obstruction, bilateral cryptorchidism, absent digits 3 and 4 on the left hand in two infants, and hypospadias, female pseudohermaphroditism, hydronephrosis with ambiguous genitalia and absent uterus and ovaries, anal atresia, clubfoot, limb-body wall complex, limb deficiencies, secondary hypospadias, and bilateral hydronephrosis and unilateral hydronephrosis with renal infarction of the contralateral kidney.

No congenital abnormalities were observed in four studies of infants born to women who used cocaine during pregnancy (Cherukuri *et al.*, 1988; Doberczak *et al.*, 1988; LeBlanc *et al.*, 1987; Townsend *et al.*, 1988). Among 114 infants born to women who used cocaine during pregnancy, the frequency of congenital anomalies (major or minor) was not increased after controlling for other substances of abuse used and maternal characteristics known to adversely affect pregnancy outcome (Zuckerman *et al.*, 1989).

Box 16.6 Perinatal complications associated with prenatal cocaine exposure

Asphyxia

Bradycardia

Brain lesions

Cardiac arrhythmias

Cerebral ischemia

Cerebrovascular infarction/hemorrhage

Congenital heart block

Congenital infections [syphilis, cytomegalovirus (CMV), human immunodeficiency virus (HIV), hepatitis]

Decreased cardiac output

Hyperbilirubinemia

Increased vascular resistance

Meconium aspiration syndrome

Myocardial infarction

Myocardial ischemia

Neurobehavioral abnormalities

Neurovascular ischemia

Respiratory depression

Seizures

Stillbirth

Tachycardia

Tachypnea

Withdrawal symptoms (unrequietable, shrill cry, opishotonic posturing, hyperirritability, hyperresponsiveness, poor feeding behavior)

Bauer et al., 2005; Chasnoff et al., 1985, 1986, 1987, 1989a; Cherukuri et al., 1988; Dixon and Bejar, 1988, 1989; Dixon and Oro, 1987; Dixon et al., 1987; Doberczak et al., 1988; Geggel et al., 1989; Hadeed and Siegel, 1989; Kapur et al., 1991; Keith et al., 1989; Kobori et al., 1989; Little et al., 1989; MacGregor et al., 1987; Madden et al., 1986; Miller et al., 1995; Neerhof et al., 1989; Oro and Dixon, 1987; Ryan et al., 1986, 1987a, 1987b; Spence et al., 1991; Sztulman et al., 1990; Telsey et al., 1988; Tenorio et al., 1988; van de Bor et al., 1990a, 1990b; Wang and Schnoll, 1987a, 1987b.

The bulk of evidence supports the association between prenatal cocaine exposure and isolated major congenital anomalies. Mechanisms of embryonic and fetal effects appear to be vascular disruption, hypoperfusion, hemorrhage, and vascular occlusion, paralleling the known effects of cocaine on adults.

Cocaine syndrome

It was suggested that a cocaine syndrome exists. Facial defects observed among 10 of 11 infants in a case series of infants exposed to cocaine during gestation included blepharophimosis, ptosis and facial diplegia, unilateral oro-orbital cleft, Pierre–Robin anomaly, cleft palate, cleft lip and palate, skin tags, and cutis aplasia (Kobori et al.,

1989). All of the infants had major brain abnormalities, cavitations, holoproscen-cephaly, and porencephaly. One additional study reported unusual facies among cocaine-exposed infants similar to fetal alcohol syndrome, and speculated whether or not a cocaine syndrome may exist (Fries *et al.*, 1993). We found no evidence of a syn-drome in a matched case–control study of 50 infants chronically exposed to cocaine pre-natally (Little *et al.*, 1996). Fetal growth retardation was the only significant finding in that study, although it is clear that an increased risk of isolated congenital anomalies occurs during the first trimester, and outside the first trimester. Recently, investigators reassessed a possible cocaine syndrome and concluded that physical growth deficits were associated with prenatal cocaine exposure. However, they confirmed our earlier study that no systematic pattern of congenital anomalies (i.e., a syndrome) characterized chil-dren who were exposed to cocaine prenatally (Minnes *et al.*, 2005). Hence, the existence of a cocaine syndrome is not generally accepted.

Perinatal distress and cerebrovascular accidents with prenatal cocaine exposure

Perinatal complications (tachycardia, bradycardia, respiratory problems, jaundice, ele-vated bilirubin, etc.) are significantly increased among infants born to cocaine abusers (Box 16.6).

Thus, maternal cocaine use is associated with major neuropathology of the fetus and newborn. The mechanisms of brain injury may be vascular accidents or ischemia, or a combination of these effects. The association of cocaine abuse and cerebral palsy has not been established, but it is a plausible association that is likely causal.

Neurobehavioral abnormalities in the perinatal period

Newborn infants exposed to cocaine *in utero* appear to have significant neurobehav-ioral impairment in the neonatal period including: increased irritability, tremulousness and muscular rigidity, vomiting, diarrhea, seizures, EEG abnormalities, and behavioral abnormalities on the Brazelton Assessment (Chasnoff *et al.*, 1985, 1987, 1989a,b, 1992; Cherukuri *et al.*, 1988; Dixon *et al.*, 1987; Doberczak *et al.*, 1988; Feng, 1993; Kandall, 1988; LeBlanc *et al.*, 1987; Little and Snell, 1991b; Little *et al.*, 1989b; Nair and Watson, 1991; Neerhof *et al.*, 1989; Oro and Dixon, 1987; Ryan *et al.*, 1986, 1987a,b)

Perinatal mortality among cocaine-exposed babies

Increased perinatal mortality in comparison to controls has been reported (Bauchner *et al.*, 1988; Chasnoff *et al.*, 1987, 1989a; Critchley *et al.*, 1988; Davidson *et al.*, 1986; Kandall *et al.*, 1993; Neerhof *et al.*, 1989; Ryan *et al.*, 1987a,b).

Neonatal hospital stay in days was significantly increased in infants born to women who used cocaine during pregnancy (Neerhof *et al.*, 1989). This may be biased because precautionary actions were taken by physicians who were knowledgeable of prenatal drug exposure.

Box 16.7 Summary of follow-up studies of cocaine-exposed infants

Decreased cognitive function (correlated with reduced head circumference)
Delayed mental and motor development
Delays in all domains (Fagan test)
Language development impairments
Lower IQ
Lower verbal reasoning
Mental and psychomotor development delay
Motor performance deficits
Poor perseverance
Reduced height and weight
School performance poor
Small head circumference

Angelilli *et al.*, 1994; Azuma and Chasnoff,1993; Chasnoff *et al.*, 1992; Ernhart *et al.*, 1987; Frank *et al.*, 2005; Griffith *et al.*, 1994; Gross *et al.*, 1991; Hack *et al.*, 1991; Hurt *et al.*, 2005; Lewis *et al.*, 2004a, 2004b; Miller-Loucar *et al.*, 2005; Nulman *et al.*, 1994; Singer *et al.*, 2004; VanBeveren *et al.*, 2000.

Postnatal follow-up of infants whose mothers used cocaine during pregnancy

The number of studies that reported long-term effects of prenatal cocaine exposure on child development is limited, but they have a common finding of growth and development delays and intellectual deficits (Box 16.7).

Animal models of cocaine

Animal models of the possible teratogenicity of cocaine have yielded inconsistent results.

Summary of cocaine during pregnancy

In summary, the epidemic use of cocaine during pregnancy has resulted in an alarming number of individuals with serious adverse outcomes in mothers, fetuses, and newborns. The use of cocaine is often compounded by frequent concomitant heavy use of other illicit drugs and alcohol. Women who use cocaine during pregnancy are at significant risk for no prenatal care, shorter gestations, premature rupture of membranes, premature labor and delivery, spontaneous abortions, abruptio placentae, decreased uterine blood flow, and death. The fetuses of these women who use cocaine are growth-retarded or severely distressed, and have an increased mortality risk. Fetal and maternal cerebrovascular accidents, with attendant profound morbidity and mortality, occur in association with maternal cocaine use during pregnancy. Major congenital anomalies involving the brain, genitourinary tract, bowel, heart, limbs, and face occur with significantly increased frequency among infants whose mothers used cocaine during gestation.

Hence, cocaine use during pregnancy is very probably teratogenic and fetotoxic. The mechanisms of cocaine's adverse effects are vascular disruption and hypoperfusion for gross abnormalities, but molecular level mechanisms are yet to be determined.

USE OF HALLUCINOGENS DURING PREGNANCY

Psychedelic drugs produce visual hallucinations through a disruption of higher central nervous system function. Most hallucinogens are actually functional analogs of neuro-transmitters (e.g., LSD resembles serotonin). Some hallucinogens are assumed to exert their effect by displacing this or other neurotransmitters, but the molecular basis for the action of hallucinogens is not established. Tolerance of hallucinogens is rapidly developed and chronic users must increase doses rapidly over the course of the drug's use to maintain desired effects (Carroll, 1990).

Hallucinogens or psychedelic drugs are not nearly as popular in 2006 as they were 30 or so years ago. Less than 2 percent of the general population uses psychedelic drugs, based upon data that are not partitioned by sex, ethnicity, or pregnancy status. Among pregnant women at a large urban hospital in Dallas, Texas, it is estimated that approx-imately 1 percent used psychedelic drugs (LSD, mescaline, psilocybin) during gestation.

Specific hallucinogens

LYSERGIC ACID DIETHYLAMIDE

Lysergic acid amides (classically known as lysergic acid diethylamide or LSD) or lysergides are amine alkaloids obtained only through chemical syntheses and have a variety of street names. Under medical supervision lysergide has been used to treat psy-chiatric illness, and ergotamine is a closely related drug. LSD stimulates the sympathetic nervous system, often producing increased heart rate and blood pressure, and a rise in body temperature. LSD used recreationally also has powerful hallucinogenic effects for which it is well known. The hallucinations usually last 8–36 h, depending upon dose. The published studies of LSD use during pregnancy are of medically unsupervised use of this class of drugs, although some clinical experiments in nonpregnant adults have been published.

Congenital anomalies among infants born to mothers who used LSD before or during pregnancy are highly heterogeneous and show no consistent pattern of anomalies (Cohen and Shiloh, 1977/78; Long, 1972). Congenital anomalies among many children reported in the literature to be associated with maternal LSD exposure are unlikely to be caused by use of the drug during pregnancy. The most frequently observed malfor-mation among exposed infants are limb defects, but the defect types were highly vari-able (i.e., lacked a pattern). Among 86 infants born to women who used LSD at unde-termined times during gestation, eight infants had a variety of congenital anomalies (Jacobson and Berlin, 1972). Of these eight infants, five had central nervous system defects, but two were exposed to LSD during embryogenesis (2/86 or 2.3 percent). No convincing evidence has been published that LSD is a human teratogen. However, lifestyle practices associated with drug abuse during pregnancy are probably harmful to intrauterine development. In one clinical series, the frequency of growth deficits and neurological impairments among children born to LSD users was not increased in frequency compared to drug-free controls (Julien, 1988).

Three investigators found increased frequencies of chromosomal breakage in somatic cells of individuals who used LSD (Cohen and Shiloh, 1977/78; Hulten et al., 1968; Long, 1972). Other investigators have reported negative results. Notably, chromosomal aberrations in somatic cells have no clinical relation to the risk of congenital anomalies in the children of parents who used LSD or to the inheritance of chromosomal abnormalities.

Importantly, illegally produced LSD may contain lysergic acid with no amination, and this can lead to peripheral neuropathy, gangrene, and necrosis that resembles toxic shock syndrome. Human toxic exposures to lysergic acid are rare, but among cattle and sheep that consumed wheat grain affected with the fungus *Claviceps pupurea*, which produces lysergic acid, peripheral neuropathy, gangrene, and necrosis were observed. As with most illegal drugs, no quality control or assurance measures are taken to assure drug purity.

MESCALINE

Mescaline is a naturally occurring hallucinogenic alkaloid that is concentrated in the 'buttons' of the peyote cactus, *Lophophora williamsii*. Flattened dried seed pods from this plant, called 'buttons' or 'peyote,' are ingested for recreational use and are used in Native American religious rituals. Members of the Native American Church use mescaline legally in their ceremonies. Naturally mescaline is often contaminated with strychnine and is associated with severe nausea and vomiting. Mescaline may also be synthesized chemically. Mescaline effects are similar to the effects of LSD, but with much more vivid and intense hallucinations. Some users report that mescaline is associated with auditory hallucinations, while LSD is reportedly not. The user also often experiences episodes of severe vomiting and nausea following ingestion of the drug. The hallucinogenic effects usually last about 12 h and sometimes much longer (20–40 hours) depending upon dose.

No published studies of congenital anomalies in infants born to mothers who used mescaline during pregnancy are available. In an animal study, neural tube defects were increased in frequency among the offspring of hamsters whose mothers were given mescaline during pregnancy at one-tenth to one-fifth the dose usually ingested by humans, but the effect was not dose related (Geber, 1967). Neonatal weight was decreased among hamsters born to mothers injected with mescaline during pregnancy (Geber and Schramm, 1974). Moreover, no such abnormalities were seen in animal studies by other investigators who employed doses three to six times those used by humans (Hirsch and Fritz, 1981). Intrauterine death was increased in exposed pregnancies in both animal studies.

PSILOCYBIN

Psilocybin is a naturally occurring hallucinogenic alkaloid present in several species of psychedelic mushrooms belonging to the genus Psilocin. *Psilocin mexicana* is the classic source of the drug and is known as the magic mushroom. It is most commonly found in Mexico, particularly in the Valley of Oaxaca. However, other species occur north of Mexico in the southern USA and elsewhere. Psilocybin typically grows in highly organic media, such as cow feces (cow patties) and usually in the springtime. Psilocybin mushrooms are eaten as an illegal recreational drug. The hallucinogenic effects usually last 6–8 h. Ingestion of these hallucinogenic mushrooms has become a popular form of substance abuse among some adolescents and young adults (Schwartz and Smith, 1988). The effects of psilocybin ingestion include hallucinogenic visions, altered states of consciousness, and a pronounced pyrogenic effect. Several surveys have indicated that mushroom use is more prevalent among high school and college students than is the use of LSD.

The frequency of congenital anomalies in the offspring of mothers who ingested psilocybin during pregnancy has not been published for human studies or animal experiments.

Summary of hallucinogens

Hallucinogen use during pregnancy is not well studied and unknown risks may exist. The purported association of LSD with limb defects found in the offspring of LSD-using women is very probably not causal. The pyrogenic effects of hallucinogens and nonmedical use of other substances may be cause for concern. However, any concern is based upon theoretical grounds and not published information.

OPIATE ABUSE DURING PREGNANCY

Opiates are a class of drugs with sedative and analgesic effects derived from white, milky secretions of the flower bud of the opium poppy plant (*Papaver somniferum*). Synthetic opiods are also available (e.g., meperidine). Opiates (natural and synthetic) are pharmacological narcotics, not to be confused with the legally defined narcotic class which includes such drugs as marijuana, amphetamines, and methamphetamines. Opiates are used medically to treat moderate to severe pain. Narcotics include opium, morphine, the codeines (hydrocodeine, oxycodeine, and codeine), meperidine, paperavine, thebaine, and heroin. Opiates act on opioid receptors to produce analgesia and euphoria. A severe opiate withdrawal syndrome occurs after discontinuation of chronic use, medical or illicit. Importantly, withdrawal occurs among both adults and neonates chronically exposed to these drugs. An increasingly more common source of opiates for abuse is prescription drugs such as oxycodone (Percocet) and hydrocodone (Vicodin), obtained either legally or illegally.

Methadone is a synthetic opioid analog and is used as an alternative to heroin.

Heroin

Heroin is a narcotic analgesic available in many countries (e.g., UK). However, in the USA it is a schedule I drug (no medically beneficial use) and cannot be prescribed for medical treatment. Heroin abuse occurs worldwide. Most population studies report the prevalence of illicit heroin use to be from 2 to 5 percent. In Amsterdam, The Netherlands, however, where illegal drug use is tolerated, an estimated 20 percent of adults use heroin. Among pregnant women in Dallas at a large public hospital, 2.5 percent reported using heroin (unpublished data).

Studies of heroin use during pregnancy are of illicit use only. The health effects of heroin use are confounded and probably compounded because often users abuse other drugs (alcohol, cocaine), use tobacco, and have poor health and nutritional status. Importantly, heroin dose, frequency, duration, and trimesters of use are usually unknown.

Numerous investigators have reported that the frequency of congenital anomalies was not increased among infants born to heroin-addicted mothers compared to the rate expected among infants born in the general population (Kandall *et al.*, 1977; Little *et al.*, 1990e; Naeye *et al.*, 1973; Stimmel and Adamsons, 1976; Stone *et al.*, 1971). No pattern of congenital anomalies that would comprise a syndrome was found among infants born to heroin users (Rothstein and Gould, 1974). One cohort study (830 heroin-exposed infants) suggested that heroin was associated with an increased frequency of congenital anomalies (3.5 percent) compared to controls (2.4 percent) (Ostrea and Chavez, 1979). However, this was because of a nonrepresentative, unrealistically low frequency of congenital anomalies among control group infants (0.5 percent). Recall from Chapter 1 that the background rate is 3.5–5 percent in human populations.

Frequencies of acquired chromosomal aberrations in peripheral blood lymphocytes were elevated above background frequency in narcotic addicts (Amarose and Norusis, 1976; Kushnick *et al.*, 1972). These findings were replicated in infants of narcotic-addicted women in one study (Amarose and Norusis, 1976), but not in another (Kushnick *et al.*, 1972). Aberrations in somatic cells and risks to reproduction are not related.

Severe infections correlated with IVDA [hepatitis B and C, syphilis, human immunodeficiency virus (HIV), gonorrhea] occur with increased frequency among pregnant heroin addicts and infants (Perez-Bescos *et al.*, 1993). Birth weight and other fetal growth measures (head circumference, birth length) are consistently decreased among infants born to heroin addicts compared to drug-free controls (Fricker and Segal, 1978; Kandall *et al.*, 1977; Lam *et al.*, 1992; Lifschitz *et al.*, 1983; Little *et al.*, 1990a, 1990e; Oleske, 1977; Zelson *et al.*, 1971). Miscarriages, perinatal death, and a variety of other perinatal complications were increased in frequency among heroin-exposed children (Fricker and Segal, 1978; Kandall *et al.*, 1977; Lifschitz *et al.*, 1983; Little *et al.*, 1990e; Oleske, 1977, Zelson *et al.*, 1971). Fetal exposure to heroin is confounded by the generally poor health status of heroin-using mothers.

Postnatal growth of children exposed to heroin prenatally seems normal compared to controls and reference data (Little *et al.*, 1991a). However, head circumference was smaller than that of children not exposed to heroin prenatally in several studies (Chasnoff *et al.*, 1986; Lifschitz *et al.*, 1985). As noted for all substances of abuse discussed in this chapter, heroin crosses the placenta freely. If the mother is addicted to heroin, her infant is also addicted because the drug rapidly enters fetal circulation. Accordingly, neonatal withdrawal symptoms (tremors, irritability, jitteriness, diarrhea, seizures, poor feeding, high-pitched, shrill cry, irregular sleep patterns, sneezing, respiratory distress, fever, vomiting) occur among 40–80 percent of infants born to heroin-using gravidas (Alroomi *et al.*, 1988; Fricker and Segal, 1978; Kandall *et al.*, 1977; Rothstein and Gould, 1974). Withdrawal symptoms may appear shortly after birth or take from 6 to 10 days to develop, depending upon the time needed for the infant to metabolize heroin at birth. These symptoms can be of prolonged duration, usually persisting for less than 3 weeks. Treatment is often with tincture of opium (paregoric) in downward tapering doses.

Ultimately, the postnatal environment of infants exposed prenatally to heroin seems to primarily determine developmental status (Ornoy *et al.*, 1996; van Baar and de Graff, 1994; van Baar *et al.*, 1994). This seems to be true for most substances of abuse, except alcohol and perhaps cocaine.

Methadone

Methadone is a synthetic opiate narcotic structurally similar to propoxyphene. The principal medical use of methadone is as a maintenance therapy for heroin addiction, but it is used illegally as a substitute for heroin. Published studies reported include only pregnant women on regimented-dose maintenance therapy who took methadone of known pharmacological purity.

Congenital anomalies were not increased in frequency compared to the background rate among infants born to heroin-addicted women treated with methadone during pregnancy (Fundaro *et al.*, 1994; Kempley, 1995; Soepatmi, 1994; Stimmel and Adamsons, 1976; van Baar *et al.*, 1994; Vering *et al.*, 1992). However, withdrawal symptoms occurred frequently (up to 80 percent) and birth weights were significantly lower (2600 g) among methadone-exposed infants (*n* = 278) (Connaughton *et al.*, 1977). Neonatal complications occur at a high rate, and include asphyxia neonatorum, transient tachypnea, aspiration pneumonia, congenital syphilis, jaundice, meconium staining, and neonatal death. Adverse maternal effects include prolonged rupture of membranes, breech presentation, abruptio placentae, preeclampsia, and postpartum hemorrhage (Naeye *et al.*, 1973). An unusually high frequency of sudden infant death syndrome (SIDS) (17) occurred among infants in a group of 688 drug-using mothers followed by Chavez and associates (1979). Of the 17 infants, 14 were born to mothers who were enrolled in a methadone treatment program, but who continued to use other drugs as well. Review of effects of methadone maintenance during pregnancy on neonatal outcome showed two consistent findings across studies: withdrawal symptoms (70–90 percent) and lowered gestational age and birth weight of infants in the drug-exposed group compared to a control group (Behnke and Eyler, 1993).

Developmental outcomes of heroin- and/or methadone-exposed children

Several researchers have been following, assessing, and reporting on the progress of children born to heroin- and methadone-using mothers. Overall, heroin- and methadone-exposed children obtained lower scores than comparison groups in the domains of motor coordination, attention and focus, activity level and behavior, emotional disturbances, and behavioral problems (aggression, anxiety, and rejection) (Behnke and Eyler, 1993; Davis and Templer, 1988; de Cubas and Field, 1993; Deren, 1986; Kaltenbach and Finnegan, 1984; Wilson *et al.*, 1979).

Summary of opiates during pregnancy

Chronic use/abuse of opiates during pregnancy does not significantly increase the risk of congenital anomalies. Adverse pregnancy outcomes are increased in frequency: abruptio placentae, neonatal withdrawal, preterm birth, and fetal growth retardation. Some differences were found in cognitive abilities, motor development and behavior between opiate-exposed children and nondrug-exposed children, but the postnatal environment with a drug-abusing mother must be considered because it is an important factor. Maternal personality traits, degrees of life stress, the quality of the mother–child relationship, and assessment of the environment must be considered.

INHALANT (ORGANIC SOLVENT) ABUSE DURING PREGNANCY

Epidemiology

Use of inhalants during pregnancy is 1 percent, somewhat lower than other substances of abuse (for example, cocaine, marijuana, and tobacco). In Dallas, it was estimated that 1 percent of women used inhalants during pregnancy, including toluene, spray paint, gasoline, freon, and other substances (Madry *et al.*, 1991). Women who use inhalants during pregnancy are primarily Hispanic or American Indian, with an age range of 20–29 years (Goodwin, 1988; Wilkins-Haug and Gabow, 1991). In Dallas, the majority of women using inhalants during pregnancy are young, 15–20 years of age, and usually Hispanic.

Fetal solvent syndrome

A collection of dysmorphic features called the 'fetal solvent syndrome' was observed among infants born to women who 'huffed' or 'sniffed' toluene, gasoline, benzene, and other aromatic liquids during pregnancy. The syndrome is characterized by prenatal growth retardation (low birth weight, microcephaly), dysmorphic facial features (facies) that resemble FAS, and digital malformations (short phalanges, nail hypoplasia). Investigators have noted that these features are reminiscent of FAS. Importantly, women who use a substance of abuse, including inhalants, during pregnancy frequently use other substances, including alcohol. Nonetheless, data from case reports seem to support the notion that inhalants such as toluene or gasoline, independently of concurrent use of other substances of abuse, may be associated with congenital anomalies consistently described as the fetal solvent syndrome. Anecdotal evidence suggests that the fetal solvent syndrome is associated with significant mental retardation. It is important to note that usual occupational exposure to organic solvents cannot be compared to inhalant abuse. The doses encountered in occupational exposure are of a lower magnitude.

Animal studies

The frequency of congenital anomalies was not increased among rats whose mothers were exposed to high levels of toluene, but growth retardation was observed (Gospe *et al.*, 1994; Ono *et al.*, 1995).

Specific inhalants

GASOLINE

Gasoline is a fuel mixture of volatile hydrocarbon and aromatic compounds possibly containing tetraethyl lead, methanol, and other agents. Gasoline is sometimes 'sniffed' by inhalant abusers to produce a euphoric effect. Acute poisoning by gasoline is associated with pneumonitis, shock, cardiac arrhythmias, convulsions, coma, and death.

A case report was published of two infants with profound mental retardation, neurological dysfunction, and minor dysmorphic features ('fetal gasoline syndrome') born to women who had abused gasoline by inhalation throughout pregnancy (Hunter *et al.*, 1979). It has not been possible to assess a causal relationship based upon two children in a case report.

TOLUENE

Toluene is an aromatic organic solvent used in paint thinner, in printing, and in adhesives. It is a substance of abuse used by 'huffing' or 'sniffing' for its euphoric effect. It has caused organic brain syndrome in adults and is associated with cerebral atrophy (Allison and Jerrom, 1984; Cooper *et al.*, 1985; Filley *et al.*, 1990; King, 1982; Larsen and Leira, 1988; Lowenstein, 1985; Pearson *et al.*, 1994). Adult brain damage suggests the same damage may be caused by toluene exposure *in utero*.

Unusual dysmorphic features suggestive of a toluene embryopathy were described in three children who were born to women who frequently inhaled large amounts of toluene throughout pregnancy (Hersh, 1989; Hersch *et al*, 1985) and these are strikingly similar to FAS (Pearson *et al.*, 1994). Among 35 infants with the toluene embryopathy phenotype, 42 percent were premature, 52 percent had low birth weight, and 32 percent were microcephalic. Postnatally, they were below the fifth percentile for all measures, including neurodevelopment and had dysmorphic facies (Arnold *et al.*, 1994). Preterm delivery, perinatal death, and prenatal growth retardation are associated with toluene use during pregnancy (Wilkins-Haug and Gabow, 1991). Two cases of renal tubular dysfunction and metabolic acidosis (including hyperchloremic acidosis and amnioaciduria) were recently reported in infants whose mothers chronically abused inhalants containing toluene (Lindemann, 1991). Early childhood growth and development were also significantly delayed among toluene-exposed infants (Wilkins-Haug and Gabow, 1991). They had the typical syndrome stigma of the toluene embryopathy at follow up (Arnold *et al.*, 1994). Four of five neonates born to women who abused toluene during pregnancy had low birth weight (< 2500 g), but only one had a congenital anomaly (Goodwin, 1988).

Summary of solvents during pregnancy

Solvent abuse during pregnancy poses significant risks to the pregnancy, endangering both the mother and the fetus. A fetal solvent syndrome probably exists and consists of dysmorphic facial features and severe growth and developmental delay (below 5th percentile).

Distal renal tubular acidosis and hyperchloremic metabolic acidosis should be expected in solvent using pregnant women and it may precipitate labor. Premature labor should be anticipated and will usually follow toluene toxicity. Fetal/neonatal metabolic acidosis (arterial pH less than or equal to 7.0), respiratory difficulties, and renal function abnormalities have been observed, in addition to the usual complications of prematurity.

TOBACCO USE IN PREGNANCY

Native Americans grew and smoked tobacco in pre-Columbian times. However, tobacco native to North America is not the tobacco used today because it was too bitter to be smoked or chewed alone, and was mixed with a variety of other substances for use, including willow bark, mushrooms, and wild lettuce. The tobacco, *Nicotiana tabacum*, is widely used by smoking, chewing, or dipping, and is a hybrid of South and North American species. Tobacco smoke comprises several-hundred different chemicals, including nicotine and carbon monoxide in greatest abundance. There are several-thousands of publications on the risks of tobacco use during pregnancy, including extensive reviews (Fredricsson and Gilljam, 1992; Landesman-Dwyer and Emanuel, 1979; McIntosh, 1984a,b; Nash and Persaud, 1988; Rosenberg, 1987; Stillman *et al.*, 1986; Streissguth, 1986; Surgeon General, 1979).

Approximately 20 percent of pregnant women smoke tobacco in some studies (Rantakallio *et al.*, 1995; Vega *et al.*, 1993), and in Dallas the rate was 15 percent. The earliest finding was increased frequencies of prematurity (estimated by lowered birth weight) among smokers (Simpson, 1957), which was later confirmed (Herriot *et al.*, 1962; Lowe, 1959; Ravenholt and Lerinski, 1965). It later became apparent that lowered birth weight was not due to prematurity, but was in fact intrauterine growth retardation (Rubin *et al.*, 1986).

Low birth weight

Several-hundred thousand women who smoked during pregnancy have been studied (Anonymous, 1993; Cnattingius *et al.*, 1993; Fox *et al.*, 1994; Hjortdal *et al.*, 1989; McIntosh, 1984a; Stillman *et al.*, 1986) and lowered birth weight was definitely associated with maternal tobacco smoking during pregnancy. Smoking more heavily during pregnancy results in infants that are more growth retarded. In addition, passive exposure to smoke was also related to reduced birth weight (Bardy *et al.*, 1993; Fortier *et al.*, 1994; Haddow *et al.*, 1989, 1993; Martinez *et al.*, 1994; Mathai *et al.*, 1992; Ogawa *et al.*, 1991; Rebagliato *et al.*, 1995; Seidman and Mashiach, 1991). However, growth is apparently not delayed when there is exposure to tobacco smoke postnatally (Day *et al.*, 1994; Jacobson *et al.*, 1994). Importantly, birth weight was unaffected in infants whose mothers ceased smoking early in pregnancy (i.e., during the early second trimester) (Ahlsten *et al.*, 1993; Li *et al.*, 1993; Olsen, 1992).

Intellectual development and behavior

Very mild, insignificant reductions in IQ (1–5 points) were found among children whose mothers smoked during pregnancy (Davie *et al.*, 1972; Dunn *et al.*, 1977; Fried, 1989, 1992, 1993; Fried *et al.*, 1992; Olds *et al.*, 1994; Rush and Callahan, 1989). However, socioeconomic status (SES) and maternal education were lower among women who smoked.

Birth defects

The purported teratogenic relationship between smoking or use of tobacco during pregnancy is unlikely, but, if it does exist, is very small (1 percent or less). The possibility that tobacco is a teratogen has been analyzed in dozens of epidemiological studies, involving over 100 000 children (McIntosh 1984a; Stillman *et al.*, 1986). The frequency of major congenital anomalies is generally not increased among mothers who smoke tobacco during pregnancy (Andrews and McGarry, 1972; Christianson, 1980; Erickson, 1991; Evans *et al.*, 1979; Hemminki *et al.*, 1983; Kullander and Kallen, 1976; Malloy *et al.*, 1989; Pradat, 1992; Seidman *et al.*, 1990; Shiono *et al.*, 1986; Tikkanen and Heinonen, 1991, 1992, 1993; Van Den Eeden *et al.*, 1990; Werler *et al.*, 1990, 1992).

Some investigators found significant associations between cigarette smoking and birth defects, such as craniosynostosis (Alderman *et al.*, 1994). A nonspecific collection of birth defects (gastroschisis, limb reduction defects, strabismus, and congenital heart disease) have been reported to be increased in frequency among infants born to smokers (Aro, 1983; Christianson, 1980; Czeizel *et al.*, 1994; Fedrick *et al.*, 1971; Goldbaum *et al.*, 1990; Haddow *et al.*, 1993; Hakim and Tielsch, 1992; Himmelberger *et al.*, 1978). Cleft palate and orofacial clefts have been reported to be increased in frequency (Andrews and McGarry, 1972; Ericson *et al.*, 1979; Hwang *et al.*, 1995; Khoury *et al.*, 1989; Shaw *et al.*, 1996). The association of tobacco with clefting remains controversial because other large studies found no such association (Frazier *et al.*, 1961; Lowe, 1959; Underwood *et al.*, 1965; Yerushalmy 1964). For example, in one study no association was found with maternal tobacco smoking among 288 067 infants, of whom 10 223 had congenital anomalies (Malloy *et al.*, 1989). In a cohort of 67 609 pregnancies, an increased frequency of anencephalic infants was found among progeny of women who smoked heavily during gestation (greater than 20 cigarettes per day) (Evans *et al.*, 1979). Notably, smoking is more prevalent in the lower social classes, as is the incidence of anencephaly. White cigarette smokers gave birth to anecephalics at 1.72 per 1000, while White nonsmokers had a rate of 1.0 per 1000 (Naeye, 1978). A similar trend was not found among Black women, who have a lower rate of anencephaly than White women, and no trend with smoking was found for smoking and anencephaly for this ethnic group. If the risk of congenital anomalies is increased above the background rate among infants whose mothers smoke tobacco during pregnancy it is very small at 1 percent or less.

Childhood cancer

Very weak evidence suggests that cancer during childhood is associated with *in utero* exposure to tobacco smoke (McKinney *et al.*, 1986; Schwartzbaum, 1992; Stjernfeldt *et al.*, 1986). These associations are equivocal and contradicted by other studies (Gold *et al.*, 1993; John *et al.*, 1991; McCredie *et al.*, 1994; Pershagen, 1989; Pershagen *et al.*, 1992).

Pregnancy complications

An increased frequency of premature rupture of membranes (Underwood *et al.*, 1965), abruptio placentae, placenta previa, and amniotic infections occurs among gravidas who are heavy smokers (Naeye, 1979). Smoking was reported to be a risk factor for gynecological diseases, ovarian cycle disturbance, spontaneous abortion, pregnancy toxicosis, premature delivery, and chronic fetal hypoxia (Sheveleva *et al.*, 1986). Preterm delivery, placenta previa, perinatal mortality, and other complications of pregnancy have shown an increase among women who smoke (Anonymous, 1993; English and Eskenzai, 1992; Guinn *et al.*, 1994; Handler *et al.*, 1994; Little and Weinberg, 1993; McIntosh, 1984b; Meis *et al.*, 1995; Raymond and Mills, 1993; Stillman *et al.*, 1986; Wilcox 1993).

Animal studies

Nicotine and cigarette smoking in animals has also been studied and reduced fetal weight was found. Notably, a very early study showed that rabbits exposed to the equivalent of 20 cigarettes per day gave birth to fetuses that were 7 percent lighter than controls (Schoeneck, 1941).

Summary of tobacco during pregnancy

Tobacco smoke adversely affects pregnancy. Passive tobacco smoke exposure negatively affects fetal growth. However, catch-up growth in the neonatal period fully compensates for fetal growth retardation for active smokers.

PHENCYCLIDINE USE IN PREGNANCY

Phencyclidine (PCP) is used as a recreational drug and is taken orally, intravenously, intranasally, or smoked. Phencyclidine is no longer available as a pharmaceutical preparation, but was formerly used as an anesthetic and analgesic in human but mainly veterinary medicine. Ketamine is a more predictable and effective medicine that is used in its place.

Among 57 infants whose mothers took PCP throughout pregnancy, including the first trimester, the frequency of congenital anomalies was not increased above background risk (3.5–5 percent) for human populations (Wachsman *et al.*, 1989). The frequency of congenital anomalies in two studies with control groups was not increased among 131 infants exposed to PCP during gestation (Golden *et al.*, 1987; Tabor *et al.*, 1990). A case report was published of an infant with intracerebral abnormalities who was exposed to PCP during gestation (Michael *et al.*, 1982), but this has no causal meaning. Birth weights and head circumferences were depressed in another report, with more than 40 percent of PCP-exposed infants falling below the tenth percentile for reference data (Lubchenco *et al.*, 1966). Postnatal follow-up at age 1 year for 36 infants exposed to PCP *in utero* found slight growth delays, with 24 percent below the tenth percentile (Wachsman *et al.*, 1989). An increased frequency of low birth weight and microcephaly was found among 505 infants exposed to cocaine and PCP during gestation (Rahbar *et al.*, 1993).

Withdrawal symptoms (tremors, jitteriness, irritability) were observed among about 50 percent of infants exposed prenatally to PCP (Wachsman *et al.*, 1989), but in none of seven infants in another case series (Chasnoff *et al.*, 1983a).

Summary of PCP in pregnancy

Phencyclidine is associated with fetal growth retardation and withdrawal symptoms. It does not seem to be a strong cause of birth defects.

USE OF TS AND BLUES IN PREGNANCY

Used as a substitute for heroin, 'Ts and blues' is a street mixture of the narcotic analgesic pentazocine (Talwin) and the over-the-counter antihistamine tripelennamine (pyribenzamine). Pentazocine is a synthetic narcotic analgesic given medically by parenteral, oral, or rectal routes to relieve moderate to severe pain. In the early 1970s it was in wide use in Chicago, and popular among inner-city drug users as a 'high' less expensive than, but similar to, heroin (Senay, 1985).

Ts and blues abuse during pregnancy has not been well studied. Data are available for 86 infants born to women who used Ts and blues during pregnancy (*n* = 13, 50, and 23, respectively) (Chasnoff *et al.*, 1983b; Little *et al.*, 1990f; von Almen and Miller, 1984). Infants born to Ts and blues abusers have fetal growth retardation and suffer from perinatal complications more frequently than controls (Chasnoff *et al.*, 1983b; Little *et al.*, 1990f; von Almen and Miller, 1984). The frequency of congenital anomalies was not increased among these 86 infants (Chasnoff *et al.*, 1983b; Little *et al.*, 1990f; von Almen and Miller, 1984).

The effect of the use of pentazocine during pregnancy on development of 39 infants whose mothers took the drug showed 21 percent were premature, 31 percent were growth retarded, 11 percent (four children) had congenital anomalies, and 28 percent had withdrawal symptoms (DeBooy *et al.*, 1993). At 68 months of age, five of 19 had failure to thrive, and eight were removed from birth mothers and placed in foster care because of abuse and neglect. Twenty-one children were tested and 81 percent (17) scored within the normal range (85 or more) and four children received scores in the subnormal (70 to 84) range. No children received scores below 70. These types of findings are difficult to assess because of other factors in the drug abusers' life style (poor diet, lack of prenatal care, and concomitant use of other substances of abuse, especially alcohol) contributed to low birth weight and other untoward outcomes among infants born to Ts and blues abusers.

Transient neonatal withdrawal symptoms were observed by several investigators in infants born to women who chronically took pentazocine in a medically supervised environment late in pregnancy (Goetz and Bain, 1974; Kopelman, 1975; Scanlon, 1974). The symptoms resembled those seen in neonatal withdrawal from other narcotics: irritability, hyperactivity, vomiting, high-pitched cry, fever, and diarrhea.

Another Ts and blues combination is also used, Alwin (pentazocine) and Ritalin (methylphenidate) (Carter and Watson, 1994), and was anecdotally associated with fetal growth retardation, but not birth defects (Debooy *et al.*, 1993). As with the other Ts and blues mixture, alcohol abuse is highly prevalent.

Ts and blues summary

Although Ts and blues use during pregnancy is associated with fetal growth retardation and withdrawal symptoms, maternal complications such as pulmonary thromboembolic disease and placental infarcts may occur secondary to intravenous injection of tablet vehicle (microcrystalline cellulose). Infants born to Ts and blues users are at increased risk for fetal alcohol syndrome because most users of this drug combination drink alcohol in abusive amounts (more than six drinks per day).

POLYDRUG USE DURING PREGNANCY

Pregnant women who use a substance of abuse usually use more than one substance. We conducted a study to analyze patterns of substance abuse and polydrug use during pregnancy at one of the largest obstetric services in the USA, providing medical care for a primarily indigent (less than 5 percent pay for their health care) patient population. The substances that were analyzed included methamphetamine, cocaine, heroin, and Ts and blues.

Among 174 pregnant women who abused drugs during their pregnancies, 83 percent had some prenatal care. Heroin users were significantly older (28.3 years) than cocaine users (24.8 years) or methamphetamine users (23.4 years) (Little *et al.*, 1990e).

Over 90 percent of gravid methamphetamine abusers were White and used tobacco (54 percent), marijuana (37 percent), and cocaine (12 percent). About one-half (55 percent) of pregnant cocaine users were Black and they also used tobacco (53 percent), alcohol (11 percent), heroin (8 percent), and marijuana (8 percent). Among White women who used cocaine, the substances they used most frequently were tobacco (46 percent), methamphetamine (42 percent), marijuana (35 percent), and alcohol (27 percent). Pregnant Black and White women heroin abusers (respectively) also used cocaine (62 and 25 percent), alcohol (38 and 25 percent), methadone (8 and 63 percent), and tobacco (62 and 35 percent). Approximately 94 percent Ts and blues users were Black and they also used alcohol (53 percent), cocaine (12 percent), marijuana (12 percent), and methamphetamine (6 percent) (Little *et al.*, 1990c).

Polydrug use (more than one drug) was reported by 130 (75 percent) of pregnant women studied. Other than tobacco, alcohol, and cocaine were the most frequently used secondary and tertiary drugs. Alcohol and/or cocaine use during pregnancy differed considerably by primary drug of abuse. Heroin and Ts and blues users drank alcohol 5.2- and 14.2-fold more often, respectively, than gravidas who abused methamphetamine. Heroin abusers used cocaine 8.9 times more frequently than abusers of methamphetamine or Ts and blues. Heroin abusers used alcohol and cocaine 5.2- and 5.2-fold, respectively, more frequently than methamphetamine abusers (Little *et al.*, 1990e).

Concomitant use of several substances of abuse that have teratogenic potential has serious implications for substance abuse during pregnancy because of the risks for mother and fetus. Growth retardation appears to be more severe, and the frequency of congenital anomalies seems to be increased in the offspring of mothers who abuse multiple substances (Oro and Dixon, 1987). The primarily intravenous use of these drugs increases the risk of maternal HIV infection and vertical transmission.

Ts and blues, heroin, and cocaine users are at greatest risk for birth defects attributable to alcohol abuse. Heroin abusers used cocaine significantly more frequently than abusers of any other drug, probably because of the popularity of a mixture called 'speedball' (cocaine and heroin, and occasionally methamphetamine). Because of polydrug use, infants born to heroin abusers are at 8.9 times greater risk for cocaine-induced damage than those born to abusers of other drugs, except for those born to cocaine abusers alone. Infants born to Ts and blues abusers are at a three to 14 times greater risk of alcohol-induced damage to the embryo or fetus than infants born to abusers of other drugs (Little *et al.*, 1990f).

It is widely known that alcohol is a leading cause of birth defects (Abel and Sokol, 1987; Jones *et al.*, 1973) and cocaine is very likely a teratogen (Chasnoff *et al.*, 1988;

Little and Snell, 1991b; Little *et al.*, 1989b; Little and VanBeveren, 1996; VanBeveren *et al.*, 2000). Infants born to heroin abusers are exposed to cocaine and alcohol five times more often than those born to methamphetamine abusers. It is clear that alcohol is a major contributor to the risk of congenital anomalies and growth retardation in infants born to drug abusers, particularly those who abuse Ts and blues or heroin. Importantly, multiple substance use increases the possibility of drug–drug and drug–alcohol interactions. Whether or not alcohol and cocaine interact to increase the severity of damage to the conceptus is not known, but this seems likely (Hofkosh *et al.*, 1995).

Cocaine and heroin increase the risk for abruptio placentae and premature birth for women who use cocaine (Acker *et al.*, 1983; Chasnoff *et al.*, 1985). Alcohol is used frequently by those who abuse cocaine, heroin, and Ts and blues, and may cause such pregnancy complications as premature labor (NIAAA, 1983).

Summary of substance abuse during pregnancy

The risk for morbidity increases with the number of substances used and the frequency of their use. Not all substances of abuse cause congenital anomalies, but most substance use is associated with the use of alcohol and/or cocaine, generally acknowledged to cause birth defects. Abuse of any substance during pregnancy is associated with fetal growth retardation and possibly with neurological dysfunction. Associated risks include sexually transmitted diseases, hepatitis, and undernutrition.

Key references

Arria AM, Derauf C, Lagasse LL *et al.* Methamphetamine and other substance use during pregnancy. Preliminary estimates from the infant development, environment, and lifestyle (IDEAL) study. *Matern Child Health J* 2006; **5**: 1.

Chomchai C, Na Manorom N, Watanarungsan P, Yossuck P, Chomchai S. Methamphetamine abuse during pregnancy and its health impact on neonates born at Siriraj Hospital, Bangkok, Thailand. *Southeast Asian J Trop Med Public Health* 2004; **35**: 228.

Dashe JS, Sheffield JS, Olscher DA, Todd SJ, Jackson GL, Wendel GD. Relationship between maternal methadone dosage and neonatal withdrawal. *Obstet Gynecol* 2002; **100**: 1244.

Frank DA, Rose-Jacobs R, Beeghly M, Wilbur M, Bellinger D, Cabral H. Level of prenatal cocaine exposure and 48-month IQ. importance of preschool enrichment. *Neurotoxicol Teratol* 2005; **27**: 15.

Hurt H, Brodsky NL, Roth H, Malmud E, Giannetta JM. School performance of children with gestational cocaine exposure. *Neurotoxicol Teratol* 2005; **27**: 203.

Kuczkowski KM. Peripartum care of the cocaine-abusing parturient. Are we ready? *Acta Obstet Gynecol Scand* 2005; **84**: 108.

Lewis BA, Singer LT, Short EJ *et al.* Four-year language outcomes of children exposed to cocaine *in utero*. *Neurotoxicol Teratol* 2004a; **26**: 617.

Lewis MW, Misra S, Johnson HL, Rosen TS. Neurological and developmental outcomes of prenatally cocaine-exposed offspring from 12 to 36 months. *Am J Drug Alcohol Abuse* 2004b; **30**: 299.

Little BB, Snell LM, VanBeveren TT, Crowell RB, Trayler S, Johnston WL. Treatment of substance abuse during pregnancy and infant outcome. *Am J Perinatol* 2003; **20**: 255.

Wolfe EL, Davis T, Guydish J, Delucchi KL. Mortality risk associated with perinatal drug and
    alcohol use in California. *J Perinatol* 2005; **25**: 93.

Further references are available on the book's website at http://www.drugsandpregnancy.com

Appendix
Alternate drug names

The drugs listed in the text are predominantly United States Adopted Names (USAN). The table below lists the alternative International Nonproprietary Names (INN), where these differ. Generic names are also provided for any brand names in the text.

Please note that individual countries may use different drug names. You can check INN and alternative names on the latest edition of the International Nonproprietary Names (INN) for Pharmaceutical Substances CD-ROM. You can also register with Mednet at http://mednet.who.int/ to access their online database.

Drug listed in text	Brand name?	INN name if different	USAN or USP name if different
5-aminosalicylic acid		Mesalazine	Mesalamine
5-FU		Fluorouracil	Fluorouracil
6-mercaptopurine		Mercaptopurine	Mercaptopurine
6-MP		Mercaptopurine	Mercaptopurine
Accutane®	Yes	Isotretinoin	Isotretinoin
Acetaminophen		Paracetamol	
Acetohexamide			
Acetyl salicylic acid		Acetylsalicylic acid	Aspirin
Achromycin®	Yes	Tetracycline	Tetracycline
Actidil®	Yes	Triprolidine	Triprolidine
Actinomycin-D		Dactinomycin	Dactinomycin
Activated charcoal			
Acyclovir	Zovirax®	Acyclovir	
Adapin	Sinequan®	Doxepin	Doxepin hydrochloride
Adenosine	Adenocard®	Adenosine phosphate	
Adriamycin	Yes	Doxorubicin	Doxorubicin
Adrucil®	Yes	Fluorouracil	Fluorouracil
Afrin®	Yes	Oxymetazoline	Oxymetazoline hydrochloride
Aftate®	Yes – also Tinactin®	Tolnaftate	Tolnaftate
Albuterol		Salbutamol	
Alclometasone	Aclovate®		Alclometasone dipropionate
Aldactone®	Yes	Spironolactone	Spironolactone
Aldomet®	Yes	Methyldopa	Methyldopate hydrochloride (ester)
Alfenta®	Yes	Alfentanil	Alfentanil hydrochloride

Drug listed in text	Brand name?	INN name if different	USAN or USP name if different
Alkeran®	Yes	Melphalan	Melphalan
Allerest®	Yes	Chlorpheniramine and phenylephrine	Chlorpheniramine and phenylephrine
Alprazolam	Xanax®		
Altretamine	Hexalen®		
Alurate		Not listed	Aprobarbital
Alwin		Not listed	Not listed
Amantadine	Symmetrel®		Amantadine hydrochloride
Ambenyl		Not listed	Not listed
Amcinonide	Cyclocort®		
Amidrin		Not listed	Not listed
Amikin			Amikacin sulfate
Amiloride	Midamor®		Amiloride hydrochloride
Aminophylline	Aminop®		
Aminopterin		Aminopterin sodium	Aminopterin sodium
Aminosalicylate		Not listed	Not listed
Amiodarone	Cordarone® or Pacerone®		
Amitril®	Yes – also Elavil®	Amitriptyline	Amitriptyline
Amlodipine	Norvasc®		Amlodipine maleate
Amobarbital	Amytal®		
Amogel-PG®	Yes	Not listed	Not listed
Amoxapine	Loxapine®		
Amoxicillin	Amoxil®		Amoxicillin sodium
Amphetamine	Adderall®	Amfetamine	Amphetamine
Amphotericin B	Fungizone®		
Ampicillin	Ampicil®		Ampicillin sodium
Amsacrine	Amsidine®		
Amyl nitrite	Amyl®	Not listed	Not listed
Amytal®	Yes	Amobarbital	Amobarbital
Anabuse	Antabuse®	Disulfiram	Disulfiram
Anafranil®	Yes	Clomipramine	Clomipramine hydrochloride
Anaspaz®, Levsin®		Not listed	Not listed
Anectine		Suxamethonium chloride	Succinylcholine chloride
Anthra-Derm®	Yes	Dithranol	Anthralin
Anthralin		Dithranol	
Antivert		Meclozine	Meclizine
Aprobarbital	Alurate®		
Aquatensen®	Enduron®	Methyclothiazide	Methyclothiazide
Ara-C		Cytarabine	Cytarabine hydrochloride
Aralen®	Yes	Chloroquine	Chloroquine
Amikacin	Amikin®	Not listed	Not listed
ASA		Acetylsalicylic acid	Aspirin
Asendin®	Yes	Amoxapine	Amoxapine
Asparaginase	Crisanaspase®/ elspar®	Not listed	Not listed

Drug listed in text	Brand name?	INN name if different	USAN or USP name if different
Aspirin		Acetylsalicylic acid	Aspirin
Atarax®	Yes – also Vistaril®	Hydroxyzine	Hydroxyzine
Atenolol	Lopressor®		
Ativan®	Yes	Lorazepam	Lorazepam
Atophen		Not listed	Not listed
Atracurium	Tracrium®	Atracurium besilate	Atracurium besylate
Atropine		Not listed	Atropine sulfate
Augmentin		Not listed	Amoxicillin/Clavulanic Acid
Aventyl®	Yes	Nortriptyline	Nortriptyline hydrochloride
Axid®	Yes	Nizatidine	Nizatidine
Azatadine	Optimine®		Azatadine maleate
Azathioprine	Imuran®		
Azithromycin	Zithromax®/ Z-pak®/Zmax		
Aztreonam	Azactam®		
Azulfidine®	Yes	Sulfasalazine	Sulfasalazine
Bactrim		Trimethoprim sulfate AND sulfamethoxazole	Trimethoprim sulfate AND sulfamethoxazole
Bactroban®	Yes	Mupirocin	Mupirocin
Banthine		Methantheline	Methantheline
Bayidy		Not listed	Not listed
Beclomethasone		Beclometasone	Beclomethasone dipropionate
Belladonna			Atropine sulfate
Benadryl®	Yes	Diphenhydramine	Diphenhydramine
Bendectin®	Yes	Pyridoxine AND doxylamine	Pyridoxine AND doxylamine
Bendroflumethiazide	Naturetin®		
Bentyl		Dicycloverine	Dicyclomine
Benzocaine	Hurricaine® spray, Americaine® spray		
Benzoin		Not listed	Tincture of Benzoin
Benzonatate	Tessalon pearls®		
Benzphetamine	Didrex®	Not listed	Not listed benzphetamine
Betamethasone	Valisone®		Betamethasone sodium phosphate
Betaxolol	Kerlone®		Betaxolol hydrochloride
Biaxin		Clarithromycin	Clarithromycin
Bio-Tabs		Not listed	Not listed
Bisacodyl			Bisacodyl
Black-Draught		Casanthranol	Casanthranol
Blenoxane®	Yes	Bleomycin	Bleomycin sulfate
Bleomycin		Bleomycin	Bleomycin sulfate
Bonine		Meclozine	Meclizine
Bretylium		Bretylium tosilate	Bretylium tosylate
Bretylol®	Yes	Bretylium tosilate	Bretylium tosylate
Bromocriptine	Parlodel®		Bromocriptine mesylate

Drug listed in text	Brand name?	INN name if different	USAN or USP name if different
Bromodiphenhydramine	Bromanyl®	Bromazine	Bromazine
Bucampicillin	Spectrobid®	Bacampicillin	Bacampicillin
Bucladin		Buclizine	Buclizine hydrochloride
Buclizine		Buclizine	Buclizine hydrochloride
Bumetanide	Bumex®		
Bumex®	Yes	Bumetanide	Bumetanide
Bupivacaine			Bupivacaine hydrochloride
Buprenorphine			Buprenorphine hydrochloride
Bupropion	Wellbutrin®		Bupropion hydrochloride
Butalbital	Fiorinal® and Fioricet® are combination drugs		
Butoconazole			Butoconazole nitrate
Butorphenol	Stadol®	Butorphanol	Butorphanol
Byclomine		Dicycloverine	Dicyclomine
Calan®	Yes	Verapramil	Verapamil
Cantil®	Yes	Mepenzolate bromide	Mepenzolate bromide
Capoten®	Yes	Captopril	Captopril
Carbamazepine	Tegretol®		
Carbenicillin			Carbenicillin disodium
Cordarone®	Yes – also Pacerone®	Amiodarone	Amiodarone
Cardioquin®	Yes	Not listed	Quinidine (USP)
Carisoprodol	Soma®	Carisoprodol	Carisoprodol
Carteolol	Ocupress®		Carteolol hydrochloride
Casanthranol		From cascara tree bark	From cascara tree bark
Cascara sagrada		From cascara tree bark	From cascara tree bark
Catapres®	Yes	Clonidine	Clonidine hydrochloride
Cefaclor	Ceclor®		
Cefazolin	Ancef®		Cefazolin sodium
Cefmenoxime			Cefmenoxime hydrochloride
Cefonicid			USAN cefonicid sodium USAN2 cefonicid monosodium
Cefoperazone			Cefoperazone sodium
Cefotaxime			Cefotaxime sodium
Cefotetan	Cefotan®		
Cefoxitin	Mefoxin®		
Cefpodoxime proxetil	Vantin®		Cefpodoxime proxetil
Ceftazidime	Fortaz®		
Ceftizoxime			Ceftizoxime sodium
Ceftriaxone	Rocephin®		Ceftriaxone sodium
Cefuroxime	Zinacef®		
Celecoxib	Celebrex®		
Celexa®	Yes	Citalopram	Citalopram hydrobromide
Celontin®	Yes	Mesuximide	Methsuximide

Drug listed in text	Brand name?	INN name if different	USAN or USP name if different
Cephalexin	Keflex®	Cefalexin	
Cephalothin		Cefalotin	Cephalothin sodium
Cephapirin		Not listed	Not listed
Cephradine		Cefradine	
Cerubidine®	Yes	Daunorubicin	Daunorubicin hydrochloride
Cetirizine	Zyrtec®		Cetirizine hydrochloride
Chloral hydrate	Noctec®	Not listed	Not listed
Chlorambucil	Leukeran®		
Chlordiazepoxide	Librium®		Chlordiazepoxide hydrochloride
Chloromycetin®	Yes	Chloramphenicol	Chloramphenicol
Chlorphenamine			Chlorpheniramine
Chlorpheniramine		Chlorphenamine	Chlorpheniramine
Chlorpromazine		Not listed	Not listed
Chloroprocaine		Chloroprocaine	Chloroprocaine
Chlorthalidone	Hygroton®	Chlortalidone	
Cholestyramine	Questran®	Colestyramine	
Chooz			
Chronulac®	Yes	Lactulose	Lactulose
Cilastatin			Cilastatin sodium
Cimetidine	Tagamet®		
Ciprofloxacin	Cipro®		
Cisapride	Propulsid®		
Cisplatin	Platinol-aq®		
Citalopram	Celexa®		Citalopram hydrobromide
Citroma®	Yes	Not listed	Not listed
Citro-Nesia®	Yes	Not listed	Not listed
Citrucel®	Yes	Methylcellulose	Methylcellulose
Clarithromycin	Biaxin®		
Clavulanic acid			Clavulanate potassium
Cleocin®	Yes	Clindamycin	Clindamycin
Clidinium		Clidinium bromide	Clidinium bromide
Clindamycin	Cleocin®		
Clioquinol			
Clistin®	Yes	Carbinoxamine	Carbinoxamine
Clobetasol			Clobetasol propionate
Clocortolone			USAN clocortolone acetate USAN2 clocortolone pivalate
Clomid®	Yes	Clomifene	Clomiphene citrate
Clomiphene		Clomifene	Clomiphene citrate
Clomipramine			Clomipramine hydrochloride
Clonazepam	Klonopin®		
Clonidine	Catapres®		
Clonazepam		Not listed	Not listed
Clorazepate		Dipotassium clorazepate	Clorazepate dipotassium
Chlorpropamide		Chlorpropamide	Chlorpropamide

Drug listed in text	Brand name?	INN name if different	USAN or USP name if different
Clotrimazole	Lotrimin®		
Cloxacillin			Cloxacillin sodium
Clozapine	Clozaril®		
Clozaril®	Yes	Clozapine	Clozapine
Cocaine			
Codeine		Not listed	Not listed
Colace®	Yes	Docusate sodium	Docusate sodium
Colchicine		Not listed	Not listed
Cologel®	Yes	Methylcellulose	Methylcellulose
Cosmegen®	Yes	Dactinomycin	Dactinomycin
Cromolyn		Cromoglicic acid	Cromolyn sodium
Cromolyn sodium		Cromoglicic acid	
Cuprimine®	Yes	Penicillamine	Penicillamine
Curare		Tubocurarine chloride	Tubocurarine chloride
Cyanocobalamin	Vitamin b12		
Cyclophosphamide	Cytoxan®		
Cyclosporine	Sandimmune®, neoral®, gengraf®	Ciclosporin	
Cyproheptadine	Periactin®		
Cystospaz®	Yes	Not listed	Not listed
Cytosar®	Yes	Cytarabine	Cytarabine
Cytosar-U®	Yes	Cytarabine	Cytarabine
Cytosine arabinoside		Cytarabine	Cytarabine
Cytoxan®	Yes	Cyclophosphamide	Cyclophosphamide
Danocrine®	Yes	Danazol	Danazol
Darbid®	Yes	Isopropamide iodide	Isopropamide iodide
Daunorubicin			Daunorubicin hydrochloride
Daxolin®	Yes	Loxapine	Loxapine
Declomycin®	Yes	Demeclocycline	Demeclocycline hydrochloride
Demeclocycline			Demeclocycline hydrochloride
Demerol®	Yes	Pethidine	Meperidine
Depakane®	Yes	Valproic acid	Valproate sodium
Depakote®	Depakote ER®	Valproate semisodium	Divalproex sodium
Depo provera®	Yes	Medroxyprogesterone	Medroxyprogesterone
Deprol®	Yes	Meprobamate and benactyzine	Meprobamate and benactyzine
Desenex®	Yes	Not listed	Not listed
Desipramine			Desipramine hydrochloride
Desloratadine	Clarinex®		
Desmopressin			Desmopressin acetate
Desyrel®	Yes	Trazodone	Trazodone hydrochloride
Dexamethasone			USAN dexamethasone
			USAN dexamethasone beloxil

Drug listed in text	Brand name?	INN name if different	USAN or USP name if different
Dexfenfluramine			Dexfenfluramine hydrochloride
Dextromethorphan		Dextromethorphan	Dextromethorphan polistirex
Dextroamphetamines	Dexedrine®, adderall®	Dexamfetamine	
Dialose® (DSS)	Yes	Docusate sodium	Docusate sodium, docusate potassium
Diazepam	Valium®		
Dibent®	Yes	Dicycloverine	Dicyclomine
Dichloralphenazone		Not listed	Not listed
Diclofenac	Voltaren®		Diclofenac
Dicyclomine	Bentyl®	Dicycloverine	
Didrex®	Yes		
Diethylpropion		Amfepramone	
Diflorasone		Not listed	Diflorasone diacetate
Dilantin®	Yes	Phenytoin	Phenytoin
Dilaudid®	Yes	Hydromorphone	Hydromorphone
Diltiazem	Cardiazem®, tiazac®		Usan diltiazem hydrochloride usan2 diltiazem malate usan3 diltiazem maleate
Diocto-K®	Yes	Docusate sodium	Docusate sodium
Diones		Not listed	Not listed
Diphenhydramine	Benadryl®		
Diphenylan®	Yes	Phenytoin	Phenytoin
Dipyramidole	Persantine®	Not listed	Not listed
Dyrenium		Triamterene	Triamterene
Di-Spaz®	Yes, also Bentyl®	Dicycloverine	Dicyclomine
Disulfiram	Antabuse®		
Diucardin®	Yes	Hydroflumethiazide	Hydroflumethiazide
Diulo®	Zaroxolyn®	Metolazone	Metolazone
Diuril®	Yes	Chlorothiazide	Chlorothiazide
Docusate		Docusate sodium	Docusate sodium
Donnagel-PG®	Yes	Not listed	Not listed
Donnapectolin-PG		Not listed	Not listed
Dormarex®	Yes	Diphenhydramine	Diphenhydramine
Doryx®	Yes	Doxycycline	Doxycycline
Doxepin			Doxepin hydrochloride
Doxorubicin	Adriamycin®		
Dristan®	Yes	Chlorphenamine, phenylephrine AND paracetamol	Chlorpheniramine, phenylephrine, AND acetaminophen
Drithocreme®	Yes	Dithranol	Anthralin
Dulcolax®	Yes	Bisacodyl	Bisacodyl tannex
Dynacin®	Yes	Minocycline	Minocycline
Econazole			Econazole nitrate
Edecrin®		Ethacrynic acid	Ethacryinic acid

Drug listed in text	Brand name?	INN name if different	USAN or USP name if different
Edrophonium	Tensilon®	Edrophonium chloride	Edrophonium chloride
Efudex®	5-fu cream	Not listed	Fluorouracil
Elavil®	Yes	Amitriptyline	Amitriptyline
Elspar®	Yes	Not listed	Asparaginase
Emitrip®	Elavil®	Amitriptyline	Amitriptyline
Enalapril	Vasotec®		Enalapril maleate
Enbrel®	Yes	Etanercept	Etanercept
Encainide			Encainide hydrochloride
Endep®	Yes	Amitriptyline	Amitriptyline
Enkaid®	Yes	Encainide	Encainide hydrochloride
Enovil®	Yes	Amitriptyline	Amitriptyline
Ephedrine		Not listed	Not listed
Epinephrine			Epinephryl borate
Equagesic®	Yes	Not listed	Not listed
Equalactin®	Yes	Polycarbophil	Polycarbophil calcium
Equanil®	Yes	Meprobamate	Meprobamate
Erythromycin			USAN erythromycin estolate USAN2 erythromycin salnacedin USP erythromycin base, erythromycin stearate
Erythromycin estolate		Erythromycin	USAN erythromycin estolate USAN2 erythromycin salnacedin
Erythromycin ethylsuccinate		Erythromycin	USAN erythromycin estolate USAN2 erythromycin salnacedin
Erythromycin gluceptate	Ilotycin gluceptate®	Not listed	erythromycin glucceptate
Erythromycin lactobionate	Erythrocin®	Erythromycin	Erythromycin
Erythromycin stearate	Erythrocin® stearate	Erythromycin	Erythromycin
Esomeprazole	Nexium®		Esomeprazole magnesium
Ethambutol	Myambutol®		Ethambutol hydrochloride
Ethanolamine	Ethamolin®	Monoethanolamine oleate	Ethanolamine oleate
ethracrynic acid	Edecrin®	Not listed	Ethacryinic acid
Ethrane®	Yes	Enflurane	Enflurane
Etodolac	Lodine®		
Etoposide	Vepesid®	Etoposide	Etoposide phosphate
Etrafon®	Yes	Perphenazine	Perphenazine
Eurax®	Yes	Crotamiton	Crotamiton
Ex-Lax®	Yes	Not listed	Not listed
Famotidine	Pepcid®		
Feen-a-Mint®	Yes	Bisacodyl	Bisacodyl tannex
Fenfluramine			Fenfluramine hydrochloride
Fenoprofen			Fenoprofen calcium

Drug listed in text	Brand name?	INN name if different	USAN or USP name if different
Fentanyl	Duragesic® patches		Fentanyl citrate
Fexofenadine	Allegra®		Fexofenadine hydrochloride
Fibercan		Not listed	Not listed
Flagyl®	Yes	Metronidazole	Metronidazole hydrochloride, metronidazole phosphate
Flecainide			Flecainide acetate
Flint SSD®	Yes	Sulfadiazine	Silver sulfadiazine
Flumethasone		Flumetasone	
Fluocinolone		Fluocinolone acetonide	Fluocinolone acetonide
Fluocionide	Lidex®	Not listed	Not listed
Fluoconazole	Diflucan®	Not listed	Not listed
Fluoroplex®	Yes, also Adrucil®	Fluorouracil	Fluorouracil
Fluothane®	Yes	Halothane	Halothane
Fluoxetine		Not listed	Not listed
Flurandrenolide		Fludroxycortide	
Flurazepam			Flurazepam hydrochloride
Fluvoxamine			Fluvoxamine maleate
Folex®	Yes	Methotrexate	Methotrexate
Forane®	Yes	Isoflurane	Isoflurane
Fosinopril		Fosinopril	Fosinopril sodium
Fosphenytoin			Fosphenytoin sodium
Ganciclovir			Ganciclovir sodium
Gantanol®	Yes	Sulfamethoxazole	Sulfamethoxazole
Gantrisin®	Yes	Sulfafurazole	Sulfisoxazole diolamine
Garamycin®	Yes	Gentamicin	Gentamicin sulfate
Gas Relief®	Yes	Not listed	Simethicone
Gas-X®	Yes	Not listed	Simethicone
Gelusil®	Yes	Not listed	Alumina, magnesia, simethicone
Genaspore®	Yes	Tolnaftate	Tolnaftate
Gentamicin			Gentamicin sulfate
Glyburide		Glibenclamide	
Glycopyrrolate		Glycopyrronium bromide	Glycopyrrolate
Gold salts		Sodium aurothiomalate	Sodium aurothiomalate
Haldol®	Yes	Haloperidol	Haloperidol decanoate
Haloperidol			Haloperidol decanoate
Heparin		Heparin sodium	Heparin sodium
Hexalen®	Yes	Altretamine	Altretamine
Hexamethylmelamine		Altretamine	Altretamine
Hexocyclium		Hexocyclium metilsulfate	Hexocyclium metilsulfate
Hexoprenaline			Hexoprenaline sulfate
Hismanal®	Yes	Astemizole	Astemizole
Hispril®	Yes	Diphenylpyraline	Diphenylpyraline
Homapin	Yes	Homatropine methylbromide	Homatropine methylbromide

Drug listed in text	Brand name?	INN name if different	USAN or USP name if different
Homatropine		Homatropine methylbromide	Homatropine methylbromide
Hydrea		Hydroxycarbamide	Hydroxyurea
Hydrocodone			USAN hydrocodone bitartrate USAN2 hydrocodone polistirex
Hydrocortisone			USAN hydrocortisone valerate USAN hydrocortisone probutrate USAN2 hydrocortisone butyrate USAN3 hydrocortisone buterate
Hydromox®	Yes	Quinethazone	Quinethazone
Hydroxyurea	Hydrea®	Not listed	Hydroxyurea
Hygroton®	Yes	Chlortalidone	Chlorthalidone
Hykinone®	Yes	Menadione sodium bisulfite	Menadione sodium bisulfite
Hyoscyamine		Not listed	Hyoscyamine Sulfate
Hyperstat®	Yes	Diazoxide	Diazoxide
Ifex®	Yes	Ifosfamide	Ifosfamide
Imitrex®	Yes	Sumatriptan	Sumatriptan succinate
Imuran®	Yes	Azathioprine	Azathioprine
Inderal®	Yes	Propranolol	Propranolol hydrochloride
Indomethacin		Indometacin	
Innovar®	Yes	Fentanyl AND droperidol	Fentanyl citrate AND droperidol
Iodine		Not listed	Not listed
Ipecacuanha			
Ipratropium		Ipratropium bromide	Ipratropium bromide
Isoetharine		Isoetarine	
Isomethertene		Isometheptene	Isometheptene
Isopropamide		Isopropamide iodide	Isopropamide iodide
Isoproterenol		Isoprenaline	
Isoptin®	Yes	Verapamil	Verapamil hydrochloride
Janimine®	Yes	Imipramine	Imipramine
Kaopectate®	Yes		
Kapectolin®	Yes	Kaolin and pectin	Kaolin and pectin
Kasof®	Yes	Docusate sodium	USAN docusate calcium USAN2 docusate potassium
Ketalar®	Yes	Ketamine	Ketamine hydrochloride
Ketamine			Ketamine hydrochloride
Ketorulac		Ketorolac	Ketorolac tromethamine
Klonopin®	Yes	Clonazepam	Clonazepam
Kondremul®	Yes		

Drug listed in text	Brand name?	INN name if different	USAN or USP name if different
Kwell®	Yes	Lindane	Lindane
Labetalol			Labetalol hydrochloride
Lamisil®	Yes	Terbinafine	Terbinafine
Leucororin		Not listed	Leucovorin
Leukeran®	Yes	Chlorambucil	Chlorambucil
Levarterenol	Levophed®	Not listed	Norepinephrine Bitartrate
Levo-alpha-acetyl-methadol	Orlaam®	Not listed	Levomethadyl
Levothyroxine	Synthroid®	Levothyroxine sodium	Levothyroxine sodium
Levsin®	Yes	L-hyosycamine	Not listed
Levsinex®	Yes	L-hyosycamine	Not listed
Librium®	Yes	Chlordiazepoxide	Chlordiazepoxide hydrochloride
Lidone®	Yes	Molindone	Molindone hydrochloride
LidoPen®	Yes	Lidocaine	Lidocaine hydrochloride
Lomotil®	Yes	Diphenoxylate	Diphenoxylate
Loperamide			Loperamide hydrochloride
Lopressor®	Yes	Metoprolol	USAN metoprolol tartrate USAN2 metoprolol fumarate USAN3 metoprolol succinate
Loratidine		Loratadine	Loratadine
Loxitane®	Yes	Loxapine	Loxapine succinate
LSD		Lysergide	Lysergide
Ludiomil®	Yes	Maprotiline	Maprotiline
Macrodantin®	Yes	Nitrofurantoin	Nitrofurantoin
Magnesium citrate		Not listed	Not listed
Magnesium hydroxide		Not listed	Not listed
Marcaine®	Yes	Bupivacaine	Bupivacaine hydrochloride
Marezine®	Yes	Meclozine	Meclizine
Marplan®	Yes	Isocarboxazid	Isocarboxazid
Matulane®	Yes	Procarbazine	Procarbazine hydrochloride
Mazanor®	Yes	Mazindol	Mazindol
Mebaral		Methylphenobarbital	Mephobarbital
Mechlorethamine		Chlormethine	
Meclizine		Meclozine	
Meclofenamate		Meclofenamic acid	Meclofenamic acid OR meclofenamate sodium
Medilax®	Yes	Phenolphthalein	Phenolphthalein
Mellaril®	Yes	Thioridazine	Thioridazine
Membendazole		Mebendazole	Mebendazole
Mepenzolate		Mepenzolate bromide	Mepenzolate bromide
Meperidine		Pethidine	Pethidine
Mephobarbital		Methylphenobarbital	
Mesantoin		Phenytoin	Phenytoin
Mescaline		Hallucinogen from peyote	Hallucinogen from peyote
Metahydrin®	Yes	Trichlormethiazide	Trichlormethiazide

Drug listed in text	Brand name?	INN name if different	USAN or USP name if different
Metoprolol			Metoprolol tartrate OR metoprolol fumarate OR metoprolol succinate
Metaproterenol		Orciprenaline	Metaproterenol sulfate
Methamphetamine		Metamfetamine	
Methantheline		Dicycloverine	Dicyclomine
Methclothiazide		Methyclothiazide	Methyclothiazide
Methicillin		Meticillin	
Methimazole		Thiamazole	
Methohexitone		Methohexital	Methohexital
Methscopolamine		Not listed	Not listed
Methsuximide		Mesuximide	
Methylaminopterin	Rheumatrex®	Methotrexate	Methotrexate
Methylene blue		Methylthioninium chloride	
Methylprednisolone			Methylprednisolone sodium phosphate
Metoclopramide		Metoclopramide	Metoclopramide hydrochloride
Metrodin®	Yes	Urofollitropin	Urofollitropin
Mexate®	Yes	Methotrexate	Methotrexate
Mexiletine		Mexiletine	Mexiletin hydrochloride
Mexiletine			Mexiletin hydrochloride
Mexitil®	Yes	Mexiletine	Mexiletin hydrochloride
Mianserin			Mianserin hydrochloride
Miconazole			Miconazole nitrate
Midazolam			Midazolam maleate
Midrin®	Yes	Acetaminophen, dichloralphenazone, and isometheptene	Acetaminophen, dichloralphenazone, and isometheptene
Migratine		Combination of Isometheptene, dichloralphenazone, and acetaminophen	Combination of Isometheptene, dichloralphenazone, and acetaminophen
Milk of Magnesia		Magnesium hydroxide	Magnesium hydroxide
Milontin®	Yes	Phensuximide	Phensuximide
Miltown®	Yes	Meprobamate	Meprobamate
Minocin®	Yes	Minocycline	Minocycline
Mintezol®	Yes	Tiabendazole	Thiabendazole
Mitomycin-C		Mitomycin	Mitomycin
Mitrolan®	Yes	Polycarbophil	Polycarbophil calcium
Moban®	Yes	Molindone	Molindone hydrochloride
Molindone			Molindone hydrochloride
Mometasone			Mometasone furoate
Monodox®	Vibramycin®	Doxycycline	Doxycycline fosfatex (usan)
M-Orexic®	Yes	Amfepramone	Diethylpropion
Morphine		Morphine glucuronide	Morphine glucuronide
Moxalactam		Latamoxef	Moxalactam disodium

Drug listed in text	Brand name?	INN name if different	USAN or USP name if different
Mupirocin			Mupirocin calcium
Mustargen®	Yes	Chlormethine	Mechlorethamine
Mutamycin®	Yes	Mitomycin	Mitomycin
Mylanta®	Yes	Aluminum hydroxide, magnesium hydroxide and simethicone	Aluminum hydroxide, magnesium hydroxide and simethicone
Myleran		Busulfan	Busulfan
Myliam	Myleran® busulfan?	Not listed	Not listed
Myochrysine®	Yes	Sodium aurothiomalate	Gold sodium thiomalate
Nafcillin			Nafcillin sodium
Naftifine			Naftifine hydrochloride
Nalbuphine			Nalbuphine hydrochloride
Naloxone			Naloxone hydrochloride
Nandrolone			Nandrolone decanoate
Naproxen			Naproxen sodium
Naqua®	Yes	Trichlormethiazide	Trichlormethiazide
Narcan®	Yes	Naloxone	Naloxone hydrochloride
Nardil®	Yes	Phenelzine	Phenelzine
Naturetin®	Yes	Bendroflumethiazide	Bendroflumethiazide
Navane®	Yes	Tiotixene	Thiothixene
Nebcin®	Yes	Tobramycin	Tobramycin
Nefazodone			Nefazodone hydrochloride
Nembutal®	Yes	Pentobarbital	Pentobarbital
Neo Synephrine®	Yes	Phenylephrine	Phenylephrine
Neomycin			Neomycin palmitate neomycin undecylenate
Neosar®	Yes	Cyclophosphamide	Cyclophosphamide
Neostigmine		Neostigmine bromide	Neostigmine bromide
Nesacaine®	Yes	Chloroprocaine	Chloroprocaine
Netilmicin			Netilmicin sulfate
Netromycin®	Yes	Netilmicin	Netilmicin sulfate
Nexium®	Yes	Esomeprazole	Esomeprazole magnesium
Niacin		Nicotinic acid	
Nicardipine			Nicardipine hydrochloride
Nipride®	Yes	Not listed	Sodium nitroprusside
Nitroglycerin		Not listed	Not listed
Nitropress®	Yes	Not listed	Sodium nitroprusside
Nitroprusside		Not listed	Not listed
Nobesine®	Yes	Amfepramone	Diethylpropion
Nolahist®	Yes	Phenindamine	Phenindamine
Nomifensine			Nomifensine maleate
Nonoxynols		Nonoxynol 9	Nonoxynol 9
Norcuron®	Yes	Vecuronium bromide	Vecuronium bromide
Norethindrone		Norethisterone	
Norethynodrel		Noretynodrel	
Normeperidine (see Meperidine)			

Drug listed in text	Brand name?	INN name if different	USAN or USP name if different
Norpace®	Yes	Disopyramide	Disopyramide
Norpanth®	Yes	Propantheline bromide	Propantheline bromide
Norplant®	Yes	Levonorgestrel	Levonorgestrel
Norpramin®	Yes	Desipramine	Desipramine hydrochloride
Nortriptyline			Nortriptyline hydrochloride
NP27		Not listed	Not listed
Numbutal®	Yes	Pentobarbital	Pentobarbital
Omeprazole			Omeprazole sodium
Oncovin®	Yes	Vincristine	Vincristine sulfate
Ondansetron			Ondansetron hydrochloride
Optimine®	Yes	Azatadine	Azatadine maleate
Oral filmtabs		Not listed	Not listed
Orthoclone OKT3®	Yes	Muromonab-CD3	Muromonab-CD3
Oxacillin			Oxacillin sodium
Oxymetazoline			Oxymetazoline hydrochloride
Oxymethalone		Oxymetholone	Oxymetholone
Oxyphenonium		Oxyphenonium bromide	Oxyphenonium bromide
Paclitaxel			Paclitaxel poliglumex
Pamelor®	Yes	Nortriptyline	Nortriptyline hydrochloride
Pamine®	Yes	Not listed	Methscopolamine bromide
Pancuronium		Pancuronium bromide	Pancuronium bromide
Pantoprazole			Pantoprazole sodium
Paperavine		Not listed	Not listed
Paracetan		Not listed	Not listed
Paradione		Paramethadione	Paramethadione
Paraplatin®	Yes	Carboplatin	Carboplatin
Paregoric		Not listed	Not listed
Parepectolin®	Yes	Attapulgite	Attapulgite
Parest®	Yes	Methaqualone	Methaqualone
Parlodel®	Yes	Bromocriptine	Bromocriptine mesylate
Parnate®	Yes	Tranylcypromine	Tranylcypromine
Paroxetine			Paroxetine mesylate
Pathilon®	Yes	Tridihexethyl iodide	Tridihexethyl iodide
Pavulen		Not listed	Not listed
Paxil®	Yes	Paroxetine	Paroxetine mesylate
PBZ®	Yes	Tripelennamine	Tripelennamine
PCM		Not listed	Not listed
PCP		Phencyclidine	Phencyclidine hydrochloride
Pefloxacin			Pefloxacin mesylate
Peganone®	Yes	Ethotoin	Ethotoin
Penbutolol			Penbutolol sulfate
Penicillin		Penicillinase	Penicillinase
Penicillin G		Benzylpenicillin	
Penicillin V		Phenoxymethylpenicillin	
Pentazocine			Pentazocine hydrochloride
Penthrane®	Yes	Methoxyflurane	Methoxyflurane
Pepcid®	Yes	Famotidine	Famotidine

Drug listed in text	Brand name?	INN name if different	USAN or USP name if different
Pergonal®	Yes	Not listed	Menotropins
Periactin®	Yes	Cyproheptadine	Cyproheptadine
Permitil®	Yes	Fluphenazine	Fluphenazine
Pertofrane®	Yes	Desipramine	Desipramine hydrochloride
Phazyme®	Yes	Not listed	Simethicone
Phencyclidine			Phencyclidine hydrochloride
Pheniramine			Pheniramine maleate
Phenobarbitone		Phenobarbital	Phenobarbital
Phenolphthalein		Phenolphthalein	Phenolphthalein
Physostigmine		Not listed	Not listed
Piperacillin			Piperacillin sodium
Piperazine		Piperazine calcium edetate	Piperazine calcium edetate
Piroxicam			Piroxicam olamine
Placidyl®	Yes	Ethchlorvynol	Ethchlorvynol
Platinol®	Yes	Cisplatin	Cisplatin
Podophyllum	Condylox®	Not listed	Not listed
Polaramine®	Yes	Dexchlorpheniramine	Dexchlorpheniramine
Polycarbophil			Polycarbophil calcium
Pontocaine®	Yes	Tetracaine	Tetracaine
Potassium iodide (SSKI)		Not listed	Not listed
Prazosin			Prazosin hydrochloride
Prednisolone			Prednival
Prelu-2®	Yes	Phendimetrazine	Phendimetrazine
Prilocaine			Prilocaine hydrochloride
Prilosec®	Yes	Omeprazole	Omeprazole
Pro-Banthine®	Yes	Propantheline bromide	Propantheline bromide
Probenecid			Probenate
Procan®	Yes	Procainamide	Procainamide
Procarbazine			Procarbazine hydrochloride
Proglycem®	Yes	Diazoxide	Diazoxide
Pro-Lax®	Yes	Macrogol	PEG 3350
Prolixin®	Yes	Fluphenazine	Fluphenazine
Proloprim®	Yes	Trimethoprim	Trimethoprim sulfate
Pronestyl®	Yes	Procainamide	Procainamide
Propantheline		Propantheline bromide	Propantheline bromide
Propoxyphene		Dextropropoxyphene	Propoxyphene napsylate
Propranolol			Propranolol hydrochloride
Propulsid®	Yes	Cisapride	Cisapride
Prostacyclin		Epoprostenol	Epoprostenol sodium
Protamine		Protamine sulfate	Protamine sulfate
Protriptyline			Protriptyline hydrochloride
Prozac®	Yes	Fluoxetine	Fluoxetine hydrochloride
Pseudoephedrine			Pseudoephedrine hydrochloride
Puri-Nethol	Purinethol®	Mercaptopurine	Mercaptopurine, 6-MP
Pyrantel pomoate		Pyrantel	

Drug listed in text	Brand name?	INN name if different	USAN or USP name if different
Pyribenzamine®	Yes	Tripelennamine	Tripelennamine
Pyridostigmine		Pyridostigmine bromide	Pyridostigmine bromide
Pyrilamine		Mepyramine	
Quaalude®	Yes	Methaqualone	Methaqualone
Quarzan®	Yes	Clidinium bromide	Clidinium bromide
Quiagel-PG®	Yes	Not listed	Not listed
Quinaglute Dura-Tabs®	Yes	Quinidine Gluconate	Quinidine Gluconate
Quinapril			Quinapril hydrochloride
Quindex Extentabs®	Yes	Quinidine	Quinidine
Quinidine		Not listed	Not listed
Quinine		Not listed	Not listed
Ranitidine			Ranitidine bismuth citrate
reglan®	Yes	Metoclopramide	Metoclopramide hydrochloride
Renese®	Yes	Polythiazide	Polythiazide
Renoquid®	Yes	Sulfacitine	Sulfacytine
Retin-A®	Yes	Tretinoin	Tretinoin
Retrovir®	Yes	Zidovudine	Zidovudine
Rhythmin	Rhythmol®	Propafenone	Propafenone hydrochloride
Ridaura®	Yes	Auranofin	Auranofin
Rifampin		Rifampicin	
Riopan®	Yes	Magaldrate	Magaldrate
Ritalin®	Yes	Methylphenidate	Methylphenidate
Robinul®	Yes	Glycopyrronium bromide	Glycopyrrolate
Rolaids®	Yes	Not listed	Not listed
Rozatidine		Not listed	Not listed
Rubex®	Yes	Doxorubicin	Doxorubicin
Salbutamol			Albuterol OR albuterol sulfate
Saluron®	Yes	Hydroflumethiazide	Hydroflumethiazide
Samdimmune®	Yes	Ciclosporin	Cyclosporine
Scabene®	Yes	Lindane	Lindane
Scopolamine	Scopace®	Hyoscine hbr	Hyoscine hbr
Seconal®	Yes	Secobarbital	Secobarbital
Sectral®	Yes	Acebutolol	Acebutolol
Seldane®	Yes	Terfenadine	Terfenadine
Senna		Not listed	Not listed
Senokot®	Yes	Not listed	Not listed
Septra®	Yes	Sulfamethoxazole and Trimethoprim	Sulfamethoxazole and Trimethoprim
Serentil®	Yes	Mesoridazine	Mesoridazine
Serex		Oxazepam	Oxazepam
Sertraline			Sertraline hydrochloride
Serutan®	Yes	Psyllium	Psyllium
Sertraline		Not listed	Not listed
Sildimac®	Yes	Sulfadiazine	Silver sulfadiazine
Silvadene®	Yes	Sulfadiazine	Silver sulfadiazine

Drug listed in text	Brand name?	INN name if different	USAN or USP name if different
Silver sulfadiazine		Sulfadiazine	
Simethicone		Not listed	Not listed
Sinequan®	Yes	Doxepin	Doxepin hydrochloride
Solbutanol		Not listed	Not listed
Solganol®	Yes	Aurothioglucose	Aurothioglucose
Sominex®	Yes	Diphenhydramine	Diphenhydramine
Sommicaps		Not listed	Not listed
Sopor®	Yes	Methaqualone	Methaqualone
Sotalol			Sotalol hydrochloride
Stavudine (d4T)		Stavudine	Stavudine
Stelazine®	Yes	Trifluoperazine	Trifluoperazine
Sublimaze®	Yes	Fentanyl	Fentanyl citrate
Succinylcholine		Suxamethonium chloride	Succinylcholine chloride
Sufenta®	Yes	Sufentanil	Sufentanil citrate
Sufentanil			Sufentanil citrate
Sulbactam			USAN sulbactam sodium USAN2 sulbactam pivoxil USAN3 sulbactam benzathine
Sulfacytine		Sulfacitine	
Sulfadiazine			Silver sulfadiazine
Sulfamylon®	Yes	Mafenide	Mafenide
Sulfisoxazole		Sulfafurazole	Sulfisoxazole diolamine
Sumatriptan			Sumatriptan succinate
Surfak®	Yes	Docusate sodium	USAN docusate calcium USAN2 docusate potassium
Tabloid®	Yes	Tioguanine	Thioguanine
Tagamet®	Yes	Cimetidine	Cimetidine hydrochloride
Talwin®	Yes	Pentazocine	USAN pentazocine hydrochloride USAN2 pentazocine lactate
Tambocor®	Yes	Flecainide	Flecainide acetate
Tonocard		Tocainide	Tocainide
Tarabine®	Yes	Cytarabine	Cytarabine hydrochloride
Tavist®	Yes	Clemastine	Clemastine fumarate
Taxol®	Yes	Paclitaxel	Paclitaxel poliglumex
Tazobactam			Tazobactam sodium
Tegison®	Yes	Etretinate	Etretinate
Tegretol®	Yes	Carbamazepine	Carbamazepine
Tenormin®	Yes	Atenolol	Atenolol
Tenuate®	Yes	Amfepramone	Diethylpropion
Terbutaline			Terbutaline sulfate
Terpin hydrate		Used with codeine in cough syrup	Used with codeine in cough syrup
Terramycin®	Yes	Oxytetracycline	Oxytetracycline
Tessalon®	Yes	Benzonatate	Benzonatate
Testosterone proprionate		Not listed	Not listed

Drug listed in text	Brand name?	INN name if different	USAN or USP name if different
Tetrahydrozoline		Tetryzoline	Tetrahydrozoline
Thalitone®	Yes	Chlortalidone	Chlorthalidone
Theophylline			
Thermazene®	Yes	Sulfadiazine	Silver sulfadiazine
Thienamycin		Not listed	Not listed
Thiethylperazine			Thiethylperazine maleate
Thiobendazole		Not listed	Not listed
Thioguanine		Tioguanine	
Thiopental	Pentothal®	Thiopental sodium	Thiopental sodium
Thiosulfil Forte®	Yes	Sulfamethizole	Sulfamethizole
Thiothixene		Tiotixene	
Thorazine®	Yes	Chlorpromazine	Chlorpromazine
Tiagabine			Tiagabine hydrochloride
Ticarcillin			USAN ticarcillin disodium USAN2 ticarcillin cresyl sodium
TIMENTIN®	Yes	Ticarcillan and clavulanic acid	Ticarcillin disodium and clavulanate potassium
Timolol			Timolol maleate
Tinactin®	Yes	Tolnaftate	Tolnaftate
Ting®	Yes	Tolnaftate	Tolnaftate
Tipramine®	Yes	Imipramine	Imipramine
Titralac®	Yes	Not listed	Not listed
Tofranil®	Yes	Imipramine	Imipramine
Tolmetin		Not listed	Tolmetin sodium
Toluene		Not listed	Not listed
Tracrium®	Yes	Atracurium besilate	Atracurium besylate
Trazodone			Trazodone hydrochloride
Trexan®	Yes	Naltrexone	Naltrexone hydrochloride
Triamcinolone			USAN triamcinolone acetonide sodium phosphate USAN2 triamcinolone diacetate
Trichlorex®	Yes	Trichlormethiazide	Trichlormethiazide
Trichloroacetic acid	Tri-chlor®		
Tridione®	Yes	Trimethadione	Trimethadione
Triethylene thiophosphoramide		Thiotepa	Thiotepa
Trilafon®	Yes	Perphenazine	Perphenazine
Trimeprazine		Alimemazine	
Trimethoprim			Trimethoprim sulfate
Trimpex®	Yes	Trimethoprim	Trimethoprim sulfate
Tums®	Yes	Not listed	Not listed
Unasyn®	Yes	Ampicillin; sulbactam	Ampicillin sodium; sulbactam sodium
Unisom®	Yes	Doxylamine	Doxylamine

Drug listed in text	Brand name?	INN name if different	USAN or USP name if different
Urobiotic®	Yes	Oxytetracycline	Oxytetracycline
Valium®	Yes	Diazepam	Diazepam
Velban®	Yes	Vinblastine	Vinblastine sulfate
Velsar®	Yes	Vinblastine	Vinblastine sulfate
Venlafaxine		Venlafaxine	Venlafaxine hydrochloride
VePesid®	Yes	Etoposide	Etoposide phosphate
Verapamil		Verapamil	Verapamil hydrochloride
Vermox®	Yes	Mebendazole	Mebendazole
Vibramycin®	Yes	Doxycycline	Doxycycline fosfatex
Vidarabine			Vidarabine phosphate, vidarabine sodium phosphate
Viloxazine			Viloxazine hydrochloride
Vinblastine			Vinblastine sulfate
Vincasar®	Yes	Vincristine	Vincristine sulfate
Vincrex®	Yes	Vincristine	Vincristine sulfate
Vincristine			Vincristine sulfate
Vioxx®	Yes	Rofecoxib	Rofecoxib
Vistaril®	Yes	Hydroxyzine	Hydroxyzine
Vivactil®	Yes	Protriptyline	Protriptyline hydrochloride
VP-16VPP	Vepesid®	Etoposide, VP-16-213	Etoposide, VP-16-213
Wellbutrin®	Yes	Bupropion	Bupropion hydrochloride
Xanax®	Yes	Alprazolam	Alprazolam
Xylocaine®	Yes	Lidocaine	Lidocaine
Zalcitabine (ddC)		Zalcitabine	Zalcitabine
Zantac®	Yes	Ranitidine	Ranitidine bismuth citrate
Zarontin®	Yes	Ethosuximide	Ethosuximide
Zaroxolyn®	Yes	Metolazone	Metolazone
Zeasorb-AF®	Yes	Miconazole	Miconazole nitrate
Zithromax®	Yes	Azithromycin	Azithromycin
Zofran®	Yes	Ondansetron	Ondansetron hydrochloride
Zoloft®	Yes	Sertraline	Sertraline hydrochloride
Zosyn®	Yes	Piperacillin, tazobactam	Piperacillin sodium, tazobactam sodium

Index

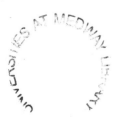